CST Study Guide

Latest CST Review and 1000+ Practice Questions with Detailed Explanation for the Certified Surgical Technologist Exam (Contains 6 Full Length Practice Tests)

Justine Walters

Elena Fraley

Vincent Wells

© 2024-2025

Printed in USA.

Disclaimer:

CONTENTS

Effective Tips to pass the CST exam:

1. Understand the Exam Structure:

Familiarize yourself with the exam structure and content breakdown to focus your study efforts efficiently.

2. Create a Study Plan:

Developing a study plan is essential to organize your review and ensure that you cover all the necessary topics. Set aside dedicated study time each day or week leading up to the exam date. Break down the content into manageable sections and prioritize areas where you need more review.

3. Practice Time Management:

The CST exam is timed, so practicing time management is crucial for success. During your study sessions, work on answering practice questions within the allotted time frame. This will help you build confidence and improve your ability to pace yourself during the actual exam.

4. Take Practice Exams:

Taking practice exams is an effective way to assess your knowledge, identify areas of weakness, and gauge your readiness for the CST exam. Practice exams can help you familiarize yourself with the format and difficulty level of the questions. Analyze your performance on practice exams to focus your review on areas that need improvement.

5. Stay Calm and Confident:

On the day of the exam, remember to stay calm and confident. Get a good night's sleep, eat a healthy breakfast, and arrive at the testing center with ample time to spare. Trust in your preparation and ability to succeed, and approach the exam with a positive mindset.

In conclusion, passing the Certified Surgical Technologist (CST®) exam requires diligent preparation, dedication, and a solid understanding of the principles. By following these tips and utilizing reliable study resources, you can increase your chances of passing the exam with ease. Good luck on your journey to becoming a CST!

Why you'll love this book for acing the CST Exam:

Up-to-Date Content:

Look no further for a comprehensive study guide tailored to the CST Exam. Packed with the latest information and a multitude of practice questions, this book ensures you're well-prepared to succeed. Regular updates guarantee alignment with the most current exam standards.

Expert Guidance:

Written by seasoned professionals who have successfully tackled the CST Exam, this book offers invaluable insights and strategies for exam success. Benefit from the authors' wealth of experience and expertise to navigate the exam with confidence.

Insightful Explanations:

Gain a deeper understanding of the material through detailed explanations provided alongside each question. By delving into the rationale behind the answers, you'll enhance your comprehension and be better equipped to tackle challenging questions on exam day.

Reflective of the Exam Format:

Experience the same question format as the actual CST Exam, allowing you to familiarize yourself with the test structure and boost your confidence. Practice with questions that mirror the exam will prepare you for success on test day.

Enhanced Critical Thinking:

Engaging with the questions, answers, and explanations in this book will sharpen your critical thinking skills and improve your ability to analyze and respond to exam questions effectively. Strengthen your cognitive abilities and enhance your problem-solving skills as you prepare for the CST Exam.

Clear and Concise Approach:

Written in a straightforward and easy-to-understand style, this CST Prep simplifies complex concepts and ensures clarity without overwhelming you with technical language. Dive into the material confidently, knowing that this resource will help you grasp key concepts and excel on the exam.

CST

GUIDE

1 PERIOPERATIVE CARE:

Perioperative care encompasses the comprehensive management of a patient throughout the surgical experience, which includes the preoperative, intraoperative, and postoperative phases. This holistic approach ensures that patients receive optimal care before, during, and after surgery, thereby enhancing outcomes and minimizing complications.

In the preoperative phase, surgical technologists and the surgical team assess the patient's medical history, perform necessary evaluations, and prepare the patient physically and psychologically for surgery. During the intraoperative phase, the surgical technologist plays a crucial role in maintaining a sterile environment, assisting the surgeon, and ensuring that all instruments and supplies are available and functioning.

Postoperatively, care continues with monitoring the patient's recovery, managing pain, and preventing infections. Effective perioperative care requires collaboration among healthcare professionals, adherence to protocols, and a focus on patient safety, ultimately leading to improved surgical outcomes and patient satisfaction.

1.1 Preoperative Preparation:

Preoperative preparation refers to the comprehensive process undertaken to ready a patient for surgical intervention. This phase is crucial for minimizing risks and ensuring optimal outcomes. It encompasses a series of assessments, including medical history evaluations, physical examinations, and necessary diagnostic tests, such as blood work or imaging studies. The surgical team, including the surgical technologist, plays a vital role in educating the patient about the procedure, addressing any concerns, and ensuring informed consent is obtained. Additionally, preoperative preparation involves the implementation of specific protocols, such as fasting guidelines, medication management, and the establishment of an intravenous (IV) line. Proper preoperative preparation not only enhances patient safety but also facilitates a smoother surgical process by ensuring that all necessary equipment and supplies are available and that the surgical environment is adequately set up. This foundational step is essential for achieving successful surgical outcomes.

1.1.1 Review surgeon's preference card:

A surgeon's preference card is a critical document that outlines the specific instruments, supplies, and techniques preferred by a surgeon for various procedures. This card serves as a personalized guide for surgical technologists, ensuring that the surgical field is prepared according to the surgeon's established protocols.

In reviewing the preference card, surgical technologists must pay close attention to details such as the types of sutures, draping materials, and any specialized instruments required. This preparation is essential for maintaining efficiency and minimizing delays during surgery. Additionally, the preference card may include information on the surgeon's preferred positioning of the patient and specific techniques for incision and closure.

By thoroughly reviewing the preference card prior to the procedure, surgical technologists can anticipate the needs of the surgeon, enhance teamwork, and contribute to optimal patient outcomes in the perioperative environment.

1.1.2 Verify availability of surgery equipment:

Verifying the availability of surgery equipment is a critical responsibility of the surgical technologist, ensuring that all necessary instruments, supplies, and devices are present and functional prior to a surgical procedure. This process involves conducting a thorough inventory check against the surgical preference card, which outlines the specific requirements for each operation. It includes inspecting equipment for cleanliness, functionality, and sterility, as well as confirming that all ancillary items, such as sutures, drapes, and medications, are readily available. Additionally, surgical technologists must communicate with the surgical team to address any discrepancies or equipment needs, ensuring that the surgical environment is prepared for optimal patient safety and efficiency. This proactive approach minimizes delays and complications during surgery, highlighting the surgical technologist's role in facilitating a successful surgical outcome.

1.1.2.1 Reserve equipment for surgery:

Reserving equipment for surgery involves the systematic process of ensuring that all necessary surgical instruments, devices, and supplies are allocated and set aside for a specific surgical procedure. This process is critical to maintaining operational efficiency and patient safety. Surgical technologists must communicate effectively with the surgical team to identify the required equipment based on the procedure type and surgeon preferences.

Once identified, the surgical technologist must confirm the availability of the equipment, checking for functionality and sterility. This may involve coordinating with the central supply department or utilizing inventory management systems. Additionally, it is essential to account for any special equipment that may need to be ordered in advance. Proper reservation of equipment minimizes delays, reduces the risk of intraoperative complications, and ensures that the surgical team is prepared to deliver optimal patient care.

1.1.3 Don personal protective equipment:

Donning personal protective equipment (PPE) is a critical procedure in maintaining safety and infection control in the surgical environment. PPE includes items such as surgical masks, gloves, gowns, and eye protection, which serve to protect both the surgical team and the patient from potential contamination. The process of donning PPE should follow a specific sequence to ensure maximum effectiveness.

First, hand hygiene must be performed thoroughly before touching any PPE. Next, the surgical gown is put on, ensuring it covers the arms and torso completely. Following this, a surgical mask is donned, covering the nose and mouth securely. Eye protection, such as goggles or face shields, should be applied next to shield against splashes. Finally, sterile gloves are donned, ensuring a proper fit and that the outer surface remains uncontaminated. Proper donning of PPE is essential for minimizing the risk of surgical site infections and maintaining a sterile field.

1.1.4 Utilize preoperative documentation:

Utilizing preoperative documentation involves the systematic collection and review of essential patient information prior to surgical procedures. This documentation typically includes the patient's medical history, physical examination findings, laboratory results, imaging studies, and any relevant consent forms. The surgical technologist plays a critical role in ensuring that all necessary documents are accurately completed and readily accessible in the operating room. This process is vital for patient safety, as it helps to confirm the surgical site, procedure, and any allergies or comorbidities that may affect anesthesia and surgical outcomes. By thoroughly reviewing preoperative documentation, surgical technologists can anticipate the needs of the surgical team, prepare appropriate instruments and supplies, and contribute to a seamless surgical experience. Ultimately, effective utilization of preoperative documentation enhances communication among the surgical team and supports optimal patient care.

1.1.4.1   Informed consent:

Informed consent is a legal and ethical process that ensures patients are fully aware of and agree to the procedures and treatments they will undergo. It involves providing patients with comprehensive information about the nature of the surgery, potential risks and benefits, alternatives to the procedure, and the likely outcomes. This process is crucial in fostering patient autonomy and trust in the healthcare system.

The surgical technologist plays a vital role in this process by ensuring that the consent form is properly completed and that the patient has had the opportunity to ask questions. It is essential that the patient understands the information provided, which may require the use of layman's terms or additional explanations. Informed consent must be obtained before any surgical intervention and is a legal requirement, protecting both the patient and the healthcare provider from potential liability.

1.1.4.2   Advanced directives:

Advanced directives are legal documents that allow patients to outline their preferences for medical treatment in the event they become unable to communicate their wishes. These directives typically include two main components: a living will and a durable power of attorney for healthcare. A living will specifies the types of medical interventions a patient desires or wishes to avoid, such as resuscitation or mechanical ventilation, under certain conditions. A durable power of attorney for healthcare designates an individual to make medical decisions on behalf of the patient if they are incapacitated. It is essential for surgical technologists to understand advanced directives, as they ensure that patient autonomy is respected and that healthcare providers adhere to the patient's wishes. Proper documentation and communication of these directives are crucial in the preoperative phase to prevent any ethical dilemmas and ensure that the surgical team is aligned with the patient's values and preferences.

1.1.4.3   Allergies:

Allergies refer to the abnormal immune response to substances that are typically harmless, known as allergens. In the surgical setting, it is crucial to identify a patient's allergies to prevent adverse reactions during and after surgery. Common allergens include medications (e.g., antibiotics, anesthetics), latex, and certain foods. The surgical technologist must meticulously review preoperative documentation to ascertain any known allergies, as this information is vital for the surgical team to select appropriate medications and materials. An allergic reaction can range from mild symptoms, such as rashes or itching, to severe anaphylactic shock, which can be life-threatening. Proper communication of a patient's allergy history to the surgical team ensures that preventive measures are taken, such as using latex-free gloves or selecting alternative medications. Thorough documentation and verification of allergies are essential components of patient safety in the perioperative environment.

1.1.4.4   Laboratory results:

Laboratory results refer to the findings obtained from various diagnostic tests performed on patient specimens, such as blood, urine, or tissue samples. These results are crucial in the preoperative phase as they provide essential information regarding the patient's health status and help identify any underlying conditions that may affect surgical outcomes. Surgical technologists must be proficient in interpreting these results to ensure that the surgical team is aware of any abnormalities, such as elevated white blood cell counts indicating infection or electrolyte imbalances that could impact anesthesia. Additionally, laboratory results guide the surgical team in making informed decisions regarding the type of procedure, anesthesia used, and the need for any additional interventions. Accurate documentation and communication of laboratory findings are vital to maintaining patient safety and optimizing surgical care, making it imperative for surgical technologists to thoroughly understand and utilize these results effectively.

1.1.5 Consider patient needs:

Considering patient needs involves a comprehensive understanding of the physical, emotional, and psychological requirements of patients undergoing surgical procedures. It encompasses assessing the patient's medical history, current health status, and individual preferences to ensure optimal care and outcomes. Surgical technologists must prioritize patient safety and comfort by anticipating needs such as pain management, anxiety reduction, and post-operative support. Effective communication with the surgical team and the patient is crucial to address any concerns and provide reassurance. Additionally, understanding cultural and personal values is essential in delivering patient-centered care. By considering these factors, surgical technologists can contribute to a positive surgical experience, enhance patient satisfaction, and promote recovery. Ultimately, recognizing and addressing patient needs is a fundamental aspect of the surgical technologist's role, ensuring that the patient is treated with dignity and respect throughout the surgical process.

1.1.5.1 Bariatrics:

Bariatrics is the branch of medicine that focuses on the treatment of obesity and related disorders through various means, including lifestyle changes, medication, and surgical interventions. Surgical technologists play a crucial role in bariatric procedures, which may include gastric bypass, sleeve gastrectomy, and adjustable gastric banding. These surgeries aim to reduce the stomach's capacity, thereby limiting food intake and promoting weight loss.

In the operating room, surgical technologists must be knowledgeable about the specific instruments and techniques used in bariatric surgery, as well as the unique anatomical considerations of obese patients. They must also be aware of potential complications, such as infection, blood clots, and nutritional deficiencies post-surgery. Understanding the psychological and physiological needs of bariatric patients is essential, as these individuals often require comprehensive support throughout their weight loss journey, including preoperative education and postoperative care.

1.1.5.2 Geriatrics:

Geriatrics is a specialized branch of medicine focused on the health care of elderly patients, addressing their unique physiological and psychological needs. As individuals age, they often experience a decline in physical function, increased comorbidities, and altered responses to medications, necessitating tailored surgical care. Surgical technologists must be adept at recognizing these factors to ensure optimal patient outcomes.

In the surgical setting, geriatric patients may present with challenges such as frailty, cognitive impairment, and increased risk of complications. It is crucial for surgical technologists to communicate effectively with the surgical team about any specific concerns related to the patient's age and health status. Additionally, understanding the importance of postoperative care and rehabilitation in geriatrics can significantly impact recovery. By prioritizing the unique needs of elderly patients, surgical technologists contribute to a safer surgical experience and improved overall health outcomes.

1.1.5.3 Pediatrics:

Pediatrics is a specialized branch of medicine that focuses on the health and medical care of infants, children, and adolescents, typically up to the age of 18. In the surgical context, understanding pediatric needs is crucial for surgical technologists. Children have unique physiological and anatomical differences compared to adults, which can affect surgical procedures and outcomes. For instance, their smaller size necessitates modifications in surgical instruments and techniques. Additionally, pediatric patients may experience heightened anxiety and require tailored communication strategies to ensure comfort and cooperation. Surgical technologists must be adept at recognizing these differences and adapting their practices accordingly. This includes preparing age-appropriate surgical environments, ensuring proper dosing of medications, and utilizing specialized equipment designed for pediatric use. Ultimately, a thorough understanding of pediatric considerations enhances patient safety and promotes positive surgical experiences for young patients.

1.1.5.4 Immunocompromised:

An immunocompromised individual is one whose immune system is weakened or not functioning optimally, rendering them more susceptible to infections and complications. This condition can arise from various factors, including congenital disorders, chronic diseases (such as diabetes or HIV/AIDS), malnutrition, or as a consequence of medical treatments like chemotherapy or immunosuppressive therapy following organ transplantation. Surgical technologists must recognize the unique needs of these patients, as their compromised immune status necessitates stringent adherence to aseptic techniques and infection control protocols during surgical procedures. Additionally, careful consideration must be given to the selection of surgical materials and the management of the surgical environment to minimize exposure to pathogens. Understanding the implications of being immunocompromised is crucial for surgical technologists to ensure optimal patient outcomes and to mitigate risks associated with surgical interventions.

1.1.5.5 Patient allergies:

Patient allergies refer to the hypersensitive reactions that occur when the immune system responds abnormally to a substance known as an allergen. Common allergens include medications, latex, food items, and environmental factors. In the surgical setting, it is crucial for surgical technologists to identify and document any known allergies prior to the procedure, as this information directly impacts patient safety and surgical outcomes. Allergic reactions can range from mild symptoms, such as rashes or itching, to severe anaphylactic responses that may lead to respiratory distress or cardiovascular collapse. Surgical technologists must be vigilant in verifying the patient's allergy history, ensuring that all team members are aware of these allergies, and utilizing alternative materials or medications as necessary. This proactive approach minimizes the risk of adverse reactions during surgery, thereby safeguarding the patient's well-being and promoting a successful surgical experience.

1.1.6 Prepare the operating room environment:

Preparing the operating room environment involves creating a sterile and organized space conducive to surgical procedures. This process begins with thorough cleaning and disinfection of all surfaces and equipment to minimize the risk of infection. Surgical technologists must ensure that all necessary instruments, supplies, and equipment are available, functional, and arranged in a manner that promotes efficiency during the procedure. This includes setting up the sterile field, which is critical for maintaining asepsis. The surgical team must also verify that the appropriate surgical drapes, sponges, and sutures are ready for use. Additionally, the operating room should be equipped with necessary technology, such as lights and monitoring devices, and the environment must be adjusted for optimal temperature and ventilation. Effective communication with the surgical team is essential to confirm that all preparations meet the specific requirements of the upcoming surgery, ensuring patient safety and procedural success.

1.1.6.1   Temperature:

Temperature in the operating room (OR) is a critical factor that influences both patient safety and surgical outcomes. The recommended temperature range for the OR is typically between 68°F to 75°F (20°C to 24°C). Maintaining this range helps to minimize the risk of hypothermia in patients, which can lead to complications such as increased blood loss, delayed wound healing, and higher infection rates. Additionally, a controlled temperature environment is essential for the comfort of the surgical team, allowing them to perform procedures efficiently without the distraction of excessive heat or cold.

It is important to monitor and adjust the temperature as necessary, considering factors such as the length of the procedure, the type of surgery, and the patient's condition. Proper temperature management, along with other environmental controls, contributes significantly to the overall success of surgical interventions and enhances patient outcomes.

1.1.6.2   Lights:

In the operating room, lights are critical for ensuring optimal visibility during surgical procedures. Surgical lights, also known as operating room lights, are designed to provide bright, shadow-free illumination directly onto the surgical site. These lights typically feature adjustable intensity and color temperature to accommodate various surgical needs and preferences of the surgical team.

They are often equipped with multiple light sources that can be positioned to minimize shadows cast by the surgeon's hands or instruments. Additionally, modern surgical lights may include features such as LED technology for energy efficiency and longevity, as well as the ability to adjust the focus and spread of light.

Proper positioning and functioning of surgical lights are essential for enhancing the precision of the procedure and ensuring patient safety. Surgical technologists must be adept at adjusting and maintaining these lights to support the surgical team effectively.

1.1.6.3   Suction:

Suction refers to the process of removing blood, fluids, and debris from the surgical site to maintain a clear operative field. It is essential for visibility and safety during surgical procedures. Suction devices typically consist of a suction pump, tubing, and various suction tips designed for specific surgical needs. The most common types of suction tips include the Yankauer, which is rigid and allows for controlled suctioning, and the Frazier, which is smaller and used for more delicate areas.

Surgical technologists must ensure that suction equipment is functioning properly before the procedure begins. This includes checking for leaks, ensuring that the collection canister is properly positioned, and verifying that the suction pressure is adequate. During surgery, the surgical technologist is responsible for anticipating the surgeon's needs for suctioning and providing the appropriate tip while maintaining a sterile environment. Proper suctioning techniques are crucial for minimizing complications and promoting optimal surgical outcomes.

1.1.6.4   Wiping down the room and furniture:

Wiping down the room and furniture refers to the process of thoroughly cleaning and disinfecting all surfaces within the operating room to ensure a sterile environment. This practice is crucial in preventing surgical site infections and maintaining patient safety. Surgical technologists must utilize appropriate cleaning agents, typically hospital-grade disinfectants, to effectively eliminate pathogens.

The procedure involves systematically cleaning high-touch areas such as operating tables, surgical lights, and instrument tables, as well as walls and floors. It is essential to follow the manufacturer's instructions for the disinfectant used, including contact time and dilution ratios. Additionally, surgical technologists should employ proper techniques, such as using single-use disposable wipes or cloths, to avoid cross-contamination. Regular wiping down of the room and furniture not only prepares the environment for surgery but also upholds the standards of infection control mandated by healthcare regulations.

1.1.7 Coordinate additional equipment:

Coordinating additional equipment involves the surgical technologist's responsibility to ensure that all necessary instruments, devices, and supplies are available and functioning prior to the surgical procedure. This includes assessing the surgical environment, understanding the specific requirements of the surgical procedure, and collaborating with the surgical team to identify any specialized equipment needed. The surgical technologist must maintain an organized and sterile field, ensuring that all equipment is properly sterilized and ready for use. This process may involve checking the functionality of electrosurgical units, suction devices, and other critical instruments. Effective communication with the surgical team is essential to anticipate needs and address any last-minute equipment requests. By meticulously coordinating additional equipment, the surgical technologist plays a vital role in enhancing surgical efficiency, minimizing delays, and ultimately contributing to patient safety and optimal surgical outcomes.

1.1.7.1 Bovie pad:

A Bovie pad, also known as an electrosurgical grounding pad, is a critical component in electrosurgery, designed to ensure patient safety during surgical procedures. This pad is typically made of a conductive material that adheres to the patient's skin and connects to the electrosurgical unit (ESU). Its primary function is to provide a return path for the electrical current generated by the ESU, which is used to cut or coagulate tissue. Proper placement of the Bovie pad is essential; it should be positioned on a fleshy area of the patient's body, away from bony prominences, to minimize the risk of burns. Additionally, the pad must be securely attached to maintain effective conductivity. Surgical technologists must verify the integrity of the Bovie pad before use, ensuring it is free from damage and properly connected to the ESU, as this is vital for both patient safety and the efficacy of the surgical procedure.

1.1.7.2 Pneumatic tourniquet:

A pneumatic tourniquet is a medical device used to control blood flow to a specific area of the body during surgical procedures. It consists of an inflatable cuff that is applied around a limb and connected to a pressure-regulating system. When inflated, the tourniquet occludes the arterial blood flow, creating a bloodless surgical field, which is particularly beneficial in orthopedic and vascular surgeries.

The application of a pneumatic tourniquet requires careful monitoring of pressure levels to prevent complications such as nerve damage or tissue ischemia. The recommended pressure varies based on the limb and procedure, typically ranging from 250 to 300 mmHg for upper extremities and 300 to 400 mmHg for lower extremities.

Additionally, the duration of inflation should be limited to minimize risks, with guidelines suggesting a maximum of 1 to 2 hours. Proper training and adherence to protocols are essential for safe and effective use.

1.1.7.3 Sequential compression devices:

Sequential compression devices (SCDs) are specialized medical equipment designed to promote venous return and prevent deep vein thrombosis (DVT) in patients undergoing surgical procedures or those with limited mobility. These devices consist of inflatable sleeves that wrap around the patient's legs and sequentially inflate and deflate to mimic the natural muscle contractions that occur during ambulation. This rhythmic compression enhances blood flow in the veins, reducing the risk of clot formation by preventing stasis. SCDs are typically used in the perioperative setting, particularly for patients at high risk for thromboembolic events. Proper application and monitoring of SCDs are crucial, as they must be adjusted to fit the patient's size and condition. Surgical technologists play a vital role in coordinating the use of SCDs, ensuring they are applied correctly before surgery and maintained throughout the procedure to optimize patient safety and outcomes.

1.1.7.4 Thermoregulatory devices:

Thermoregulatory devices are essential tools used in the surgical environment to maintain a patient's core body temperature during procedures. These devices help prevent hypothermia, which can lead to complications such as increased blood loss, prolonged recovery, and heightened risk of infection. Common thermoregulatory devices include forced-air warming blankets, conductive warming blankets, and warming cabinets for intravenous fluids. Forced-air warming blankets circulate warm air around the patient, effectively raising their temperature. Conductive warming blankets utilize heated gel or pads to provide direct warmth. Additionally, warming cabinets are employed to keep IV fluids and blood products at optimal temperatures before administration. Surgical technologists must be proficient in the setup and monitoring of these devices, ensuring they are functioning correctly throughout the procedure. Proper use of thermoregulatory devices is crucial for patient safety and comfort, highlighting the surgical technologist's role in the surgical team.

1.1.7.5 Positioning devices:

Positioning devices are specialized tools and equipment used in the surgical environment to support and stabilize patients during procedures. These devices ensure that the patient is positioned safely and comfortably, minimizing the risk of injury and optimizing access for the surgical team. Common types of positioning devices include foam pads, armboards, and various types of surgical tables that can be adjusted for height and tilt. Additionally, devices such as safety straps, headrests, and gel pads are utilized to secure the patient and protect pressure points. Proper use of positioning devices is critical, as it not only enhances the surgical field visibility but also aids in maintaining the patient's physiological stability throughout the procedure. Surgical technologists must be knowledgeable about the different types of positioning devices and their appropriate applications to facilitate effective teamwork and ensure patient safety during surgery.

1.1.8 Obtain instruments and supplies needed for surgery:
This process involves the systematic gathering and preparation of all necessary surgical instruments and supplies required for a specific procedure. Surgical technologists must possess a thorough understanding of the surgical instruments, their functions, and the specific needs of the surgical team. This includes selecting the appropriate surgical instruments, sutures, drapes, and other materials based on the surgical procedure being performed.

The surgical technologist must ensure that all items are sterile and in proper working condition, adhering to strict infection control protocols. Additionally, they must organize instruments in a manner that facilitates efficient access during surgery, often using instrument trays or caddies. Effective communication with the surgical team is essential to confirm that all required items are available and to anticipate any additional needs that may arise during the procedure. This preparation is crucial for ensuring a smooth surgical process and optimal patient outcomes.

1.1.9 Perform medical hand wash:
Medical hand washing is a critical infection control practice that involves thoroughly cleaning hands to remove dirt, organic material, and microorganisms. This process is essential in preventing the transmission of pathogens in healthcare settings, particularly in surgical environments. The procedure typically includes the use of soap and water or an alcohol-based hand sanitizer.

To perform a medical hand wash, begin by wetting hands with clean, running water. Apply soap and lather by rubbing hands together, ensuring to clean all surfaces, including between fingers, under nails, and around wrists. Scrub for at least 20 seconds, then rinse thoroughly under running water. Dry hands with a clean towel or air dryer.

This practice is vital before and after patient contact, after handling instruments, and before any sterile procedures to maintain a sterile environment and protect both patient and healthcare worker from infections.

1.1.10 Check package integrity of sterile supplies:
Checking the package integrity of sterile supplies is a critical step in ensuring patient safety and preventing surgical site infections. This process involves inspecting the packaging for any signs of damage, such as tears, holes, or moisture, which can compromise the sterility of the contents. A sterile package should be intact, sealed, and free from any contamination. Additionally, the expiration date must be verified to ensure that the supplies are still within their usable timeframe. If any abnormalities are detected, the package should not be used, and the contents must be discarded or re-sterilized as necessary. Proper handling and storage of sterile supplies are also essential to maintain their integrity. Surgical technologists must be vigilant in this practice, as the integrity of sterile supplies directly impacts surgical outcomes and patient health. Regular training and adherence to protocols further enhance the effectiveness of this crucial task.

1.1.11 Open sterile supplies/instruments while maintaining aseptic technique:
Opening sterile supplies and instruments is a critical process in surgical procedures that ensures the prevention of infection. Aseptic technique refers to the methods used to create and maintain a sterile environment. When opening sterile supplies, surgical technologists must first ensure that their hands are clean and that they are wearing appropriate personal protective equipment (PPE). Supplies should be opened in a manner that avoids contamination; this typically involves using a sterile field and adhering to the principles of asepsis.

The outer packaging is opened first, allowing the inner sterile contents to remain untouched. Instruments should be handled with sterile gloves, and any items that fall outside the sterile field must be discarded. It is essential to maintain visual awareness of the sterile field throughout the process, ensuring that no non-sterile items come into contact with sterile instruments or supplies. This meticulous approach is vital for patient safety and successful surgical outcomes.

1.1.12 Perform surgical scrub:
The surgical scrub is a critical aseptic technique performed by surgical technologists and other operating room personnel to reduce the risk of surgical site infections. This process involves thorough hand and forearm cleansing using an antimicrobial soap or surgical scrub solution. The scrub typically lasts for 3 to 5 minutes, ensuring that all surfaces of the hands, wrists, and forearms are meticulously cleaned. The technique includes the use of a brush or sponge to remove debris and microorganisms, followed by rinsing with sterile water.

After the scrub, hands are dried with a sterile towel, and a sterile gown and gloves are donned to maintain a sterile field. The surgical scrub not only protects the patient but also the surgical team by minimizing the transfer of pathogens. Mastery of this technique is essential for surgical technologists to uphold the highest standards of patient safety and infection control in the operating room.

1.1.12.1 Initial:
The term "Initial" in the context of performing a surgical scrub refers to the first step in the hand hygiene process that surgical technologists must undertake before entering the sterile field. This initial scrub is crucial for reducing the risk of surgical site infections by effectively removing dirt, debris, and transient microorganisms from the hands and forearms.

During the initial scrub, surgical technologists typically use an antimicrobial soap or surgical scrub solution, applying it to all surfaces of the hands and forearms, including between fingers and under nails. The scrub should last a minimum of 2-5 minutes, depending on the facility's protocols. It is essential to follow a systematic approach, ensuring that all areas are thoroughly cleaned. After the initial scrub, hands must be rinsed without touching any non-sterile surfaces, and a sterile towel or hand dryer should be used to dry the hands, maintaining sterility before donning surgical gloves.

1.1.12.2 Waterless:

Waterless surgical scrub refers to the use of alcohol-based hand sanitizers or antiseptic solutions that do not require water for application. These products are designed to effectively reduce the microbial load on the skin before surgical procedures. Waterless scrubs typically contain a high concentration of alcohol (usually 60-95%) along with emollients to prevent skin irritation. The application process involves dispensing the product onto dry hands and rubbing it thoroughly, ensuring that all surfaces, including between fingers and under nails, are covered.

The advantages of waterless scrubs include a quicker application time, reduced risk of skin irritation compared to traditional soap and water scrubs, and the ability to maintain sterility in environments where water access is limited. Additionally, waterless scrubs have been shown to be effective against a broad spectrum of pathogens, making them a valuable tool in maintaining aseptic technique in surgical settings.

1.1.13 Don gown and gloves:

Donning a surgical gown and gloves is a critical step in maintaining a sterile environment during surgical procedures. The process begins with selecting an appropriate gown, typically made of a fluid-resistant material, which provides a barrier against contamination. The surgical technologist should ensure that the gown is the correct size to allow for ease of movement while providing full coverage.

To don the gown, the surgical technologist should first perform hand hygiene, then open the gown package without touching the inner surface. The gown is then put on by allowing it to unfold and slipping the arms into the sleeves, ensuring that the back of the gown remains closed.

Next, sterile gloves are donned, usually using the closed-glove technique to prevent contamination. This involves grasping the cuff of one glove with the opposite hand and pulling it on, followed by the same process for the other glove. Properly donning gown and gloves is essential for infection control and patient safety.

1.1.14 Assemble and set up sterile instruments and supplies for surgical procedures:

Assembling and setting up sterile instruments and supplies for surgical procedures is a critical responsibility of the surgical technologist. This process involves selecting the appropriate instruments, ensuring they are sterile, and arranging them systematically on the sterile field to facilitate the surgeon's access during the operation. The surgical technologist must verify that all instruments are functioning properly and that the necessary supplies, such as sutures, drapes, and sponges, are available and sterile. Proper organization is essential; instruments are typically arranged in the order of use, which enhances efficiency and minimizes the risk of contamination. Additionally, the surgical technologist must adhere to strict aseptic techniques to maintain the sterile environment, preventing surgical site infections. This meticulous preparation is vital to the success of the surgical procedure and the safety of the patient.

1.1.15 Transport the patient to and from operating room:

Transporting the patient to and from the operating room is a critical responsibility of the surgical technologist. This process involves safely moving the patient from the preoperative area to the operating room and back post-surgery, ensuring patient comfort and security throughout. Prior to transport, the surgical technologist must verify the patient's identity, surgical procedure, and any specific needs, such as mobility restrictions or the use of assistive devices. During transport, the surgical technologist should monitor the patient's vital signs and maintain communication with the surgical team to address any immediate concerns. Proper techniques, including the use of stretchers or wheelchairs, must be employed to prevent injury to both the patient and staff. Additionally, ensuring that all necessary equipment and supplies are ready in the operating room is essential for a smooth transition, thereby promoting a safe and efficient surgical environment.

1.1.16 Transfer patient to operating room table:

Transferring a patient to the operating room table is a critical procedure that ensures patient safety and comfort while facilitating surgical access. This process involves several key steps: first, the surgical technologist must verify the patient's identity and surgical site, adhering to the "time-out" protocol to prevent errors. The patient is then carefully positioned on a stretcher or transport device, ensuring that all monitoring equipment is secure.

Once in the operating room, the surgical technologist, along with the surgical team, assists in transferring the patient onto the operating table using proper body mechanics to prevent injury. The patient should be positioned appropriately, often supine or in a specific position based on the procedure, with safety straps applied to prevent movement. Finally, the surgical team must ensure that the patient is comfortable and that all necessary equipment is within reach before proceeding with the surgery.

1.1.17 Apply patient safety devices:

Applying patient safety devices refers to the implementation of various tools and equipment designed to protect patients from harm during surgical procedures. These devices include safety belts, armboards, and positioning devices that ensure patient stability and prevent falls or injury while on the operating table. The surgical technologist must assess the patient's specific needs, considering factors such as age, mobility, and the type of procedure being performed. Proper application of these devices is crucial to maintaining the patient's safety and comfort, as well as facilitating optimal surgical access for the surgical team. Additionally, it is essential to follow institutional protocols and manufacturer guidelines when applying these devices to ensure they are used effectively and safely. The surgical technologist plays a vital role in monitoring the patient's condition throughout the procedure, ensuring that safety devices remain in place and adjusting them as necessary to accommodate changes in the patient's status.

1.1.17.1 Bovie pad:

A Bovie pad, also known as an electrosurgical grounding pad, is a critical component used in electrosurgery to ensure patient safety during surgical procedures. It is designed to disperse the electrical current generated by the electrosurgical unit (ESU) throughout the patient's body, preventing burns and ensuring effective cutting or coagulation of tissue. The pad is typically made of a conductive material, often aluminum or a similar metal, and is adhered to the patient's skin, usually on a non-operative site. Proper placement of the Bovie pad is essential; it should be positioned close to the surgical site and away from bony prominences to minimize resistance and maximize current flow. Surgical technologists must verify that the pad is securely attached and functioning correctly, as improper use can lead to complications such as thermal injuries. Regular inspection and adherence to manufacturer guidelines are crucial for maintaining patient safety during electrosurgical procedures.

1.1.17.2 Safety strap:

A safety strap is a medical device used to secure a patient to the operating table during surgical procedures. Its primary purpose is to prevent patient movement, which could lead to injury or complications during surgery. The safety strap is typically made of durable, adjustable materials that can accommodate various body sizes and shapes. It is positioned across the patient's body, usually at the thighs or lower abdomen, and is fastened securely but comfortably to avoid restricting circulation.

Proper application of the safety strap is critical; it should be checked for tightness and positioning to ensure it does not interfere with the surgical site or the patient's comfort. Additionally, surgical technologists must remain vigilant to monitor the patient's condition and ensure that the strap does not cause any undue pressure or discomfort. Effective use of safety straps is essential for maintaining patient safety and enhancing the overall surgical experience.

1.1.17.3 Protective padding:

Protective padding refers to specialized materials used to cushion and support patients during surgical procedures, minimizing the risk of pressure injuries and ensuring patient comfort. This padding is typically made from soft, durable materials such as foam, gel, or air-filled structures that conform to the body's contours. The primary purpose of protective padding is to distribute pressure evenly across the body, particularly in areas prone to injury, such as bony prominences. Proper application of protective padding is crucial in maintaining skin integrity and preventing complications such as pressure ulcers, which can arise from prolonged immobility during surgery. Additionally, protective padding can help secure the patient in the surgical position, reducing the risk of accidental movement that could compromise the procedure. Surgical technologists must be knowledgeable about the various types of protective padding available and their appropriate use to enhance patient safety and comfort throughout the surgical experience.

1.1.17.4 X-ray safety:

X-ray safety refers to the protocols and practices designed to protect patients, surgical staff, and the environment from unnecessary exposure to ionizing radiation during radiographic procedures. It encompasses the use of protective equipment, such as lead aprons, thyroid shields, and lead glasses, to minimize radiation exposure. Proper positioning of the patient and the X-ray machine is essential to ensure that only the targeted area is exposed, thereby reducing scatter radiation.

Additionally, the use of shielding devices, such as lead barriers, can further protect personnel in the operating room. It is crucial for surgical technologists to understand the principles of ALARA (As Low As Reasonably Achievable) to limit radiation exposure. Regular maintenance and calibration of X-ray equipment are also vital to ensure accurate imaging and safety. Adhering to these safety measures not only safeguards health but also enhances the quality of patient care during surgical procedures involving X-ray imaging.

1.1.18 Apply patient monitoring devices as directed:

Applying patient monitoring devices involves the correct placement and operation of equipment that tracks vital signs and physiological parameters during surgical procedures. This includes devices such as electrocardiograms (ECGs), pulse oximeters, blood pressure monitors, and capnographs. Surgical technologists must ensure that these devices are properly calibrated and functioning before use.

The process begins with selecting appropriate monitoring devices based on the patient's condition and the type of surgery being performed. Proper application includes securing electrodes or sensors to the patient's skin, ensuring good contact for accurate readings, and connecting the devices to the appropriate monitors.

Surgical technologists must also be familiar with interpreting the data these devices provide, recognizing normal versus abnormal readings, and understanding when to alert the surgical team of any concerning changes. Adhering to protocols for patient safety and comfort is paramount during this process.

1.1.19 Participate in positioning the patient:

Participating in positioning the patient involves the surgical technologist's active role in ensuring the patient is placed correctly on the operating table to facilitate optimal surgical access and safety. This process requires a thorough understanding of various positioning techniques, the specific surgical procedure being performed, and the patient's individual needs, including any pre-existing conditions or mobility limitations.

The surgical technologist must collaborate with the surgical team to select appropriate positioning devices, such as foam pads, safety straps, or headrests, to maintain patient comfort and prevent injury. Proper positioning also minimizes the risk of pressure ulcers and nerve damage during surgery. Additionally, the surgical technologist should be aware of the principles of body mechanics to safely assist in moving and positioning the patient. Effective communication with the surgical team is essential to ensure that all members are aware of the positioning plan and any necessary adjustments during the procedure.

1.1.20 Prepare surgical site:

Preparing the surgical site involves a series of critical steps aimed at ensuring a sterile environment for the surgical procedure. This process begins with the proper positioning of the patient, followed by the application of antiseptic solutions to cleanse the skin and reduce microbial flora. The surgical technologist must meticulously drape the area to maintain sterility and prevent contamination. This includes using sterile drapes that cover not only the surgical site but also the surrounding area to create a controlled field. Additionally, the surgical technologist must ensure that all necessary instruments and supplies are readily available and organized for the surgeon's use. Effective communication with the surgical team is essential during this phase to confirm that all preparations meet the required standards. Ultimately, the goal of preparing the surgical site is to minimize the risk of infection and facilitate a safe and efficient surgical procedure.

1.1.20.1 Hair removal:

Hair removal is a critical component of preparing the surgical site, aimed at minimizing the risk of infection and ensuring optimal visibility for the surgical team. The process typically involves shaving or clipping hair from the designated surgical area, following established protocols to maintain patient safety and comfort.

Shaving is often discouraged due to the potential for micro-abrasions, which can increase the risk of surgical site infections. Instead, clippers are preferred as they effectively reduce hair without compromising the skin's integrity.

The surgical technologist must assess the surgical site and determine the appropriate method of hair removal, taking into account the type of procedure and the patient's skin condition. Additionally, hair removal should be performed as close to the time of the procedure as possible to minimize the risk of contamination. Proper technique and adherence to infection control measures are essential during this preparatory step.

1.1.20.2 Surgical preparation:

Surgical preparation refers to the systematic process of readying the patient and the surgical site for an operative procedure. This includes thorough skin antisepsis to minimize the risk of postoperative infections, which is typically achieved through the application of antiseptic solutions such as chlorhexidine or iodine-based agents. The surgical technologist must ensure that the area is properly draped to maintain a sterile field, using sterile drapes to cover the surrounding skin and prevent contamination. Additionally, the surgical team must verify the correct surgical site and procedure through a preoperative checklist, often referred to as a "time-out," to enhance patient safety. Proper positioning of the patient is also crucial, ensuring comfort and access for the surgical team while preventing pressure injuries. Overall, surgical preparation is vital for creating a sterile environment, safeguarding patient health, and facilitating a successful surgical outcome.

1.1.21 Gown and glove sterile team members:

Gown and glove sterile team members refer to the surgical personnel who are responsible for maintaining a sterile environment during surgical procedures. This includes the surgeon, surgical assistants, and scrub nurses or technologists who don sterile gowns and gloves before entering the operating room. The gown serves as a barrier to prevent the transfer of microorganisms from the surgical team to the sterile field, while gloves protect both the patient and the surgical team from contamination.

Proper technique in donning these garments is crucial; gowns should be put on in a manner that prevents contact with non-sterile surfaces, and gloves should be applied without touching the outer surface of the gloves with bare hands. Adherence to these protocols ensures the integrity of the sterile field, minimizing the risk of surgical site infections and promoting patient safety throughout the surgical process.

1.1.22   Participate in draping the patient:

Draping the patient is a critical step in the surgical process, ensuring both the sterility of the surgical field and the comfort of the patient. This procedure involves covering the patient with sterile drapes to create a barrier that minimizes the risk of contamination during surgery. The surgical technologist plays a vital role in this process by selecting appropriate drapes, ensuring they are sterile, and positioning them correctly to expose only the surgical site.

The technologist must be aware of the surgical procedure being performed to drape the patient effectively, as different surgeries may require specific draping techniques. Proper draping not only protects the patient from infection but also provides the surgical team with a clear and organized workspace. Additionally, the surgical technologist must communicate effectively with the surgical team to ensure that the draping process is performed efficiently and safely, maintaining a sterile environment throughout the procedure.

1.1.23   Secure cords/tubing to drapes and apply light handles:

Securing cords and tubing to drapes is a critical practice in maintaining a sterile environment during surgical procedures. This involves using appropriate methods, such as adhesive tape or surgical clips, to fasten electrical cords and tubing to the surgical drapes, preventing them from becoming tangled or accidentally pulled during the operation. This practice not only enhances the safety of the surgical team and the patient but also minimizes the risk of contamination.

Applying light handles is equally important, as these handles allow for the manipulation of surgical lights without compromising sterility. Light handles should be covered with sterile covers and secured to ensure they remain clean and functional throughout the procedure. Properly managing cords, tubing, and light handles contributes to an organized surgical field, facilitating efficient workflow and reducing the likelihood of surgical errors or delays.

1.1.24   Drape specialty equipment:

Drape specialty equipment refers to the various surgical drapes and accessories specifically designed to cover and protect surgical instruments, the surgical field, and the patient during operative procedures. These drapes are made from materials that are sterile, fluid-resistant, and designed to minimize the risk of infection. They come in various sizes and shapes to accommodate different surgical specialties and procedures, ensuring that the surgical site remains sterile and that the surrounding areas are protected from contamination.

Proper draping techniques are crucial in maintaining a sterile environment, as they help to prevent the introduction of pathogens during surgery. Additionally, drape specialty equipment may include adhesive drapes, which secure the drape in place, and fenestrated drapes, which have openings to expose the surgical site while still providing coverage around it. Understanding the appropriate use and application of these drapes is essential for surgical technologists to ensure patient safety and optimal surgical outcomes.

1.1.24.1   C-arm:

A C-arm is a mobile imaging device that provides real-time fluoroscopic imaging during surgical procedures. It consists of an X-ray source and a detector positioned in a C-shaped configuration, allowing for a wide range of motion and flexibility. The primary function of the C-arm is to assist surgeons by providing continuous imaging of the surgical site, enabling precise navigation and verification of anatomical structures.

C-arms are commonly used in orthopedic, vascular, and pain management procedures, as they allow for minimally invasive techniques while ensuring accurate placement of instruments and implants. The surgical technologist plays a crucial role in preparing and draping the C-arm, ensuring it is sterile and positioned correctly to avoid contamination. Additionally, they must be knowledgeable about the equipment's operation, including adjusting settings for optimal imaging quality and understanding radiation safety protocols to protect both the surgical team and the patient.

1.1.24.2   Da Vinci:

The Da Vinci Surgical System is a state-of-the-art robotic surgical platform that enhances the capabilities of surgeons during minimally invasive procedures. It consists of a surgeon's console, a patient-side robotic cart, and advanced imaging technology. The system allows for precise manipulation of surgical instruments through robotic arms, which translates the surgeon's hand movements into smaller, more precise movements of the instruments inside the patient's body.

The Da Vinci system provides a three-dimensional view of the surgical site with high-definition visualization, improving depth perception and clarity. It is commonly used in urological, gynecological, and general surgeries. Surgical technologists play a crucial role in preparing and draping the Da Vinci equipment, ensuring sterile conditions, and assisting the surgical team throughout the procedure. Understanding the functionality and setup of the Da Vinci system is essential for surgical technologists to facilitate efficient and safe surgical interventions.

1.1.24.3   Microscope:

A microscope is an optical instrument used to magnify and visualize small structures that are not visible to the naked eye, commonly employed in various surgical procedures. It consists of a series of lenses that enhance the visibility of tissues, cells, and other microscopic entities, allowing for precise examination and manipulation during surgery. In the surgical setting, particularly in neurosurgery and ophthalmology, microscopes provide high-resolution images and depth perception, facilitating intricate tasks such as suturing and tissue dissection. The surgical technologist plays a crucial role in draping the microscope to maintain a sterile field, ensuring that the lenses and surrounding components are protected from contamination. Proper draping techniques involve using sterile covers and ensuring that the equipment is positioned correctly for optimal surgeon access. Understanding the functionality and maintenance of the microscope is essential for surgical technologists to support the surgical team effectively.

1.1.25 Participate in Universal Protocol (Time Out):

The Universal Protocol, established by The Joint Commission, is a critical safety measure designed to prevent wrong-site, wrong-procedure, and wrong-person surgeries. The "Time Out" is a standardized pause taken immediately before the surgical procedure begins. During this time, the surgical team, including the surgeon, surgical technologist, and anesthesia provider, collectively verifies essential information. This includes confirming the patient's identity, the surgical site, the procedure to be performed, and any relevant allergies or medical conditions.

The surgical technologist plays a vital role in this process by facilitating communication among team members and ensuring that all necessary documentation is accurate and available. The Time Out serves as a final check to enhance patient safety and foster a culture of teamwork and accountability within the operating room. Adherence to the Universal Protocol is essential for minimizing surgical errors and ensuring optimal patient outcomes.

1.2 Intraoperative Procedures:

Intraoperative procedures refer to the series of actions and protocols performed during the surgical intervention, encompassing all activities from the moment the patient is positioned on the operating table until the conclusion of the surgery. These procedures are critical for ensuring patient safety, maintaining sterile conditions, and facilitating the surgeon's work. Surgical technologists play a vital role in this phase, assisting the surgical team by preparing instruments, managing the sterile field, and anticipating the needs of the surgeon. Key components include the verification of surgical site and patient identity, the application of aseptic techniques, and the monitoring of the patient's vital signs. Intraoperative procedures also involve the use of various surgical instruments and technologies, as well as the management of specimens for pathology. Mastery of these procedures is essential for surgical technologists to contribute effectively to positive surgical outcomes and enhance patient care.

1.2.1 Maintain aseptic technique throughout the procedure:

Maintaining aseptic technique throughout the surgical procedure is crucial for preventing surgical site infections and ensuring patient safety. Aseptic technique refers to the practices and procedures that prevent contamination by pathogens. This involves meticulous hand hygiene, the use of sterile instruments, and the proper draping of the surgical field. Surgical technologists must ensure that all team members adhere to sterile protocols, including wearing appropriate personal protective equipment (PPE) such as gloves, gowns, and masks. During the procedure, it is essential to monitor the sterile field continuously, avoiding any breaches that could introduce microorganisms. Additionally, any items that come into contact with the sterile field must be sterile, and non-sterile items should be kept at a safe distance. By rigorously applying these principles, surgical technologists play a vital role in maintaining a sterile environment, thereby minimizing the risk of infection and promoting optimal surgical outcomes.

1.2.2 Follow Standard and Universal Precautions:

Standard and Universal Precautions are essential infection control practices designed to prevent the transmission of infectious agents in healthcare settings. These precautions require that all blood and certain body fluids be treated as if they are infectious, regardless of the patient's known status. Surgical technologists must consistently apply these precautions to protect themselves, patients, and the surgical team. This includes the use of personal protective equipment (PPE) such as gloves, masks, gowns, and eye protection when exposure to blood or body fluids is anticipated. Additionally, proper hand hygiene, safe handling of sharps, and the appropriate disposal of contaminated materials are critical components. By adhering to these guidelines, surgical technologists can minimize the risk of healthcare-associated infections and ensure a safer surgical environment, ultimately contributing to better patient outcomes and maintaining the integrity of the surgical process.

1.2.3 Anticipate the steps of surgical procedures:

Anticipating the steps of surgical procedures involves the surgical technologist's ability to foresee the sequence of actions required during surgery, ensuring a smooth and efficient operation. This skill is critical as it allows the surgical team to maintain a sterile environment, prepare necessary instruments, and anticipate the surgeon's needs. A surgical technologist must be familiar with various surgical techniques, instruments, and the specific procedure being performed. This includes understanding the anatomy involved, potential complications, and the expected outcomes. By anticipating the steps, the surgical technologist can prepare the sterile field, organize instruments in the order they will be used, and assist the surgical team effectively. This proactive approach minimizes delays, enhances patient safety, and contributes to optimal surgical outcomes. Continuous education and experience in different surgical specialties further enhance this essential skill.

1.2.4 Perform counts with circulator at appropriate intervals:

Performing counts with the circulator at appropriate intervals is a critical safety protocol in the surgical setting. This process involves the systematic verification of all surgical instruments, sponges, and other items used during a procedure to prevent retained foreign objects within the patient. The surgical technologist collaborates closely with the circulator to conduct these counts before the incision, during the procedure, and prior to closure.

The initial count establishes a baseline, while subsequent counts are performed at designated stages, such as after significant tissue manipulation or when items are added or removed. Accurate counting is essential for patient safety, as discrepancies can lead to severe complications, including infection or additional surgeries. Effective communication and meticulous attention to detail are vital during this process to ensure that all items are accounted for, fostering a culture of safety and accountability within the surgical team.

1.2.5 Verify, receive, mix, and label all medications and solutions:

This process involves several critical steps to ensure patient safety and effective surgical outcomes. Verification begins with confirming the medication's identity, dosage, and expiration date against the surgeon's orders. Upon receiving medications and solutions, the surgical technologist must inspect them for any signs of contamination or damage. Mixing solutions requires adherence to specific protocols, including using aseptic techniques to prevent infection and ensuring accurate measurements to maintain therapeutic efficacy. Proper labeling is essential; each medication and solution must be clearly marked with the name, concentration, and expiration date to avoid confusion during the procedure. This meticulous approach not only safeguards the patient but also enhances the surgical team's efficiency, ensuring that the correct medications are readily available and administered as intended during the operation. Adhering to these practices is a fundamental responsibility of the surgical technologist in the intraoperative environment.

1.2.6 Provide intraoperative assistance under the direction of the surgeon:

Providing intraoperative assistance under the direction of the surgeon involves a surgical technologist's active role in the operating room during surgical procedures. This includes preparing and maintaining the sterile field, passing instruments, and ensuring that all necessary supplies are readily available. The surgical technologist must anticipate the surgeon's needs, demonstrating a thorough understanding of the surgical procedure and the instruments involved. Effective communication is crucial, as the technologist must respond promptly to the surgeon's requests, whether it be for specific instruments or adjustments in the surgical setup. Additionally, the surgical technologist is responsible for monitoring the patient's condition and maintaining a safe environment throughout the procedure. This role requires a high level of attention to detail, teamwork, and the ability to remain calm under pressure, ultimately contributing to the overall success of the surgical intervention.

1.2.7 Identify different types of operative incisions:

Operative incisions are surgical cuts made in the skin and underlying tissues to access the surgical site. Understanding the various types of incisions is crucial for surgical technologists, as they influence the surgical approach, healing, and potential complications. Common types of incisions include:

1. Midline Incision: A vertical cut along the midline of the abdomen, providing access to abdominal organs.

2. Paramedian Incision: A vertical incision made parallel to the midline, often used for lateral access to the abdominal cavity.

3. Transverse Incision: A horizontal incision, typically used in procedures like cesarean sections.

4. Oblique Incision: A diagonal cut, often used in procedures involving the gallbladder or appendix.

5. Laparoscopic Incisions: Small incisions made for minimally invasive procedures, allowing for the insertion of trocars.

Each incision type has specific indications and implications for patient recovery and surgical outcomes.

1.2.8 Identify instruments by:

Identifying surgical instruments is a critical skill for surgical technologists, as it ensures the correct tools are available during procedures. This process involves recognizing instruments based on their physical characteristics, such as shape, size, and function. Surgical instruments can be categorized into various groups, including cutting, grasping, clamping, and suturing tools. Each instrument serves a specific purpose, and familiarity with their design is essential for efficient surgical practice.

Additionally, surgical technologists must understand the materials used in instrument construction, such as stainless steel, which impacts durability and sterilization. Knowledge of instrument names, both common and technical, is vital for effective communication within the surgical team. This identification process not only enhances patient safety but also contributes to the overall efficiency of surgical operations, allowing for quick retrieval and proper handling of instruments during procedures.

1.2.8.1   Function:

The function of surgical instruments refers to their specific purpose and role during surgical procedures. Each instrument is designed to perform a particular task, which can include cutting, grasping, clamping, suturing, or retracting tissues. Understanding the function of each instrument is crucial for surgical technologists, as it ensures the correct instrument is selected and utilized at the appropriate time during surgery. For example, scissors are primarily used for cutting tissues, while forceps are designed for grasping and holding structures. Additionally, clamps are employed to occlude blood vessels or tissues, and retractors are used to hold back tissues for better visibility of the surgical site. Mastery of instrument functions enhances the surgical technologist's ability to assist the surgical team efficiently, contributing to patient safety and optimal surgical outcomes. Proper identification and understanding of instrument functions are foundational skills for effective surgical practice.

1.2.8.2   Application:

In the context of surgical instruments, "Application" refers to the specific use or function of each instrument during surgical procedures. Understanding the application of surgical instruments is crucial for surgical technologists, as it ensures that the correct instrument is selected and utilized effectively in the operating room. Each instrument is designed with a particular purpose, such as cutting, grasping, suturing, or retracting tissues. For example, a scalpel is applied for incisions, while forceps are used for grasping tissues or objects. Knowledge of instrument application also includes recognizing the appropriate timing and technique for their use, which can significantly impact patient outcomes. Mastery of instrument application not only enhances the efficiency of surgical procedures but also contributes to the overall safety and effectiveness of patient care. Thus, surgical technologists must be well-versed in the application of various instruments to support the surgical team proficiently.

1.2.8.3   Classification:

Classification in surgical instrumentation refers to the systematic categorization of surgical tools based on their design, function, and intended use in surgical procedures. Instruments are typically classified into several categories, including cutting and dissecting instruments (e.g., scalpels, scissors), grasping and holding instruments (e.g., forceps, clamps), and suturing instruments (e.g., needle holders). This classification aids surgical technologists in quickly identifying the appropriate instruments required for specific surgical tasks, enhancing efficiency and patient safety during procedures. Additionally, understanding the classification of instruments allows surgical technologists to anticipate the needs of the surgical team, ensuring that the correct instruments are readily available. Familiarity with instrument classification is crucial for maintaining an organized surgical field and contributes to the overall success of surgical interventions. Mastery of this classification system is essential for those preparing for the Certified Surgical Technologist (CST) exam.

1.2.9 Assemble, test, operate, and disassemble specialty equipment:

Assembling specialty equipment involves the systematic arrangement of components according to manufacturer specifications, ensuring that all parts are correctly fitted and secured. Testing is crucial to verify that the equipment functions properly before use, which includes checking for electrical connections, mechanical movements, and safety features. Operating the equipment requires a thorough understanding of its functions, settings, and protocols to ensure safe and effective use during surgical procedures. This includes monitoring performance and making adjustments as necessary. Finally, disassembling specialty equipment must be conducted with care to prevent damage and ensure safe storage or maintenance. This process often involves reversing the assembly steps while adhering to safety protocols. Mastery of these skills is essential for surgical technologists, as they directly impact patient safety and the overall success of surgical interventions.

1.2.9.1   Microscopes:

Microscopes are essential optical instruments used in surgical procedures that require magnification of small structures, such as tissues and cells. They enhance the surgeon's ability to visualize intricate anatomical details, facilitating precision in delicate operations. There are various types of microscopes, including surgical microscopes, which are specifically designed for use in the operating room. These microscopes often feature adjustable magnification, illumination systems, and ergonomic designs to ensure optimal viewing angles and comfort for the surgeon.

Surgical technologists must be proficient in assembling, testing, operating, and disassembling these devices. This includes ensuring proper calibration, adjusting light intensity, and confirming the clarity of the optics. Additionally, technologists should be aware of the sterile techniques required to maintain the microscope's cleanliness during procedures. Understanding the functionality and maintenance of microscopes is crucial for supporting surgical teams and ensuring successful patient outcomes.

1.2.9.2   Computer navigation systems:

Computer navigation systems are advanced technological tools utilized in surgical procedures to enhance precision and accuracy during operations. These systems integrate imaging technologies, such as CT scans or MRI, with real-time data to create a three-dimensional representation of the surgical site. This allows surgeons to visualize anatomical structures in detail, facilitating better planning and execution of complex procedures.

The system typically consists of software that processes imaging data and hardware components, including tracking devices and displays. Surgical technologists must be proficient in assembling, testing, operating, and disassembling these systems to ensure optimal functionality. Proper calibration and maintenance are crucial, as any discrepancies can lead to surgical errors. Additionally, understanding the interface and navigation tools is essential for assisting the surgical team effectively. Overall, computer navigation systems significantly improve surgical outcomes by providing enhanced visualization and guidance throughout the procedure.

1.2.9.3   Thermal technology:

Thermal technology in the surgical setting refers to the use of heat-based devices and techniques to facilitate surgical procedures and enhance patient safety. This includes equipment such as electrosurgical units, which utilize high-frequency electrical currents to cut tissue and coagulate blood vessels, minimizing bleeding during surgery. Thermal technology also encompasses devices like diathermy machines, which generate heat to promote hemostasis and tissue healing.

Surgical technologists must be proficient in assembling, testing, operating, and disassembling these devices to ensure optimal functionality and patient safety. Proper understanding of thermal technology includes knowledge of temperature settings, safety precautions to prevent burns, and the importance of maintaining sterile conditions. Additionally, awareness of the specific applications and limitations of thermal devices is crucial for effective surgical assistance, as improper use can lead to complications. Mastery of thermal technology is essential for the surgical technologist's role in the operating room.

1.2.9.4   Laser technology:
Laser technology refers to the use of focused light energy produced by a laser (Light Amplification by Stimulated Emission of Radiation) for various medical applications, particularly in surgical procedures. Lasers emit light that can be precisely controlled in terms of intensity, wavelength, and duration, allowing for targeted tissue interaction. This technology is utilized for cutting, coagulating, and vaporizing tissue with minimal damage to surrounding structures, enhancing surgical precision and reducing recovery time. Different types of lasers, such as CO_2, Nd:YAG, and diode lasers, are employed based on the specific tissue characteristics and surgical requirements. The application of laser technology in surgery includes dermatological procedures, ophthalmic surgeries, and minimally invasive techniques. Understanding the principles of laser operation, safety protocols, and the biological effects of laser energy is crucial for surgical technologists to effectively assist in procedures utilizing this advanced technology.

1.2.9.4.1   Helium:
Helium is a noble gas that is colorless, odorless, and non-toxic, primarily used in laser technology as a component of certain laser systems, particularly helium-neon (HeNe) lasers. In these systems, helium serves as a gas that, when electrically stimulated, produces a coherent light beam. The HeNe laser emits light at a wavelength of 632.8 nanometers, which is in the visible red spectrum. This type of laser is known for its stability, low divergence, and ability to produce a continuous wave of light, making it ideal for applications such as surgical procedures, where precision is crucial. In surgical settings, helium-neon lasers are often utilized for tissue cutting, coagulation, and photocoagulation, providing minimal thermal damage to surrounding tissues. Understanding the properties and applications of helium in laser technology is essential for surgical technologists to ensure safe and effective use during surgical interventions.

1.2.9.4.2   Argon:
Argon is an inert gas that is commonly used in laser technology, particularly in surgical applications. As a noble gas, it does not react chemically with other substances, making it an ideal choice for procedures requiring precision and minimal tissue damage. Argon lasers emit a blue-green light, which is absorbed by hemoglobin and melanin, allowing for effective coagulation and cutting of soft tissues. This characteristic enables surgeons to perform delicate procedures, such as retinal surgery and dermatological treatments, with enhanced control over bleeding and tissue preservation. The argon laser's ability to focus energy on specific tissues while minimizing collateral damage is crucial in surgical settings. Additionally, the gas can be used in conjunction with other laser types to optimize treatment outcomes. Understanding the properties and applications of argon lasers is essential for surgical technologists to ensure safe and effective use in the operating room.

1.2.9.4.3   CO2 beam coagulators:
CO2 beam coagulators are specialized surgical instruments that utilize a focused beam of carbon dioxide (CO_2) laser light for precise tissue cutting and coagulation. The CO_2 laser operates at a wavelength of 10,600 nanometers, which is highly absorbed by water, making it particularly effective for soft tissue procedures. The laser energy is delivered through a handpiece and can be adjusted for various settings, allowing for controlled incision depth and hemostasis.

During surgical procedures, CO_2 beam coagulators minimize thermal damage to surrounding tissues, reducing postoperative complications and promoting faster healing. They are commonly used in dermatological surgeries, gynecological procedures, and otolaryngology, among others. The ability to simultaneously cut and coagulate tissue enhances surgical efficiency and precision, making CO_2 beam coagulators an essential tool in modern surgical practice. Proper training and understanding of laser safety protocols are crucial for surgical technologists working with these devices.

1.2.9.5   Ultrasound technology:
Ultrasound technology is a diagnostic imaging technique that utilizes high-frequency sound waves to create images of internal body structures. It operates on the principle of echolocation, where sound waves emitted by a transducer penetrate the body and reflect off tissues, organs, and fluids. The reflected sound waves are then captured and converted into visual images displayed on a monitor. This non-invasive method is widely used in various medical fields, including obstetrics, cardiology, and abdominal imaging, due to its ability to provide real-time visualization without exposure to ionizing radiation. Ultrasound is particularly valuable in guiding surgical procedures, assessing organ function, and detecting abnormalities such as tumors or cysts. The technology is portable and can be

performed at the bedside, making it an essential tool in both emergency and routine medical care. Its safety profile and versatility contribute to its prominence in modern medical diagnostics.

1.2.9.5.1 Harmonic scalpel:

The harmonic scalpel is a surgical instrument that utilizes ultrasonic technology to cut and coagulate tissue simultaneously. It operates at a frequency of approximately 55.5 kHz, which generates ultrasonic vibrations that create a rapid oscillation of the blade. This oscillation allows for precise cutting of tissue while minimizing thermal damage to surrounding structures. The harmonic scalpel is particularly advantageous in procedures requiring delicate dissection, such as in laparoscopic surgeries, as it reduces blood loss and promotes faster healing. The device's ability to seal blood vessels up to 5 mm in diameter further enhances its utility in various surgical settings. Additionally, the harmonic scalpel is designed to be user-friendly, with a lightweight and ergonomic design that allows for improved maneuverability. Its effectiveness in achieving hemostasis and reducing operative time makes it a valuable tool in the surgical technologist's arsenal.

1.2.9.5.2 Phacoemulsification:

Phacoemulsification is a modern cataract surgery technique that utilizes ultrasound technology to break up cloudy lenses in the eye, allowing for their removal and replacement with an artificial intraocular lens (IOL). During the procedure, a small incision is made in the cornea, and a phacoemulsification probe is inserted. This probe emits high-frequency ultrasound waves that emulsify the cataractous lens into tiny fragments. These fragments are then aspirated out of the eye through the same probe. The advantages of phacoemulsification include reduced recovery time, minimal tissue trauma, and the ability to perform the procedure under local anesthesia. Surgical technologists play a crucial role in this process by preparing the sterile field, ensuring the proper functioning of the ultrasound equipment, and assisting the surgeon with instrument handling and patient positioning. Mastery of phacoemulsification techniques is essential for surgical technologists involved in ophthalmic surgeries.

1.2.9.6 Endoscopic technology:

Endoscopic technology refers to the use of specialized instruments, known as endoscopes, to visualize and access the interior of a body cavity or organ. This minimally invasive technique allows for both diagnostic and therapeutic procedures, reducing the need for larger incisions associated with traditional surgery. Endoscopes are equipped with a light source and camera, transmitting real-time images to a monitor, enabling surgeons to assess conditions such as tumors, ulcers, or bleeding. Various types of endoscopes exist, including flexible and rigid models, tailored for specific applications like gastrointestinal, respiratory, or urological procedures. The advantages of endoscopic technology include decreased postoperative pain, shorter recovery times, and reduced risk of infection. Surgical technologists play a crucial role in preparing and maintaining endoscopic equipment, ensuring sterility, and assisting the surgical team during procedures, thereby enhancing patient outcomes and procedural efficiency.

1.2.9.7 Power equipment:

Power equipment in the surgical setting refers to electrically or battery-operated devices that assist in performing surgical procedures. This includes tools such as surgical drills, saws, electrosurgical units, and powered retractors. These instruments enhance precision, efficiency, and safety during surgery by providing consistent power and control. Surgical drills, for instance, are used for bone cutting or drilling, while electrosurgical units facilitate cutting and coagulation of tissue through high-frequency electrical currents.

Proper use and maintenance of power equipment are critical to prevent malfunctions and ensure patient safety. Surgical technologists must be proficient in setting up, operating, and troubleshooting these devices, as well as understanding their indications and contraindications. Familiarity with the equipment's components, including power sources, foot pedals, and attachments, is essential. Additionally, adherence to manufacturer guidelines and institutional protocols is vital for effective and safe surgical outcomes.

1.2.10 Assemble and maintain retractors:

Retractors are surgical instruments used to hold back tissues, providing the surgeon with a clear view and access to the surgical site. Assembling retractors involves selecting the appropriate type and size based on the procedure and anatomical area. Common types include hand-held retractors, self-retaining retractors, and specific retractors designed for particular surgeries.

To maintain retractors, surgical technologists must ensure they are clean, functional, and properly sterilized before use. This includes inspecting for any damage, ensuring smooth operation of mechanical parts, and confirming that all components are present. During surgery, retractors should be adjusted as needed to optimize exposure while minimizing tissue trauma. After the procedure, retractors must be carefully cleaned and sterilized according to established protocols to prevent infection and ensure readiness for future use. Proper assembly and maintenance of retractors are crucial for surgical efficiency and patient safety.

1.2.11 Pass instruments and supplies:

Passing instruments and supplies is a critical responsibility of the surgical technologist during a surgical procedure. This task involves the timely and efficient transfer of surgical instruments, sutures, and other necessary supplies to the surgeon and surgical team. The surgical technologist must possess a thorough understanding of the instruments used in the procedure, including their names, functions, and proper handling techniques.

Effective communication and anticipation of the surgeon's needs are essential, as the technologist must be prepared to pass instruments without delay, ensuring the surgical workflow remains uninterrupted. Proper technique includes maintaining a sterile field, passing instruments in a way that minimizes the risk of contamination, and providing the correct instrument based on the surgeon's requests. Mastery of this skill enhances patient safety and contributes to the overall success of the surgical procedure, making it a fundamental aspect of the surgical technologist's role.

1.2.12   Identify appropriate usage of sutures/needles and stapling devices:

The appropriate usage of sutures, needles, and stapling devices is critical in surgical procedures for wound closure and tissue approximation. Sutures are classified into absorbable and non-absorbable types, with absorbable sutures being used for internal tissues that do not require removal, while non-absorbable sutures are utilized for skin closure or areas needing prolonged support. The choice of needle—such as cutting, tapered, or reverse cutting—depends on the tissue type being sutured; for example, tapered needles are ideal for soft tissues, while cutting needles are suited for tougher tissues. Stapling devices offer a rapid and efficient method for closing wounds, particularly in gastrointestinal and thoracic surgeries, providing consistent tension and minimizing tissue trauma. Understanding the specific indications, advantages, and limitations of each device ensures optimal outcomes and promotes patient safety during surgical interventions.

1.2.13   Prepare, pass, and cut suture material as directed:

Preparing, passing, and cutting suture material are critical tasks in surgical procedures that ensure effective wound closure and tissue approximation. Preparation involves selecting the appropriate suture type, size, and needle based on the surgical site and tissue characteristics. The surgical technologist must ensure that the suture is sterile and ready for use, often by checking the packaging and expiration date.

Passing suture material to the surgeon requires skill and precision, as it must be handed over in a manner that allows for seamless continuation of the procedure. This may involve using a needle holder or forceps to maintain sterility and control.

Cutting suture material is performed with sterile scissors, ensuring that the cut is clean and precise to avoid tissue damage. Proper technique in these tasks is essential for optimal surgical outcomes and patient safety.

1.2.14   Provide assistance with stapling devices:

Providing assistance with stapling devices involves the surgical technologist's role in the preparation, operation, and maintenance of various stapling instruments used during surgical procedures. Stapling devices are critical for approximating tissues and securing anastomoses, particularly in gastrointestinal, thoracic, and vascular surgeries. The surgical technologist must ensure that these devices are sterile, functioning correctly, and readily available during the procedure.

This includes understanding the different types of staplers, such as linear, circular, and endoscopic staplers, and their specific applications. The technologist assists the surgeon by passing the stapler, ensuring proper placement, and activating the device as directed. Post-operation, the surgical technologist is responsible for the safe disposal of used stapling devices and maintaining an organized surgical field. Knowledge of the mechanisms and potential complications associated with stapling devices is essential for effective assistance and patient safety.

1.2.15   Differentiate among the various methods and applications of hemostasis:

Hemostasis is the physiological process that prevents and stops bleeding, maintaining blood in a fluid state within the vascular system. Various methods of achieving hemostasis can be categorized into mechanical, thermal, and chemical techniques. Mechanical methods include direct pressure, sutures, and clamps, which physically occlude blood vessels. Thermal methods utilize heat to coagulate proteins and seal tissues, such as with electrocautery or laser devices. Chemical methods involve the application of hemostatic agents, like topical thrombin or gelatin sponges, which promote clot formation. Each method has specific applications based on the surgical context, the type of tissue involved, and the extent of bleeding. Understanding these methods is crucial for surgical technologists to assist effectively in surgical procedures, ensuring optimal patient outcomes and minimizing complications related to excessive blood loss.

1.2.15.1   Mechanical:

Mechanical hemostasis refers to the physical methods employed to control bleeding during surgical procedures. This approach involves the use of instruments and devices to achieve hemostasis without the need for chemical agents or thermal energy. Common mechanical techniques include the application of clamps, ligatures, and sutures to occlude blood vessels and tissues. Additionally, the use of hemostatic devices, such as staples or clips, can effectively secure tissue and prevent blood loss. Mechanical methods are often favored for their immediate effectiveness and the ability to provide direct control over bleeding sites. Surgical technologists must be proficient in the selection and application of these techniques, as well as in the handling of instruments that facilitate mechanical hemostasis. Understanding the principles of mechanical hemostasis is crucial for ensuring patient safety and optimal surgical outcomes.

1.2.15.2   Thermal:

Thermal hemostasis refers to the use of heat to achieve hemostasis during surgical procedures. This method employs devices such as electrosurgical units, lasers, or thermal coagulators to coagulate blood vessels and tissues, thereby minimizing blood loss. The application of heat causes protein denaturation and tissue contraction, leading to the formation of a coagulum that seals the vessel.

Electrosurgery, for instance, utilizes high-frequency electrical currents to generate heat, allowing for precise cutting and coagulation of tissues. Laser technology, on the other hand, focuses light energy to achieve similar effects, providing a more controlled and less invasive approach.

Thermal hemostasis is particularly advantageous in delicate surgeries where precision is paramount, as it reduces the risk of collateral damage to surrounding tissues. Understanding the principles and applications of thermal hemostasis is essential for surgical technologists to assist effectively in maintaining hemostasis during surgical interventions.

1.2.15.3   Chemical:

Chemical hemostasis refers to the use of pharmacological agents to promote blood clotting and control bleeding during surgical procedures. This method involves the application of substances such as topical hemostatic agents, which can include absorbable gelatin sponges, oxidized cellulose, and thrombin. These agents work by enhancing the natural coagulation process, either by providing a scaffold for platelet aggregation or by directly stimulating the clotting cascade.

Chemical hemostatic agents are particularly useful in areas where traditional mechanical methods may be ineffective or impractical. They can be applied directly to the bleeding site, allowing for rapid action. Additionally, some agents are designed to be absorbed by the body over time, minimizing the risk of foreign body reactions. Understanding the appropriate use of chemical hemostatic agents is crucial for surgical technologists, as it ensures effective management of intraoperative bleeding and contributes to patient safety and optimal surgical outcomes.

1.2.16   Irrigate, suction, and sponge operative site:

Irrigation, suction, and sponging are critical components in maintaining a clear and controlled surgical field during procedures. Irrigation involves the introduction of a sterile fluid to wash away debris, blood, or contaminants from the operative site, enhancing visibility and promoting healing. Common irrigants include saline and antiseptic solutions, selected based on the procedure and tissue type.

Suctioning is the process of removing excess fluids, blood, or tissue debris using a suction device, which helps maintain a dry and unobstructed view of the surgical area. This is essential for preventing complications and ensuring the surgeon can perform with precision.

Sponging refers to the use of sterile sponges to absorb blood and fluids, further aiding in the cleanliness of the surgical field. Surgical technologists must be adept at these techniques to support the surgical team effectively and ensure patient safety throughout the procedure.

1.2.17   Monitor medication and solution use:

Monitoring medication and solution use is a critical responsibility of the surgical technologist during surgical procedures. This involves the careful oversight of all medications and solutions administered to the patient, ensuring their proper preparation, labeling, and administration. Surgical technologists must be familiar with various medications, including anesthetics, antibiotics, and analgesics, as well as intravenous solutions used for hydration and electrolyte balance.

They must verify dosages, routes of administration, and the timing of medication delivery, adhering to established protocols and safety guidelines. Additionally, surgical technologists are responsible for observing the patient's response to medications, identifying any adverse reactions or complications, and communicating these observations to the surgical team promptly. Accurate documentation of medication use is also essential for maintaining patient safety and ensuring continuity of care. This vigilance helps prevent medication errors and enhances overall surgical outcomes.

1.2.18   Verify with surgeon the correct type and/or size of specialty specific implantable items:

This process involves confirming with the surgeon the specific requirements for implantable items, such as prosthetics, grafts, or devices that will be used during a surgical procedure. It is crucial for surgical technologists to ensure that the correct type and size of these items are available and prepared prior to surgery. This verification minimizes the risk of complications, such as implant rejection or surgical delays, which can arise from using incorrect or incompatible items. The surgical technologist should reference the surgeon's preferences, the patient's anatomy, and the surgical plan. This may include consulting surgical records, implant catalogs, and manufacturer specifications. Effective communication with the surgical team is essential to confirm that all items meet the necessary standards and specifications, ensuring patient safety and optimal surgical outcomes.

1.2.19   Prepare bone and tissue grafts:

Preparing bone and tissue grafts involves the meticulous process of obtaining, processing, and sterilizing graft materials for surgical use. Bone grafts can be autografts (from the patient), allografts (from a donor), or synthetic materials, while tissue grafts may include skin, fascia, or muscle. The surgical technologist plays a crucial role in ensuring that grafts are appropriately prepared to promote healing and integration. This includes selecting the correct type of graft based on the surgical procedure, ensuring sterility, and maintaining the viability of the graft material.

Techniques such as debridement, shaping, and soaking in sterile solutions may be employed to enhance graft compatibility. Proper preparation is essential to minimize the risk of infection and rejection, ultimately contributing to successful surgical outcomes. Understanding the properties and handling of graft materials is vital for surgical technologists in facilitating effective surgical interventions.

1.2.19.1   Allograft:

An allograft is a type of graft that involves the transplantation of tissue from one individual to another of the same species but with a different genetic makeup. This procedure is commonly utilized in surgical interventions such as orthopedic surgeries, dental implants, and reconstructive procedures. Allografts can include bone, cartilage, skin, and other tissues. The primary advantage of allografts is their ability to provide a scaffold for new tissue growth, facilitating healing and regeneration in the recipient. Allografts are typically procured from deceased donors and processed in tissue banks to ensure sterility and safety. They undergo rigorous screening to minimize the risk of disease transmission and rejection. The use of allografts can significantly reduce the need for harvesting autografts, which involve taking tissue from the patient's own body, thereby minimizing additional surgical sites and associated complications.

1.2.19.2   Autograft:

An autograft is a type of tissue graft that is harvested from the same individual who will receive the graft. This method is commonly utilized in surgical procedures to promote healing and tissue regeneration, as it minimizes the risk of rejection and disease transmission. Autografts can be taken from various sites in the body, including skin, bone, and cartilage, depending on the surgical requirements.

The primary advantage of autografts is their biocompatibility, as the tissue is genetically identical to the recipient, facilitating better integration and healing. For instance, in orthopedic surgeries, bone autografts are often used to fill defects or enhance fusion in spinal procedures. The harvesting process requires careful technique to ensure the donor site heals properly while providing sufficient graft material. Overall, autografts are a critical component in reconstructive and orthopedic surgeries, offering optimal outcomes for patients.

1.2.19.3   Synthetic:

Synthetic bone and tissue grafts are man-made materials designed to mimic the properties of natural bone and tissue. These grafts are often composed of biocompatible substances such as polymers, ceramics, or composites that promote cellular growth and integration with the host tissue. Common synthetic materials include hydroxyapatite, calcium phosphate, and bioactive glass, which provide a scaffold for new tissue formation.

The primary advantage of synthetic grafts is their availability and consistency in quality, reducing the risk of disease transmission associated with allografts (donor tissues). Additionally, synthetic grafts can be engineered to possess specific mechanical properties and degradation rates, allowing for tailored solutions based on the surgical requirements.

In surgical procedures, synthetic grafts are utilized in various applications, including orthopedic surgeries, dental implants, and reconstructive surgeries, facilitating effective healing and restoration of function.

1.2.20   Verify, prepare, and label specimen(s):

Verifying, preparing, and labeling specimens is a critical responsibility of the surgical technologist. This process begins with the verification of the specimen type and its intended analysis, ensuring it aligns with the surgeon's documentation and the surgical procedure performed. Accurate preparation involves handling the specimen with care to prevent contamination or damage, which may include rinsing, cutting, or placing it in appropriate containers.

Labeling is equally vital; each specimen must be clearly labeled with essential information such as the patient's name, date of the procedure, type of specimen, and any relevant identifiers. This ensures proper tracking and reduces the risk of errors in specimen handling. The surgical technologist must adhere to strict protocols to maintain specimen integrity and facilitate accurate diagnosis, making this process essential for patient safety and effective surgical outcomes.

1.2.21   Prepare drains, catheters, and tubing for insertion:

Preparing drains, catheters, and tubing for insertion involves a systematic approach to ensure sterility, functionality, and patient safety. This process begins with selecting the appropriate type and size of drain or catheter based on the surgical procedure and patient anatomy. All equipment must be inspected for integrity and expiration dates. Sterile techniques are paramount; surgical technologists must don appropriate personal protective equipment (PPE) and work within a sterile field.

The items are then assembled, ensuring that all necessary components, such as connectors and securing devices, are included. Lubrication may be applied to facilitate smooth insertion, particularly for catheters. Additionally, the surgical technologist must be prepared to assist the surgeon during the insertion process, providing necessary instruments and maintaining a clear view of the surgical site. Proper preparation is crucial to minimize complications and enhance patient outcomes.

1.2.22 Observe patient's intraoperative status:

Observing a patient's intraoperative status involves continuously monitoring the patient's physiological and psychological condition during surgical procedures. This includes assessing vital signs such as heart rate, blood pressure, oxygen saturation, and respiratory rate, which provide critical information regarding the patient's stability. Surgical technologists must also be vigilant for any signs of distress or adverse reactions to anesthesia, as these can indicate complications. Additionally, monitoring the surgical field for excessive bleeding or changes in tissue color is essential for ensuring patient safety. Effective communication with the surgical team is vital, as any abnormalities observed must be promptly reported to the surgeon or anesthesiologist. This proactive approach not only enhances patient care but also contributes to the overall success of the surgical procedure. Understanding the importance of this observation helps surgical technologists play a crucial role in maintaining intraoperative patient safety and well-being.

1.2.22.1 Monitor color of blood:

Monitoring the color of blood during surgical procedures is a critical aspect of assessing a patient's intraoperative status. Blood color can provide immediate insights into the patient's oxygenation and overall hemodynamic stability. Arterial blood, typically bright red, indicates adequate oxygenation, while darker red or purple venous blood suggests deoxygenation. Surgical technologists must be vigilant in observing these changes, as variations in blood color can signal complications such as hypoxia, hemorrhage, or inadequate perfusion. Additionally, the presence of abnormal colors, such as a brownish hue, may indicate the presence of methemoglobinemia or other pathological conditions. Regularly assessing blood color, alongside other vital signs, allows surgical teams to respond promptly to any intraoperative changes, ensuring patient safety and optimal surgical outcomes. This monitoring is integral to maintaining a clear understanding of the patient's physiological status throughout the surgical procedure.

1.2.22.2 Blood loss:

Blood loss refers to the loss of blood volume during surgical procedures, which can significantly impact a patient's hemodynamic stability. It is crucial for surgical technologists to monitor and assess blood loss to ensure patient safety. Blood loss can occur due to various factors, including surgical technique, injury to blood vessels, or underlying medical conditions.

During surgery, the surgical technologist is responsible for observing the surgical field for signs of excessive bleeding, such as pooling of blood or saturation of sponges. Accurate estimation of blood loss is essential for timely interventions, such as fluid resuscitation or blood transfusions.

The surgical team must maintain awareness of the patient's vital signs, including blood pressure and heart rate, as these can indicate the severity of blood loss. Effective communication with the surgeon and anesthesiologist is vital to address any concerns related to blood loss promptly, ensuring optimal patient outcomes.

1.2.22.3 Patient position:

Patient positioning is a critical aspect of surgical procedures that involves placing the patient in a specific posture to facilitate optimal access to the surgical site while ensuring safety and comfort. Proper positioning is essential to prevent complications such as pressure ulcers, nerve injuries, and respiratory issues. The surgical technologist must be knowledgeable about various positions, including supine, prone, lateral, and lithotomy, and their implications for different types of surgeries.

Each position requires careful consideration of the patient's anatomy and the surgical approach. For instance, the supine position is commonly used for abdominal and thoracic surgeries, while the prone position is often employed for spinal or posterior cranial procedures. Additionally, the surgical team must ensure proper padding and support to maintain circulation and nerve function. Continuous monitoring of the patient's vital signs and overall condition during positioning is crucial to ensure intraoperative safety and effectiveness.

1.2.23 Perform appropriate actions during an emergency:

Performing appropriate actions during an emergency involves a series of critical steps that surgical technologists must be prepared to execute efficiently and effectively. This includes recognizing the nature of the emergency, such as a patient's sudden deterioration, equipment failure, or environmental hazards. Surgical technologists should maintain a calm demeanor, as panic can exacerbate the situation. Immediate actions may involve alerting the surgical team, initiating emergency protocols, and providing necessary assistance, such as administering first aid or managing sterile fields. It is essential to have a clear understanding of the facility's emergency procedures, including evacuation routes and the location of emergency equipment. Additionally, maintaining effective communication with the surgical team and other healthcare personnel is crucial for ensuring patient safety. Regular training and simulation exercises can enhance preparedness, enabling surgical technologists to respond swiftly and appropriately during emergencies, ultimately safeguarding patient outcomes.

1.2.24 Initiate preventative actions in potentially harmful situations:

Initiating preventative actions in potentially harmful situations refers to the proactive measures taken by surgical technologists to mitigate risks that could compromise patient safety, staff well-being, or the sterile environment. This involves recognizing hazards such as equipment malfunction, contamination, or unsafe practices. Surgical technologists must be vigilant in monitoring the surgical field and surrounding environment, ensuring that all instruments are functioning correctly and that sterile techniques are maintained.

In practice, this may include double-checking the integrity of sterile supplies, promptly reporting any equipment issues, and adhering to established protocols for infection control. Additionally, surgical technologists should engage in effective communication with the surgical team to address any concerns immediately. By anticipating and addressing potential threats, surgical technologists play a critical role in fostering a safe surgical environment, ultimately enhancing patient outcomes and minimizing the risk of complications.

1.2.25   Connect and activate drains to suction apparatus:
Connecting and activating drains to a suction apparatus is a critical procedure in surgical settings, ensuring the effective removal of fluids from surgical sites. Drains, such as Jackson-Pratt or Hemovac, are utilized to prevent fluid accumulation, which can lead to complications like infection or delayed healing. To connect a drain to a suction apparatus, the surgical technologist must first ensure that the suction device is functioning properly and set to the appropriate pressure level. The drain's tubing is then securely attached to the suction port, ensuring a tight seal to prevent leaks. Once connected, the technologist activates the suction by turning on the apparatus, monitoring the system for proper drainage and any potential obstructions. This process is vital for maintaining a clear surgical field and promoting optimal patient outcomes postoperatively. Proper technique and vigilance during this procedure are essential for patient safety and effective surgical care.

1.2.26   Prepare dressings and wound site:
Preparing dressings and the wound site is a critical responsibility of a surgical technologist, ensuring optimal healing and infection prevention. This process involves selecting appropriate dressing materials based on the type of wound, surgical procedure, and patient needs. The surgical technologist must first assess the wound site for any signs of infection, such as redness, swelling, or discharge. After cleansing the area with antiseptic solutions, the technologist applies sterile dressings, ensuring they are securely placed to protect the wound while allowing for necessary drainage. It is essential to maintain a sterile field throughout this procedure to prevent contamination. Additionally, the surgical technologist must document the dressing type, application date, and any observations related to the wound site, facilitating ongoing patient care and monitoring. Proper preparation of dressings and the wound site is vital for promoting healing and minimizing complications post-surgery.

1.2.27   Assist in the application of casts, splints, braces, and similar devices:
Assisting in the application of casts, splints, braces, and similar devices involves supporting the surgical team in immobilizing and stabilizing injured or post-operative areas of the body. This process is crucial for promoting healing and preventing further injury. Surgical technologists must be knowledgeable about the various types of immobilization devices, including fiberglass and plaster casts, as well as soft and rigid splints.

During the application, the surgical technologist prepares the materials, ensuring they are sterile and ready for use. They assist the surgeon by positioning the patient correctly and providing necessary instruments and supplies. Additionally, they may help monitor the patient's comfort and circulation during the procedure. Understanding the principles of anatomy and the specific indications for each device is essential for effective assistance, ensuring optimal patient outcomes and adherence to safety protocols.

1.3   Postoperative Procedures:
Postoperative procedures refer to the series of actions and protocols implemented following surgical interventions to ensure patient safety, promote healing, and prevent complications. These procedures encompass a range of activities, including monitoring vital signs, managing pain, and assessing the surgical site for signs of infection or abnormality. Surgical technologists play a crucial role in the postoperative phase by assisting in the transfer of patients to recovery, ensuring that all surgical instruments and materials are accounted for, and maintaining a sterile environment. Additionally, they may assist in educating patients and their families about postoperative care, including wound care, activity restrictions, and signs of potential complications. Effective communication with the surgical team and adherence to established protocols are essential to facilitate a smooth recovery process and enhance patient outcomes. Understanding these procedures is vital for surgical technologists as they contribute significantly to patient care and safety in the postoperative setting.

1.3.1 Report medication and solution amount used:
Reporting the medication and solution amounts used during surgical procedures is a critical component of postoperative care. This process involves accurately documenting the types and quantities of medications and solutions administered to the patient, which is essential for ensuring patient safety and continuity of care. Surgical technologists must meticulously record these details in the patient's medical record, as they provide vital information for the postoperative team, including anesthesiologists and nursing staff. Accurate reporting helps in monitoring the patient's response to medications, managing potential side effects, and preventing complications related to medication errors. Furthermore, this documentation serves as a legal record of the care provided and is crucial for compliance with healthcare regulations. Surgical technologists should be familiar with the specific medications and solutions used in various procedures, as well as the appropriate methods for calculating and reporting these amounts.

1.3.2 Participate in case debrief:

Participating in a case debrief is a critical component of the surgical process, aimed at evaluating and improving surgical outcomes. A case debrief is a structured discussion that occurs after a surgical procedure, involving the surgical team, including surgeons, nurses, and surgical technologists. During this debrief, team members review the case, discussing what went well, any complications encountered, and areas for improvement. This process fosters open communication, enhances teamwork, and promotes a culture of safety. It allows surgical technologists to share their observations and insights, contributing to collective learning and professional development. By actively participating in case debriefs, surgical technologists can help identify best practices, reinforce protocols, and ultimately improve patient care. Engaging in this reflective practice is essential for continuous quality improvement within the surgical environment.

1.3.3 Remove drapes and other equipment from patient:

Removing drapes and other equipment from the patient is a critical step in the postoperative phase of surgical procedures. This process involves carefully lifting and disposing of sterile drapes that were used to maintain a sterile field during surgery, ensuring that no contaminants are introduced to the surgical site. It is essential to follow proper protocols to prevent infection and maintain patient safety. The surgical technologist must assess the surgical site for any remaining instruments, sponges, or other materials that may have been used during the procedure. Once the area is deemed safe, the surgical technologist should systematically remove all equipment, ensuring that the patient is comfortable and protected during the transition from the operating room to recovery. This task requires attention to detail and adherence to infection control practices, as it directly impacts patient outcomes and overall surgical success.

1.3.3.1   Suction:

Suction refers to the process of removing blood, fluids, and debris from the surgical site to maintain a clear operative field. This is crucial for visibility and safety during surgical procedures. Surgical suction devices, such as handheld suction or wall-mounted systems, are employed to facilitate this process. The suction tip, often referred to as a suction catheter, is designed to effectively evacuate fluids without damaging surrounding tissues.

The surgical technologist is responsible for ensuring the suction equipment is functioning properly, including checking for blockages and ensuring that the suction canister is appropriately placed and secured. Additionally, the technologist must anticipate the surgeon's needs for suction throughout the procedure, providing it promptly to enhance visibility and control. Proper suction technique also involves maintaining sterile conditions and handling the equipment in a manner that minimizes the risk of contamination.

1.3.3.2   Cautery:

Cautery refers to the process of using heat to destroy tissue, control bleeding, or remove unwanted growths during surgical procedures. There are two primary types of cautery: thermal and electrocautery. Thermal cautery utilizes direct heat from a heated instrument to achieve tissue destruction, while electrocautery employs electrical currents to generate heat, allowing for precise tissue manipulation.

Electrocautery is further divided into monopolar and bipolar techniques. Monopolar cautery involves a single active electrode, with the current passing through the patient to a grounding pad, whereas bipolar cautery uses two electrodes, allowing for localized tissue destruction without affecting surrounding areas.

Cautery is essential in minimizing blood loss during surgery, reducing the risk of infection, and facilitating the removal of lesions. Surgical technologists must be adept at handling cautery instruments, ensuring proper settings, and maintaining safety protocols to protect both the patient and the surgical team.

1.3.3.3   Instrumentation:

Instrumentation in the surgical setting refers to the array of surgical tools and devices utilized during procedures to facilitate various tasks, including cutting, grasping, suturing, and cauterizing. Surgical instruments are categorized based on their function: cutting instruments (e.g., scalpels, scissors), grasping instruments (e.g., forceps, clamps), and suturing instruments (e.g., needle holders). Each instrument is designed with specific characteristics to enhance precision and efficiency.

Proper handling and maintenance of these instruments are crucial for patient safety and surgical success. Surgical technologists must be proficient in identifying, organizing, and managing instruments, ensuring they are sterile and ready for use. Additionally, understanding the appropriate use of each instrument aids in anticipating the surgeon's needs during the procedure. Mastery of instrumentation is essential for surgical technologists, as it directly impacts the workflow and outcomes of surgical interventions.

1.3.3.4   Nondisposable items:

Nondisposable items, also known as reusable surgical instruments and equipment, are tools that can be sterilized and used multiple times in surgical procedures. These items include surgical instruments such as scalpels, forceps, scissors, and retractors, as well as equipment like electrosurgical units and suction devices. Their design allows for thorough cleaning and sterilization, ensuring they are safe for patient use in subsequent surgeries. Proper handling and maintenance of nondisposable items are critical to prevent cross-contamination and ensure patient safety. Surgical technologists must be proficient in identifying, organizing, and preparing these instruments for use, as well as understanding the specific sterilization protocols required for each item. Following surgical procedures, it is essential to correctly remove and process nondisposable items to maintain a sterile environment and adhere to infection control standards. This knowledge is vital for ensuring the efficiency and safety of surgical operations.

1.3.4 Report abnormal postoperative findings:

Reporting abnormal postoperative findings involves the systematic identification and communication of any deviations from expected recovery patterns following surgical procedures. Surgical technologists play a crucial role in monitoring patients postoperatively, as they are trained to recognize signs of complications such as infection, hemorrhage, or adverse reactions to anesthesia. Abnormal findings may include elevated vital signs, unusual drainage from surgical sites, or changes in the patient's level of consciousness. It is essential for surgical technologists to document these observations accurately and relay them promptly to the surgical team or nursing staff. Effective communication ensures that appropriate interventions can be initiated swiftly, thereby minimizing potential risks to the patient's health. Understanding the significance of these findings and the protocols for reporting them is vital for maintaining patient safety and enhancing overall surgical outcomes.

1.3.4.1   Bleeding at surgical site:

Bleeding at the surgical site refers to the loss of blood from blood vessels that may occur during or after a surgical procedure. This can manifest as external bleeding, where blood is visible on the surface, or internal bleeding, where blood accumulates within the body cavity. It is crucial for surgical technologists to monitor for signs of bleeding, as it can indicate complications such as inadequate hemostasis, damage to blood vessels, or the presence of underlying conditions. The assessment of bleeding involves observing the surgical site for excessive drainage, changes in vital signs, and the patient's overall condition. Immediate reporting of abnormal findings to the surgical team is essential, as timely intervention can prevent significant blood loss and associated complications. Effective management may include applying pressure, utilizing hemostatic agents, or preparing for potential reoperation to control the source of bleeding.

1.3.4.2   Hematoma:

A hematoma is a localized collection of blood outside of blood vessels, typically resulting from trauma or surgical intervention. It occurs when blood leaks from damaged vessels into surrounding tissues, leading to swelling, pain, and discoloration. Hematomas can develop in various anatomical locations, including subcutaneous tissues, muscles, and organs. Postoperatively, they may arise due to inadequate hemostasis, excessive movement, or underlying coagulopathy.

Clinically, hematomas can present as firm, tender masses that may be palpable upon examination. The color may vary from red to purple and eventually changes to yellow as the blood is reabsorbed. Complications include infection, pressure on adjacent structures, and, in severe cases, compartment syndrome. Surgical technologists must be vigilant in monitoring for signs of hematoma formation and report any abnormal findings to the surgical team promptly, ensuring timely intervention and management to prevent further complications.

1.3.4.3   Rash:

A rash is a noticeable change in the texture or color of the skin, often characterized by redness, swelling, and irritation. In the postoperative context, rashes can indicate allergic reactions, infections, or other complications. Surgical technologists must be vigilant in monitoring patients for rashes, as they may arise from various factors, including surgical materials, medications, or underlying health conditions.

Rashes can manifest in different forms, such as maculopapular, vesicular, or urticarial, each requiring specific assessment and intervention. The presence of a rash may signal an allergic response to latex gloves, antiseptics, or sutures. Additionally, rashes can be indicative of infections, such as cellulitis or surgical site infections, necessitating immediate medical evaluation. Prompt identification and reporting of rashes are crucial in ensuring patient safety and effective postoperative care, as they may lead to further complications if not addressed appropriately.

1.3.5 Dispose of contaminated waste and drapes after surgery in compliance with Standard Precautions:

The disposal of contaminated waste and drapes post-surgery is a critical component of infection control and patient safety. Standard Precautions, established by the Centers for Disease Control and Prevention (CDC), dictate that all blood, body fluids, and contaminated materials should be treated as potentially infectious. Contaminated drapes, sponges, and instruments must be placed in designated biohazard bags or containers immediately after use to prevent exposure and cross-contamination. These containers should be clearly labeled and puncture-resistant. Surgical technologists must ensure that waste is segregated appropriately, with sharps disposed of in designated sharps containers. Following institutional protocols, waste disposal should occur in compliance with local regulations and guidelines to minimize environmental impact. Proper training and adherence to these procedures are essential for maintaining a safe surgical environment and protecting healthcare workers and patients from potential infections.

1.3.6 Transfer patient from operating table to stretcher:

Transferring a patient from the operating table to a stretcher is a critical procedure that requires careful coordination and attention to patient safety. This process involves the surgical team, typically including the surgical technologist, anesthesiologist, and nursing staff. The primary goal is to ensure the patient is moved without causing discomfort or injury, particularly if they are under anesthesia or have undergone significant surgical intervention.

Before the transfer, the surgical technologist should ensure that the stretcher is positioned appropriately and locked in place. The surgical team should communicate effectively, using clear verbal cues to synchronize their movements. The patient should be supported adequately, with one team member stabilizing the head and another managing the lower body. It is essential to maintain the patient's privacy and dignity throughout the transfer. Proper body mechanics should be employed to prevent injury to both the patient and the healthcare providers involved in the transfer.

1.3.7 Dispose of contaminated sharps after surgery in compliance with Standard Precautions:

The disposal of contaminated sharps refers to the proper handling and disposal of instruments that can puncture or cut skin, such as needles, scalpel blades, and other sharp objects used during surgical procedures. Compliance with Standard Precautions is critical to prevent the transmission of bloodborne pathogens and ensure the safety of healthcare workers and patients.

Sharps must be placed immediately into designated, puncture-resistant containers that are clearly labeled and located in accessible areas within the surgical environment. These containers should be sealed and disposed of according to local regulations and institutional policies. It is essential to avoid overfilling sharps containers and to never attempt to recap needles or manipulate sharps by hand after use. Adhering to these protocols minimizes the risk of needlestick injuries and promotes a safe surgical environment, ultimately protecting both healthcare personnel and patients from potential infections.

1.3.8 Perform room clean up and restock supplies:

Performing room clean-up and restocking supplies is a critical responsibility of the surgical technologist, ensuring that the operating room (OR) is prepared for subsequent procedures. This process involves the systematic removal of all used instruments, drapes, and other materials from the surgical field, followed by thorough cleaning of surfaces to maintain a sterile environment. The surgical technologist must adhere to infection control protocols, utilizing appropriate disinfectants and techniques to eliminate contaminants.

After cleaning, the surgical technologist restocks essential supplies, including sterile instruments, sutures, and dressings, ensuring that all items are organized and readily accessible for the next surgical team. This task requires attention to detail and knowledge of the specific needs of various surgical procedures. Effective room clean-up and restocking contribute to patient safety, operational efficiency, and the overall success of surgical interventions.

2   ANCILLARY DUTIES:

Ancillary duties refer to the supportive tasks and responsibilities that surgical technologists perform to ensure the smooth operation of the surgical environment. These duties extend beyond the core responsibilities of preparing the operating room and assisting the surgical team during procedures. They encompass a range of activities, including maintaining sterile fields, managing surgical instruments, and ensuring the availability of necessary supplies. Additionally, ancillary duties may involve assisting with patient positioning, monitoring vital signs, and participating in the cleaning and sterilization of instruments post-surgery. Effective execution of these duties is crucial for patient safety and optimal surgical outcomes. Surgical technologists must demonstrate proficiency in these ancillary tasks, as they contribute significantly to the overall efficiency of surgical procedures and the functioning of the healthcare team. Understanding and performing these duties is essential for certification and professional practice in the surgical field.

2.1 Administrative and Personnel:

Administrative and personnel duties in the surgical setting encompass the management of both operational and human resources aspects essential for effective surgical services. This includes scheduling surgical procedures, maintaining accurate patient records, and ensuring compliance with regulatory standards. Surgical technologists may assist in the recruitment, training, and evaluation of staff, contributing to a cohesive team environment. They also play a crucial role in inventory management, ensuring that surgical supplies and equipment are adequately stocked and maintained. Effective communication with surgeons, nurses, and other healthcare professionals is vital for the smooth operation of the surgical suite. Additionally, understanding policies related to patient confidentiality and safety protocols is imperative. By managing these administrative and personnel tasks efficiently, surgical technologists support the overall functionality of the surgical team, enhancing patient care and operational efficiency within the healthcare facility.

2.1.1 Revise surgeon's preference card as necessary:

The surgeon's preference card is a vital document that outlines the specific instruments, supplies, and techniques preferred by a surgeon for various procedures. It serves as a reference for surgical technologists to ensure that the correct items are prepared and available during surgery. Revising this card as necessary is crucial for maintaining accuracy and efficiency in the operating room. Changes may arise due to updates in surgical techniques, new instruments, or alterations in the surgeon's preferences based on recent experiences or evolving practices. Regularly reviewing and updating the preference card helps prevent delays, enhances patient safety, and ensures that the surgical team is well-prepared. Surgical technologists should collaborate with the surgeon to confirm any modifications and ensure that the card reflects the most current practices, thereby optimizing surgical outcomes and streamlining the workflow in the operating room.

2.1.2 Follow proper cost containment processes:

Cost containment processes refer to strategies and practices implemented to control and reduce expenses within a surgical setting without compromising patient care quality. Surgical technologists play a crucial role in these processes by ensuring efficient use of supplies and resources. This includes accurately tracking inventory, minimizing waste, and adhering to protocols for the use of surgical instruments and materials.

By participating in regular audits of surgical supplies and equipment, surgical technologists can identify areas where costs can be reduced, such as eliminating unnecessary items from surgical trays or optimizing sterilization processes. Additionally, they should be aware of the financial implications of their actions, such as the costs associated with overtime or the use of premium supplies. Effective communication with the surgical team about resource utilization and potential savings can foster a culture of cost efficiency, ultimately benefiting the healthcare institution and enhancing patient care.

2.1.3 Utilize computer technology for:

Utilizing computer technology in the surgical setting involves the application of various digital tools and systems to enhance surgical procedures and improve patient outcomes. This includes the use of electronic health records (EHR) for accurate documentation and easy access to patient information, which facilitates better communication among the surgical team. Computer technology also encompasses surgical planning software that aids in preoperative assessments and simulations, allowing for more precise surgical strategies. Additionally, intraoperative monitoring systems provide real-time data on patient vitals, ensuring timely interventions when necessary. Furthermore, computer-assisted surgical devices, such as robotic systems, enhance the precision of surgical techniques. Overall, the integration of computer technology in surgical practice streamlines workflows, reduces the likelihood of errors, and ultimately contributes to improved efficiency and safety in the operating room.

2.1.3.1 Surgeon's preference cards:

Surgeon's preference cards are essential tools used in the surgical environment to document and communicate a surgeon's specific preferences for surgical procedures. These cards typically include detailed information such as the types of instruments, sutures, and supplies preferred by the surgeon, as well as any special techniques or positioning requirements. The cards serve as a reference for surgical technologists and other operating room staff, ensuring that all necessary items are prepared and available before the procedure begins. By utilizing these cards, surgical teams can enhance efficiency, minimize delays, and reduce the risk of errors during surgery. Additionally, preference cards can be updated regularly to reflect any changes in a surgeon's preferences, promoting continuous improvement in surgical practices. Overall, they play a critical role in facilitating effective communication and collaboration within the surgical team, ultimately contributing to better patient outcomes.

2.1.3.2 Interdepartmental communication:

Interdepartmental communication refers to the exchange of information and collaboration between different departments within a healthcare facility, such as surgery, anesthesia, nursing, and administration. Effective interdepartmental communication is crucial for ensuring patient safety, optimizing surgical outcomes, and enhancing overall operational efficiency. Surgical technologists play a vital role in facilitating this communication by utilizing computer technology, such as electronic health records (EHRs), messaging systems, and scheduling software. These tools enable real-time updates on patient status, surgical schedules, and resource availability, allowing for timely decision-making and coordination among team members. Additionally, clear communication protocols and documentation practices help prevent misunderstandings and errors, ultimately fostering a cohesive working environment. By leveraging technology, surgical technologists can enhance interdepartmental collaboration, ensuring that all team members are informed and aligned in their efforts to provide high-quality patient care.

2.1.3.3 Continuing education:

Continuing education refers to the ongoing professional development and training that surgical technologists engage in after obtaining their initial certification. This process is essential for maintaining competency, staying current with technological advancements, and adhering to evolving surgical protocols and standards. Continuing education can encompass a variety of formats, including workshops, seminars, online courses, and conferences, all designed to enhance knowledge and skills relevant to surgical technology.

The National Board of Surgical Technology and Surgical Assisting (NBSTSA) mandates that certified surgical technologists complete a specific number of continuing education units (CEUs) within a designated period to renew their certification. This requirement ensures that professionals remain informed about best practices, new surgical techniques, and innovations in equipment and technology. Engaging in continuing education not only fosters personal growth but also contributes to improved patient care and safety in the surgical environment.

2.1.3.4 Research:

Research in the context of surgical technology involves the systematic investigation and analysis of medical literature, clinical practices, and technological advancements to enhance patient care and surgical outcomes. Surgical technologists utilize computer technology to access databases, journals, and online resources to gather evidence-based information relevant to surgical procedures, instruments, and techniques. This process includes reviewing studies on surgical outcomes, infection control protocols, and innovations in surgical equipment. By staying informed through research, surgical technologists can contribute to the development of best practices, improve procedural efficiency, and ensure adherence to safety standards. Additionally, research findings can guide the selection of appropriate surgical instruments and techniques tailored to specific patient needs. Ultimately, the integration of research into daily practice empowers surgical technologists to support the surgical team effectively and advocate for patient safety and quality care in the operating room.

2.1.4 Follow hospital and national disaster plan protocol:

Following hospital and national disaster plan protocols involves adhering to established guidelines and procedures designed to ensure the safety and well-being of patients, staff, and visitors during emergencies. These protocols are developed in accordance with local, state, and federal regulations and are essential for effective response to disasters, such as natural calamities, pandemics, or mass casualty incidents.

As a surgical technologist, it is crucial to be familiar with the specific disaster response plan of your healthcare facility, including evacuation routes, triage procedures, and communication strategies. Training sessions and drills are often conducted to prepare staff for various scenarios, ensuring that everyone understands their roles and responsibilities. By following these protocols, surgical technologists contribute to a coordinated response, minimizing chaos and enhancing patient care during critical situations. Adherence to these plans is vital for maintaining operational continuity and safeguarding lives.

2.1.5 Fire:

Fire in the surgical setting refers to the rapid oxidation of materials that can lead to combustion, posing a significant risk to patients and surgical staff. The primary components necessary for fire to occur are heat, fuel, and oxygen, often referred to as the fire triangle. In the operating room, potential sources of ignition include electrosurgical devices, lasers, and heat-producing equipment. Flammable substances, such as alcohol-based antiseptics and drapes, serve as fuel. Oxygen is abundant in the surgical environment, especially when supplemental oxygen is used for patients.

To mitigate fire risks, surgical technologists must adhere to strict protocols, including proper draping techniques, maintaining a safe distance from ignition sources, and ensuring that flammable materials are adequately dried before procedures. Additionally, staff should be trained in fire response procedures, including the use of fire extinguishers and the evacuation of patients, ensuring a safe surgical environment.

2.1.6 Chemical spill:

A chemical spill refers to the unintended release of hazardous substances, which can occur in various healthcare settings, including surgical environments. These spills may involve chemicals such as disinfectants, anesthetics, or other surgical agents that can pose risks to personnel, patients, and the environment.

In the event of a chemical spill, immediate action is crucial to mitigate potential harm. Surgical technologists must follow established protocols, including notifying the appropriate personnel, containing the spill, and utilizing personal protective equipment (PPE) to ensure safety. Proper training in spill response procedures is essential, as it enables surgical technologists to act swiftly and effectively.

Additionally, understanding the Material Safety Data Sheets (MSDS) for chemicals used in the surgical setting is vital, as these documents provide critical information on handling, exposure risks, and emergency measures. Prompt and efficient management of chemical spills is essential for maintaining a safe surgical environment.

2.1.7 Laser:

A laser (Light Amplification by Stimulated Emission of Radiation) is a device that emits a focused beam of light through a process of optical amplification. In surgical applications, lasers are utilized for cutting, coagulating, and vaporizing tissue with precision. The key characteristics of lasers include monochromaticity, coherence, and directionality, which allow for minimal damage to surrounding tissues and enhanced visibility during procedures.

Different types of lasers, such as CO_2, Nd:YAG, and argon lasers, are employed based on the specific surgical requirements and tissue types. For instance, CO_2 lasers are effective for soft tissue procedures due to their ability to cut and coagulate simultaneously. Surgical technologists must understand the operational principles, safety protocols, and proper handling of lasers to ensure patient safety and optimal outcomes. Knowledge of laser settings, wavelengths, and applications is essential for effective collaboration in the surgical team.

2.1.8 Smoke:

Surgical smoke is a byproduct generated during the use of thermal devices, such as lasers, electrosurgical pencils, and other heat-producing instruments, in surgical procedures. It consists of vaporized tissue, cellular debris, and various toxic chemicals, which can pose health risks to surgical staff and patients. The composition of surgical smoke can include harmful substances such as benzene, hydrogen cyanide, and formaldehyde, making it essential for surgical technologists to be aware of its dangers. Inhalation of smoke can lead to respiratory issues and other long-term health complications. To mitigate these risks, effective smoke evacuation systems should be employed during procedures to capture and filter smoke at the source. Additionally, surgical technologists should be trained in the proper use of these systems and understand the importance of maintaining a smoke-free environment to ensure the safety of the surgical team and the patient.

2.1.9 Understand basic principles of electricity and electrical safety:

Electricity is the flow of electric charge, typically through conductors, and is fundamental in powering surgical instruments and equipment. Understanding the basic principles involves recognizing voltage (the potential difference), current (the flow of electric charge), and resistance (the opposition to current flow). Electrical safety is paramount in the surgical environment to prevent hazards such as electrical shock or equipment malfunction. Key safety practices include ensuring proper grounding of equipment, using circuit breakers, and adhering to the "three-prong" plug standard. Surgical technologists must also be aware of the risks associated with wet environments, as moisture can increase conductivity. Regular inspection of electrical equipment for frayed cords or damaged plugs is essential. Additionally, understanding the importance of using equipment as intended and following manufacturer guidelines can significantly reduce the risk of electrical accidents in the operating room, ensuring a safe surgical environment for both patients and staff.

2.1.10   Apply ethical and legal practices related to surgical patient care:

Applying ethical and legal practices in surgical patient care involves adhering to established standards that govern the conduct of healthcare professionals. Ethically, surgical technologists must prioritize patient autonomy, beneficence, non-maleficence, and justice. This means respecting patients' rights to make informed decisions about their care, ensuring that interventions benefit the patient while minimizing harm, and providing equitable treatment regardless of personal characteristics. Legally, surgical technologists must comply with laws and regulations, such as obtaining informed consent, maintaining patient confidentiality as mandated by HIPAA, and adhering to institutional policies. Documentation is also critical, as it serves as a legal record of care provided. By integrating ethical principles and legal requirements into their practice, surgical technologists contribute to a safe and respectful surgical environment, ultimately enhancing patient outcomes and fostering trust in the healthcare system.

2.1.11   Use interpersonal skills and group dynamics:

Interpersonal skills refer to the abilities that facilitate effective communication and interaction with others, crucial in a surgical setting. These skills include active listening, empathy, conflict resolution, and the ability to provide constructive feedback. Group dynamics, on the other hand, involve the study of how individuals behave and interact within a team. In the context of surgical technology, understanding group dynamics is essential for fostering collaboration and ensuring optimal patient outcomes. Surgical technologists must navigate diverse personalities and roles, adapting their communication styles to promote teamwork and efficiency. Effective use of interpersonal skills enhances trust and respect among team members, leading to improved morale and reduced stress in high-pressure environments. Mastery of these skills enables surgical technologists to contribute positively to the surgical team, ensuring that all members work cohesively towards a common goal: patient safety and successful surgical procedures.

2.1.11.1   Listening:

Listening is a critical interpersonal skill that involves actively receiving and interpreting verbal and non-verbal messages during communication. In the surgical environment, effective listening is essential for ensuring patient safety, enhancing team collaboration, and minimizing misunderstandings. It requires the surgical technologist to focus intently on the speaker, demonstrating attentiveness through body language, eye contact, and appropriate feedback. Active listening also involves processing the information conveyed, asking clarifying questions, and reflecting on the content to ensure comprehension. This skill fosters a supportive atmosphere where team members feel valued and understood, ultimately contributing to better surgical outcomes. Additionally, listening aids in recognizing non-verbal cues, such as a surgeon's urgency or a colleague's concerns, which can be pivotal during high-pressure situations. By honing listening skills, surgical technologists can enhance communication, build trust within the surgical team, and promote a culture of safety and efficiency in the operating room.

2.1.11.2   Diplomacy:

Diplomacy in the context of surgical technology refers to the ability to communicate effectively and tactfully with colleagues, patients, and other healthcare professionals. It involves navigating complex interpersonal dynamics while maintaining professionalism and fostering a collaborative environment. Surgical technologists often work in high-pressure situations where emotions can run high; therefore, employing diplomacy is crucial for conflict resolution and team cohesion. This skill enables surgical technologists to articulate their thoughts clearly, listen actively, and respond appropriately to diverse perspectives. By demonstrating empathy and respect, they can build trust and rapport with team members, which is essential for optimal patient care. Additionally, diplomacy aids in addressing misunderstandings or disagreements constructively, ensuring that the surgical team remains focused on the common goal of patient safety and successful outcomes. Overall, effective diplomacy enhances communication, promotes teamwork, and contributes to a positive surgical environment.

2.1.11.3   Responsiveness:

Responsiveness in the surgical environment refers to the ability of surgical technologists to react promptly and effectively to the needs of the surgical team and the patient. This includes being attentive to verbal and non-verbal cues, anticipating the needs of the surgeon, and adapting to the dynamic nature of the operating room. A responsive surgical technologist maintains a high level of situational awareness, which is crucial for ensuring patient safety and the smooth progression of surgical procedures. This skill involves active listening, clear communication, and the ability to prioritize tasks efficiently. By demonstrating responsiveness, surgical technologists contribute to a collaborative atmosphere, fostering trust and teamwork among all members of the surgical team. Ultimately, responsiveness enhances the overall surgical experience, minimizes the risk of errors, and supports optimal patient outcomes.

2.1.12 Understand the importance of cultural diversity:

Cultural diversity refers to the variety of cultural or ethnic groups within a society. In the context of surgical technology, understanding cultural diversity is crucial for delivering effective patient care. It encompasses recognizing and respecting the differences in beliefs, values, practices, and communication styles among patients from various backgrounds. This understanding fosters an inclusive environment that enhances patient trust and satisfaction.

Surgical technologists must be aware of how cultural factors can influence a patient's response to medical procedures, pain management, and recovery. For instance, some cultures may have specific rituals or preferences regarding surgical interventions. By being culturally competent, surgical technologists can improve teamwork in the operating room, minimize misunderstandings, and ensure that all patients receive equitable care. Ultimately, embracing cultural diversity leads to better health outcomes and a more harmonious healthcare environment.

2.1.13 Understand concepts of death and dying:

The concepts of death and dying encompass the biological, psychological, and sociocultural dimensions of the end-of-life process. Biologically, death is defined as the irreversible cessation of all vital functions, including cardiac and respiratory activity. Psychologically, individuals experience a range of emotions, such as denial, anger, bargaining, depression, and acceptance, often referred to as the stages of grief, as proposed by Elisabeth Kübler-Ross. Socioculturally, beliefs and rituals surrounding death vary significantly across different cultures, influencing how individuals and families cope with loss. For surgical technologists, understanding these concepts is crucial as they often interact with patients and families facing terminal conditions. This knowledge fosters empathy and enhances communication, allowing surgical technologists to provide compassionate care and support during challenging times. Recognizing the emotional and ethical implications of death and dying is essential for promoting a holistic approach to patient care in the surgical setting.

2.1.14 Participate in organ and tissue procurement:

Participating in organ and tissue procurement involves the surgical technologist's role in the process of obtaining organs and tissues for transplantation. This process is critical for saving lives and enhancing the quality of life for patients with organ failure or severe tissue damage. Surgical technologists assist in preparing the operating room, ensuring that all necessary instruments and supplies are sterile and ready for use. They also collaborate with the surgical team to maintain a sterile field during the procedure, which is essential for preventing infections. Additionally, surgical technologists may be involved in the documentation of the procurement process, ensuring compliance with legal and ethical standards. Their understanding of anatomy, surgical procedures, and the specific requirements for organ preservation is vital. By participating in this process, surgical technologists contribute significantly to the success of organ transplantation and the overall healthcare system.

2.1.15 Serve as preceptor to perioperative personnel:

Serving as a preceptor to perioperative personnel involves mentoring and guiding surgical technologists, nurses, and other healthcare professionals within the surgical environment. A preceptor is an experienced practitioner who provides hands-on training, support, and evaluation of the skills and knowledge of less experienced staff. This role is crucial in fostering a culture of safety and excellence in the operating room. The preceptor is responsible for orienting new team members to protocols, procedures, and equipment, ensuring they understand their roles and responsibilities. Additionally, the preceptor assesses the learner's competencies, offering constructive feedback to enhance their performance. This mentorship not only aids in the professional development of the preceptee but also contributes to improved patient outcomes by ensuring that all team members are well-prepared and proficient in their tasks. Ultimately, serving as a preceptor reinforces the collaborative nature of the surgical team.

2.2 Equipment Sterilization and Maintenance:

Equipment sterilization and maintenance refer to the processes and practices employed to ensure that surgical instruments and devices are free from all forms of microbial life, thereby preventing infections during surgical procedures. Sterilization can be achieved through various methods, including steam sterilization (autoclaving), ethylene oxide gas, and hydrogen peroxide plasma. Each method has specific protocols regarding temperature, pressure, and exposure time, which must be meticulously followed to achieve effective sterilization.

Maintenance involves routine inspections, cleaning, and repairs of surgical instruments to ensure their functionality and safety. This includes checking for wear and tear, ensuring proper alignment, and replacing any damaged components. Proper sterilization and maintenance are critical in upholding patient safety, minimizing the risk of surgical site infections, and extending the lifespan of surgical equipment. Adherence to established guidelines and protocols is essential for surgical technologists to ensure optimal outcomes in the operating room.

2.2.1 Troubleshoot equipment malfunctions:

Troubleshooting equipment malfunctions involves systematically identifying and resolving issues that arise with surgical instruments and devices during procedures. This process begins with recognizing the symptoms of malfunction, such as unusual noises, failure to operate, or inconsistent performance. Surgical technologists must be familiar with the operational protocols of each piece of equipment to effectively diagnose problems.

Once a malfunction is suspected, the technologist should perform a series of checks, including verifying power sources, inspecting connections, and ensuring that all components are properly assembled. If the issue persists, consulting the equipment's manual or manufacturer guidelines is essential for further troubleshooting steps.

In some cases, it may be necessary to escalate the issue to a biomedical technician or other qualified personnel. Effective troubleshooting not only minimizes delays in surgical procedures but also ensures patient safety and optimal outcomes.

2.2.2 Decontaminate and clean instruments and equipment:
Decontamination and cleaning of surgical instruments and equipment are critical processes aimed at reducing the risk of infection and ensuring patient safety. Decontamination involves the removal of visible soil and the reduction of microbial load through physical or chemical means. This process typically includes rinsing instruments to remove blood and debris, followed by the application of an appropriate cleaning solution.

Cleaning is the next step, which involves using ultrasonic cleaners or manual scrubbing with brushes to ensure all surfaces are free from contaminants. It is essential to follow manufacturer guidelines for cleaning agents and techniques to prevent damage to instruments. After cleaning, instruments should be thoroughly rinsed, dried, and inspected for functionality. Proper decontamination and cleaning protocols are vital for maintaining the integrity of surgical instruments and preventing cross-contamination during surgical procedures.

2.2.3 Inspect, test, and assemble instruments and equipment:
Inspecting, testing, and assembling instruments and equipment are critical tasks for surgical technologists to ensure patient safety and optimal surgical outcomes. Inspection involves a thorough visual examination of surgical instruments for defects, such as rust, cracks, or improper alignment, which could compromise their functionality. Testing includes functional assessments, such as checking the sharpness of cutting instruments and the operation of mechanical devices like clamps and retractors. Proper assembly requires knowledge of the specific instruments needed for each surgical procedure, ensuring that they are organized and ready for use in a sterile environment. This process also involves verifying that all necessary equipment, such as electrosurgical units and suction devices, are in working order. By meticulously inspecting, testing, and assembling instruments and equipment, surgical technologists play a vital role in maintaining a safe and efficient surgical setting.

2.2.4 Sterilize instruments for immediate use:
Sterilizing instruments for immediate use, often referred to as "flash sterilization," is a critical process in surgical settings where time-sensitive procedures necessitate the rapid availability of sterile instruments. This method involves the use of steam under pressure to eliminate all forms of microbial life, including spores, in a short time frame, typically 3 to 10 minutes, depending on the instrument type and sterilizer used.

The process requires meticulous preparation, including thorough cleaning of instruments to remove organic matter, proper packaging to allow steam penetration, and adherence to specific parameters such as temperature and exposure time. Flash sterilization is generally reserved for emergency situations or when instruments are needed unexpectedly, as it may not provide the same level of assurance as traditional sterilization methods. Therefore, surgical technologists must understand the protocols and limitations associated with this practice to ensure patient safety and compliance with regulatory standards.

2.2.4.1   Short cycle:
A short cycle refers to the rapid sterilization process of surgical instruments intended for immediate use in the operating room. This method is crucial when there is a need for sterile instruments that have not been pre-sterilized or when additional instruments are required during a procedure. The short cycle typically employs steam sterilization in a specialized device known as a rapid sterilizer or a flash sterilizer.

In this process, instruments are subjected to high-pressure steam at elevated temperatures for a brief period, usually ranging from 3 to 10 minutes, depending on the type of instruments and the manufacturer's guidelines. It is essential to ensure that the instruments are thoroughly cleaned and dried prior to sterilization to achieve effective results. Proper monitoring and documentation of the sterilization cycle are critical to ensure compliance with safety standards and to minimize the risk of infection during surgical procedures.

2.2.5 Package and sterilize instruments and equipment:
Packaging and sterilization of surgical instruments and equipment are critical processes to ensure the safety and efficacy of surgical procedures. Proper packaging involves using materials that maintain sterility, such as sterilization pouches, wraps, or containers, which must be labeled with pertinent information, including the contents and date of sterilization. The choice of packaging material is essential, as it must withstand the sterilization process while preventing contamination.

Sterilization methods include steam (autoclaving), ethylene oxide gas, and hydrogen peroxide plasma, each suitable for different types of instruments. The autoclave is the most common method, utilizing high-pressure steam to eliminate all microorganisms. It is crucial to monitor sterilization cycles with indicators and biological tests to verify efficacy. Following sterilization, instruments should be handled with sterile technique to maintain their sterility until use in the operating room. This meticulous process is vital for preventing surgical site infections and ensuring patient safety.

3 BASIC SCIENCE:

Basic science refers to the foundational principles and concepts that underpin the biological and physical sciences, particularly as they relate to human anatomy, physiology, and the mechanisms of disease. In the context of surgical technology, basic science encompasses the study of the structure and function of the human body, including cellular biology, histology, and organ systems. It provides essential knowledge that informs surgical procedures, patient care, and the understanding of surgical pathology. Mastery of basic science is crucial for surgical technologists, as it enables them to comprehend the implications of surgical interventions, anticipate potential complications, and assist in the safe and effective delivery of surgical care. This knowledge base is integral to the CST certification exam, ensuring that candidates possess the necessary scientific understanding to perform their roles competently in the operating room environment.

3.1 Anatomy and Physiology:

Anatomy is the branch of biology that studies the structure of organisms, including their systems, organs, and tissues. It provides a detailed understanding of the physical layout of the body and its components. Physiology, on the other hand, focuses on the functions and processes of these anatomical structures, explaining how they work individually and in concert to maintain homeostasis. Together, anatomy and physiology form the foundation of medical knowledge, allowing surgical technologists to comprehend the complexities of the human body. This understanding is crucial for anticipating the needs during surgical procedures, recognizing normal versus abnormal conditions, and facilitating effective communication within the surgical team. Mastery of anatomy and physiology enables surgical technologists to assist in operations with precision, ensuring patient safety and optimal outcomes. A thorough grasp of these concepts is essential for success in the Certified Surgical Technologist (CST) certification exam.

3.1.1 Use appropriate medical terminology and abbreviations:

Medical terminology is a standardized language used by healthcare professionals to ensure clear and precise communication. It comprises specific terms that describe anatomical structures, conditions, procedures, and treatments. Abbreviations are shortened forms of words or phrases that enhance efficiency in documentation and verbal communication. For instance, "BP" stands for blood pressure, and "OR" refers to the operating room.

In surgical technology, the use of appropriate terminology and abbreviations is crucial for ensuring patient safety and effective teamwork. Miscommunication can lead to errors in patient care, so surgical technologists must be proficient in these terms to accurately interpret and relay information. Familiarity with medical terminology also aids in understanding surgical procedures, anatomy, and the instruments used, thereby enhancing the surgical technologist's role in the operating room. Mastery of this language is essential for successful certification and practice in the surgical field.

3.1.2 Demonstrate knowledge of anatomical systems as they relate to the surgical procedure:

Demonstrating knowledge of anatomical systems involves understanding the structure and function of the human body as it pertains to surgical interventions. This knowledge is critical for surgical technologists, as it enables them to anticipate the needs of the surgical team and ensure patient safety. Familiarity with anatomical landmarks, organ systems, and their relationships is essential for effective instrument handling, patient positioning, and sterile technique. For instance, recognizing the vascular supply to an organ can influence surgical approaches and techniques. Additionally, understanding variations in anatomy, such as congenital anomalies, is vital for adapting procedures. This knowledge not only aids in the execution of the surgical procedure but also enhances communication among team members, ultimately contributing to successful surgical outcomes. Mastery of anatomical systems is, therefore, a foundational component of a surgical technologist's role in the operating room.

3.1.2.1 Cardiovascular:

The cardiovascular system, also known as the circulatory system, comprises the heart, blood vessels, and blood. Its primary function is to transport oxygen, nutrients, hormones, and waste products throughout the body, maintaining homeostasis and supporting cellular metabolism. The heart, a muscular organ, pumps oxygenated blood from the left ventricle into the aorta, distributing it to various tissues via arteries. Deoxygenated blood returns to the heart through veins, entering the right atrium and subsequently the right ventricle, where it is pumped to the lungs for oxygenation. Surgical technologists must understand the anatomy of the cardiovascular system, including major vessels like the aorta, pulmonary arteries, and veins, as well as the heart's chambers and valves. This knowledge is crucial during cardiovascular surgeries, such as coronary artery bypass grafting (CABG) or valve replacement, where precise manipulation and monitoring of these structures are essential for patient safety and successful outcomes.

3.1.2.2 Endocrine:

The endocrine system is a complex network of glands that produce and secrete hormones directly into the bloodstream, regulating various physiological processes throughout the body. Key glands include the pituitary, thyroid, adrenal, pancreas, and gonads (ovaries and testes). Hormones act as chemical messengers, influencing growth, metabolism, reproduction, and mood. In surgical procedures, understanding the endocrine system is crucial, as it can impact patient management and outcomes. For instance, conditions such as diabetes mellitus require careful monitoring of blood glucose levels during surgery, while thyroid disorders may necessitate preoperative assessment of hormone levels. Surgical technologists must be familiar with the implications of endocrine dysfunction, including potential complications like adrenal crisis or thyroid storm, and be prepared to assist the surgical team in managing these risks. Knowledge of the endocrine system enhances the surgical technologist's ability to contribute effectively to patient care and surgical success.

3.1.2.3   Gastrointestinal:

The gastrointestinal (GI) system comprises a complex network of organs responsible for the digestion and absorption of nutrients, as well as the elimination of waste. It includes the mouth, esophagus, stomach, small intestine, large intestine, rectum, and anus. Each component plays a vital role in the digestive process. The mouth initiates digestion through mechanical and enzymatic breakdown of food. The esophagus transports food to the stomach, where gastric juices further digest it. The small intestine is crucial for nutrient absorption, utilizing villi and microvilli to maximize surface area. The large intestine absorbs water and electrolytes, forming solid waste for excretion. Understanding the anatomy and physiology of the GI system is essential for surgical technologists, as it aids in anticipating surgical procedures, managing instruments, and recognizing potential complications during operations involving the digestive tract. Knowledge of this system enhances patient safety and surgical efficiency.

3.1.2.4   Genitourinary:

The genitourinary system encompasses the organs involved in reproduction and the urinary tract. It includes the kidneys, ureters, bladder, urethra, and the reproductive organs, such as the testes, prostate, ovaries, and uterus. This system plays a crucial role in the elimination of waste products through urine and the regulation of fluid balance, electrolytes, and blood pressure. In surgical procedures, understanding the anatomy and physiology of the genitourinary system is essential for surgical technologists, as they assist in operations like nephrectomy, cystectomy, and prostatectomy. Knowledge of relevant anatomical landmarks, vascular supply, and potential complications is vital for ensuring patient safety and optimal surgical outcomes. Surgical technologists must also be familiar with the instruments and techniques specific to genitourinary surgeries, as well as the sterile field management to prevent infection and maintain a safe environment during procedures.

3.1.2.5   Integumentary:

The integumentary system comprises the skin, hair, nails, and associated glands, serving as the body's first line of defense against environmental hazards. It plays a crucial role in protecting underlying tissues from pathogens, chemicals, and physical trauma. The skin itself is composed of three primary layers: the epidermis, dermis, and subcutaneous tissue. The epidermis provides a waterproof barrier and is involved in the production of melanin, which protects against ultraviolet radiation. The dermis contains connective tissue, blood vessels, and nerve endings, facilitating sensation and thermoregulation. The subcutaneous layer anchors the skin to underlying structures and stores fat for insulation and energy. Understanding the integumentary system is essential for surgical technologists, as it influences wound healing, infection control, and the overall management of surgical sites, ensuring optimal patient outcomes during and after surgical procedures.

3.1.2.6   Lymphatic:

The lymphatic system is a crucial component of the immune system, consisting of a network of lymphatic vessels, lymph nodes, and lymphoid organs. Its primary function is to transport lymph, a clear fluid containing white blood cells, throughout the body, facilitating the removal of waste products and pathogens. Lymphatic vessels collect excess interstitial fluid from tissues, which is then filtered through lymph nodes, where immune responses can be initiated against foreign substances. This system plays a vital role in maintaining fluid balance and supporting the body's defense mechanisms. In surgical procedures, understanding the lymphatic system is essential, as it can influence the spread of infections and the healing process. Surgeons must be aware of lymphatic drainage patterns to avoid complications, such as lymphedema, and to ensure effective removal of malignant tissues during oncological surgeries. Knowledge of the lymphatic system is integral to surgical technologists in providing optimal patient care.

3.1.2.7   Muscular:

The muscular system is composed of specialized tissues that enable movement and stability in the human body. It consists of three types of muscle tissue: skeletal, cardiac, and smooth. Skeletal muscles are under voluntary control and are responsible for body movements, while cardiac muscle is involuntary and makes up the heart, facilitating blood circulation. Smooth muscle, also involuntary, lines hollow organs such as the intestines and blood vessels, aiding in processes like digestion and blood flow regulation.

In surgical procedures, understanding the muscular system is crucial for several reasons. Surgeons must consider muscle location and function to avoid damage during operations. Additionally, knowledge of muscle anatomy aids in the proper positioning of patients and the selection of appropriate surgical approaches. Surgical technologists must be familiar with muscle groups relevant to specific procedures to assist effectively, ensuring optimal outcomes and patient safety.

3.1.2.8   Neurological:

The neurological system encompasses the brain, spinal cord, and peripheral nerves, playing a crucial role in controlling bodily functions and facilitating communication between different body parts. Understanding the anatomy of the neurological system is essential for surgical technologists, particularly in procedures involving neurosurgery, spinal surgery, or interventions for neurological disorders. Key components include the central nervous system (CNS), which consists of the brain and spinal cord, and the peripheral nervous system (PNS), which includes all other neural elements. Surgical procedures may involve the removal of tumors, repair of traumatic injuries, or decompression of nerves. Knowledge of cranial nerves, spinal anatomy, and the blood supply to the brain is vital for anticipating complications and ensuring patient safety. Additionally, awareness of neurological assessments and postoperative care is essential for monitoring the patient's recovery and neurological function post-surgery.

3.1.2.9   Ophthalmic:

Ophthalmic refers to the branch of medicine and surgery that deals with the diagnosis and treatment of eye disorders and conditions. Surgical technologists must possess a thorough understanding of the anatomy of the eye, including the cornea, lens, retina, and optic nerve, as well as the surrounding structures such as the eyelids and lacrimal glands. In ophthalmic surgery, procedures may include cataract extraction, glaucoma surgery, and retinal repair. Knowledge of specialized instruments, such as microscopes, phacoemulsifiers, and various forceps, is crucial. Surgical technologists must also be familiar with sterile techniques specific to the ophthalmic field, as the eye is particularly susceptible to infection. Understanding the physiological responses of the eye during surgery, including intraocular pressure changes, is essential for maintaining patient safety and ensuring successful outcomes. This expertise enables surgical technologists to effectively assist the surgical team in providing optimal care for patients undergoing ophthalmic procedures.

3.1.2.10   Otorhinolaryngology:

Otorhinolaryngology, commonly referred to as ENT (Ear, Nose, and Throat), is a medical specialty that focuses on the diagnosis and treatment of disorders related to the ear, nose, throat, and related structures of the head and neck. This field encompasses a wide range of conditions, including hearing loss, sinusitis, allergies, voice disorders, and sleep apnea. Surgical technologists in this specialty must possess a thorough understanding of the anatomy and physiology of the otorhinolaryngological systems, as well as the various surgical procedures performed, such as tonsillectomy, adenoidectomy, and endoscopic sinus surgery. Knowledge of instrumentation specific to ENT surgeries, such as microscopes, endoscopes, and specialized surgical tools, is essential. Additionally, familiarity with patient positioning and the surgical environment is crucial for ensuring optimal outcomes and patient safety during procedures. Understanding these elements is vital for effective collaboration within the surgical team.

3.1.2.11   Peripheral vascular:

Peripheral vascular refers to the network of blood vessels located outside the heart and brain, primarily comprising arteries, veins, and capillaries that supply blood to the limbs and organs. This system is crucial for maintaining adequate blood flow, oxygen delivery, and nutrient transport throughout the body. Surgical technologists must understand the anatomy and physiology of peripheral vascular structures, including the femoral, popliteal, and radial arteries, as well as the accompanying veins. Knowledge of peripheral vascular anatomy is essential during surgical procedures such as bypass grafting, endarterectomy, or vascular access for dialysis. Understanding the potential complications, such as thrombosis or embolism, is also vital for ensuring patient safety. Furthermore, familiarity with surgical instruments and techniques used in peripheral vascular surgeries enhances the surgical technologist's ability to assist effectively in the operating room, ensuring optimal outcomes for patients undergoing vascular procedures.

3.1.2.12   Pulmonary:

The pulmonary system, also known as the respiratory system, is responsible for the exchange of gases between the body and the environment. It comprises the lungs, airways, and associated structures that facilitate the intake of oxygen and the expulsion of carbon dioxide. During surgical procedures, understanding the pulmonary system is crucial, as anesthesia and surgical positioning can significantly impact respiratory function.

The lungs are divided into lobes, with the right lung having three lobes and the left lung having two. The trachea branches into bronchi, leading to bronchioles and alveoli, where gas exchange occurs. Surgical technologists must be aware of conditions such as pneumothorax, atelectasis, and pulmonary embolism, which can arise during surgery. Knowledge of pulmonary anatomy and physiology aids in monitoring respiratory status, ensuring proper ventilation, and responding to emergencies, thereby enhancing patient safety throughout the surgical process.

3.1.2.13   Reproductive:

The reproductive system is a complex network of organs and structures responsible for the production of gametes (sperm and eggs), fertilization, and the development of offspring. In males, it includes the testes, vas deferens, prostate gland, and penis, which facilitate sperm production and delivery. In females, the system comprises the ovaries, fallopian tubes, uterus, and vagina, which are essential for egg production, fertilization, and gestation. Understanding the anatomy and physiology of the reproductive system is crucial for surgical technologists, as they assist in various procedures such as cesarean sections, hysterectomies, and prostatectomies. Knowledge of the vascular supply, nerve innervation, and potential complications related to reproductive surgeries is vital for ensuring patient safety and effective surgical outcomes. Surgical technologists must be adept at recognizing anatomical landmarks and variations to provide optimal support during these intricate procedures.

3.1.2.14   Skeletal:

The skeletal system comprises all the bones and cartilage in the human body, providing structure, support, and protection for vital organs. It consists of 206 bones in adults, categorized into two main groups: the axial skeleton (skull, vertebral column, and rib cage) and the appendicular skeleton (limbs and pelvic girdle). This system plays a critical role in facilitating movement by serving as attachment points for muscles and acting as levers during locomotion. Additionally, the skeletal system is vital for hematopoiesis, the production of blood cells, which occurs in the bone marrow. It also serves as a reservoir for minerals, particularly calcium and phosphorus, essential for various physiological functions. Understanding the anatomy and physiology of the skeletal system is crucial for surgical technologists, as it directly influences surgical approaches, techniques, and the management of conditions such as fractures, arthritis, and tumors.

3.1.3 Demonstrate knowledge of human physiology as they relate to the surgical procedure:

Demonstrating knowledge of human physiology in relation to surgical procedures involves understanding the normal functions and structures of the human body, as well as how these may be altered during surgery. This knowledge is critical for surgical technologists, as it informs their role in maintaining patient safety and optimizing surgical outcomes. For instance, understanding the circulatory system enables the surgical technologist to anticipate blood loss and assist in managing hemostasis. Knowledge of the respiratory system is essential for monitoring ventilation and oxygenation during anesthesia. Furthermore, comprehending the anatomy of the surgical site allows for effective instrument handling and positioning of the patient. Ultimately, a solid grasp of human physiology equips surgical technologists to support the surgical team effectively, ensuring that interventions are performed with precision and that patient care is prioritized throughout the surgical process.

3.1.3.1   Cardiovascular:

The cardiovascular system, comprising the heart, blood vessels, and blood, is essential for transporting oxygen, nutrients, hormones, and waste products throughout the body. The heart functions as a muscular pump, maintaining blood circulation through two primary circuits: the pulmonary circuit, which carries deoxygenated blood to the lungs for oxygenation, and the systemic circuit, which distributes oxygen-rich blood to the body's tissues. Surgical technologists must understand cardiovascular anatomy, including the chambers of the heart (atria and ventricles), major blood vessels (aorta, vena cavae, pulmonary arteries, and veins), and the conduction system that regulates heart rhythm. Knowledge of cardiovascular physiology is crucial during surgical procedures, particularly those involving the heart or major blood vessels, as it informs the management of hemodynamics, anesthesia considerations, and potential complications such as bleeding or cardiac arrest. This understanding enables surgical technologists to anticipate the needs of the surgical team and ensure patient safety.

3.1.3.2   Endocrine:

The endocrine system is a complex network of glands that produce and secrete hormones directly into the bloodstream, regulating various bodily functions. Key glands include the pituitary, thyroid, adrenal, pancreas, and gonads (ovaries and testes). Hormones act as chemical messengers, influencing metabolism, growth, development, tissue function, and mood. For surgical technologists, understanding the endocrine system is crucial, as many surgical procedures can impact hormonal balance and function. For example, thyroid surgeries can affect metabolism and calcium levels, while adrenal gland surgeries may influence stress response and electrolyte balance. Surgical technologists must be aware of the implications of endocrine disorders, such as diabetes or hyperthyroidism, on surgical outcomes and patient care. Knowledge of hormone interactions and their physiological effects is essential for anticipating complications and ensuring optimal patient management during and after surgical procedures.

3.1.3.3   Gastrointestinal:

The gastrointestinal (GI) system encompasses the organs involved in the digestion and absorption of food, including the mouth, esophagus, stomach, small intestine, large intestine, rectum, and anus. It plays a crucial role in breaking down food into nutrients, which are then absorbed into the bloodstream for energy, growth, and cell repair. Surgical technologists must understand the anatomy and physiology of the GI tract to assist effectively during surgical procedures such as appendectomies, cholecystectomies, and bowel resections. Knowledge of GI physiology includes recognizing the functions of digestive enzymes, the role of the liver in metabolism, and the importance of the microbiome in maintaining gut health. Additionally, awareness of common GI disorders, such as inflammatory bowel disease and diverticulitis, is essential for anticipating potential complications during surgery. This understanding enables surgical technologists to provide optimal support to the surgical team and ensure patient safety throughout the procedure.

3.1.3.4   Genitourinary:

The genitourinary system encompasses the organs involved in the production and excretion of urine, as well as those associated with reproduction. This system includes the kidneys, ureters, bladder, urethra, and the reproductive organs such as the testes, ovaries, and associated structures. Understanding the anatomy and physiology of the genitourinary system is crucial for surgical technologists, as many surgical procedures involve these organs, including nephrectomy, cystectomy, and prostatectomy. The kidneys filter blood to produce urine, while the ureters transport urine to the bladder for storage. The bladder serves as a reservoir until urination occurs through the urethra. In males, the reproductive system includes the prostate and seminal vesicles, while in females, it includes the ovaries and uterus. Knowledge of this system aids in anticipating surgical needs, managing instruments, and understanding potential complications during genitourinary surgeries.

3.1.3.5   Integumentary:

The integumentary system comprises the skin, hair, nails, and associated glands, serving as the body's first line of defense against environmental hazards. It plays a crucial role in protecting underlying tissues from pathogens, chemical exposure, and physical trauma. The skin, the largest organ, consists of three primary layers: the epidermis, dermis, and subcutaneous tissue. The epidermis provides a waterproof barrier and contains melanocytes, which produce melanin for pigmentation. The dermis houses blood vessels, nerves, and connective tissue, facilitating thermoregulation and sensation. The subcutaneous layer, composed of adipose tissue, provides insulation and energy storage. Understanding the integumentary system is essential for surgical technologists, as it influences wound healing, infection control, and surgical site preparation. Proper knowledge of integumentary anatomy and physiology ensures effective patient care and minimizes complications during surgical procedures.

3.1.3.6   Lymphatic:

The lymphatic system is a crucial component of the immune system, consisting of a network of lymphatic vessels, lymph nodes, and lymphoid organs. It is responsible for the transportation of lymph, a clear fluid containing white blood cells, proteins, and waste products, throughout the body. This system plays a vital role in maintaining fluid balance by collecting excess interstitial fluid and returning it to the bloodstream. Lymph nodes act as filters, trapping pathogens and foreign substances, which are then destroyed by lymphocytes, a type of white blood cell. Additionally, the lymphatic system facilitates the absorption of dietary fats through specialized lymphatic vessels called lacteals, located in the intestines. Understanding the lymphatic system's anatomy and function is essential for surgical technologists, as it can influence surgical procedures, particularly those involving oncological surgeries, where lymph node involvement is critical for staging and treatment planning.

3.1.3.7   Muscular:

The muscular system comprises all the muscles in the body, which are responsible for movement, stability, and posture. Muscles are classified into three types: skeletal, smooth, and cardiac. Skeletal muscles are voluntary and attached to bones, facilitating movement through contraction and relaxation. Smooth muscles are involuntary and found in the walls of hollow organs, such as the intestines and blood vessels, controlling functions like digestion and blood flow. Cardiac muscle, also involuntary, is unique to the heart, enabling it to pump blood throughout the body.

Understanding the muscular system is crucial for surgical technologists, as it directly relates to surgical procedures involving muscle manipulation, repair, or removal. Knowledge of muscle anatomy, including origins, insertions, and innervations, is essential for anticipating surgical challenges and ensuring proper patient positioning. Additionally, awareness of muscle physiology aids in understanding the implications of surgical interventions on overall mobility and recovery.

3.1.3.8   Neurological:

The neurological system encompasses the brain, spinal cord, and peripheral nerves, playing a critical role in controlling bodily functions and responding to stimuli. Understanding the neurological system is essential for surgical technologists, as many surgical procedures involve the nervous system, including neurosurgery, orthopedic surgery, and procedures addressing trauma or tumors. The central nervous system (CNS) processes information and coordinates actions, while the peripheral nervous system (PNS) transmits signals between the CNS and the rest of the body. Surgical technologists must be familiar with neurological anatomy, such as the cerebrum, cerebellum, brainstem, and spinal cord, as well as the functions of various cranial nerves. Knowledge of neurological physiology is crucial for recognizing potential complications during surgery, such as nerve damage or impaired motor function, and for ensuring proper positioning and sterile technique to protect the nervous system throughout the surgical process.

3.1.3.9   Ophthalmic:

Ophthalmic surgery pertains to surgical procedures involving the eye and its surrounding structures. This specialty encompasses a range of interventions, including cataract extraction, corneal transplants, and retinal surgeries. Understanding the anatomy and physiology of the eye is crucial for surgical technologists, as they must be familiar with the intricate structures such as the cornea, lens, retina, and optic nerve. The surgical technologist plays a vital role in preparing the sterile field, handling delicate instruments, and assisting the surgeon during procedures. Knowledge of common ophthalmic instruments, such as the phacoemulsifier, forceps, and speculum, is essential. Additionally, awareness of potential complications, such as infection or hemorrhage, and the physiological responses of the eye to surgical manipulation is critical. Overall, proficiency in ophthalmic procedures ensures patient safety and optimal surgical outcomes.

3.1.3.10   Otorhinolaryngology:

Otorhinolaryngology, commonly referred to as ENT (Ear, Nose, and Throat), is a specialized field of medicine that focuses on the diagnosis and treatment of disorders related to the ear, nose, throat, and related structures of the head and neck. This discipline encompasses a wide range of conditions, including hearing loss, sinusitis, allergies, voice disorders, and sleep apnea. Surgical technologists in this field must possess a thorough understanding of the anatomy and physiology of the head and neck, as well as the specific surgical procedures involved, such as tonsillectomy, adenoidectomy, and tympanoplasty. Knowledge of the intricate relationship between these structures is crucial, as they often influence one another in both health and disease. Additionally, surgical technologists must be familiar with the instruments and techniques used in ENT surgeries to ensure optimal patient outcomes and assist the surgical team effectively.

3.1.3.11   Peripheral vascular:
Peripheral vascular refers to the network of blood vessels located outside the heart and brain, including arteries, veins, and capillaries that supply blood to the limbs and organs. This system is crucial for maintaining adequate blood flow, oxygen delivery, and nutrient supply to tissues. Understanding peripheral vascular physiology is essential for surgical technologists, as it directly impacts surgical procedures involving the extremities or vascular interventions.

Conditions such as peripheral artery disease (PAD) can lead to reduced blood flow, necessitating surgical interventions like bypass grafts or angioplasty. Surgical technologists must be familiar with the anatomy of peripheral vessels, including the femoral, popliteal, and tibial arteries, as well as the venous return system. Knowledge of peripheral vascular physiology aids in anticipating complications, ensuring proper positioning during surgery, and facilitating effective communication with the surgical team regarding patient status and potential risks associated with vascular procedures.

3.1.3.12   Pulmonary:
The pulmonary system refers to the organs and structures involved in the process of respiration, primarily the lungs, airways, and associated blood vessels. Its primary function is to facilitate gas exchange, allowing oxygen to enter the bloodstream and carbon dioxide to be expelled. During surgical procedures, understanding pulmonary physiology is crucial, as anesthesia and positioning can significantly impact respiratory function. The lungs are divided into lobes, with the right lung having three lobes and the left lung having two, accommodating the heart's position. The alveoli, tiny air sacs within the lungs, are the sites of gas exchange, where oxygen diffuses into the blood, and carbon dioxide is removed. Surgical technologists must be aware of conditions such as obstructive lung disease, which can complicate anesthesia and recovery, and ensure that proper ventilation techniques are employed to maintain adequate oxygenation throughout the surgical process.

3.1.3.13   Reproductive:
The reproductive system is a complex network of organs and structures responsible for the production of gametes (sperm and eggs), the facilitation of fertilization, and the nurturing of developing offspring. In males, the primary components include the testes, vas deferens, seminal vesicles, and prostate gland, which work together to produce and transport sperm. In females, the ovaries, fallopian tubes, uterus, and vagina play crucial roles in ovulation, fertilization, and gestation. Understanding the anatomy and physiology of the reproductive system is essential for surgical technologists, as many surgical procedures, such as hysterectomies, cesarean sections, and prostatectomies, directly involve these structures. Knowledge of hormonal regulation, reproductive cycles, and potential complications is vital for anticipating surgical needs and ensuring patient safety. Surgical technologists must be adept at recognizing the implications of reproductive health on surgical interventions and postoperative care.

3.1.3.14   Skeletal:
The skeletal system comprises 206 bones in the adult human body, providing structure, support, and protection to vital organs. It serves as a framework for the body, facilitating movement by acting as levers for muscles. The skeletal system is divided into two main categories: the axial skeleton, which includes the skull, vertebral column, and rib cage, and the appendicular skeleton, which consists of the limbs and their attachments.

Bone tissue is dynamic, undergoing continuous remodeling through the processes of osteogenesis and resorption, influenced by factors such as nutrition, hormones, and mechanical stress. Additionally, the skeletal system plays a crucial role in hematopoiesis, the production of blood cells, occurring primarily in the bone marrow. Understanding the anatomy and physiology of the skeletal system is essential for surgical technologists, as it directly impacts surgical procedures involving fractures, joint replacements, and spinal surgeries.

3.1.4 Identify the following surgical pathologies:
Identifying surgical pathologies involves recognizing various medical conditions that may necessitate surgical intervention. Surgical pathologies can range from benign tumors to malignant cancers, infectious processes, and traumatic injuries. Understanding these pathologies is crucial for surgical technologists, as it aids in anticipating the needs of the surgical team and preparing the appropriate instruments and supplies. For instance, conditions such as appendicitis, cholecystitis, and hernias require specific surgical approaches and techniques. Additionally, knowledge of surgical pathologies assists in understanding the underlying anatomy and physiology, which is essential during surgical procedures. Accurate identification ensures that the surgical team can effectively plan and execute interventions, ultimately contributing to patient safety and positive outcomes. Mastery of this topic enhances a surgical technologist's ability to function in a dynamic operating room environment, making it a fundamental aspect of surgical education and practice.

3.1.4.1 Abnormal anatomy:

Abnormal anatomy refers to structural deviations from the typical anatomical organization of the body. These deviations can arise from congenital anomalies, trauma, disease processes, or surgical alterations. Understanding abnormal anatomy is crucial for surgical technologists, as it impacts surgical planning, technique, and patient safety. For instance, congenital conditions such as situs inversus, where organs are mirrored from their normal positions, require surgeons to adapt their approach. Similarly, acquired abnormalities, such as tumors or inflammatory changes, can distort normal anatomical relationships, complicating surgical access and technique. Surgical technologists must be adept at recognizing these variations to assist effectively during procedures, ensuring that instruments are used correctly and that the surgical field is maintained. Knowledge of abnormal anatomy enhances the surgical team's ability to anticipate challenges, communicate effectively, and provide optimal patient care throughout the surgical process.

3.1.4.2 Disease processes:

Disease processes refer to the series of biological and physiological changes that occur in the body as a result of a pathological condition. These processes can be classified into several categories, including inflammatory, infectious, neoplastic, degenerative, and metabolic disorders. Each category represents a different mechanism through which disease manifests. For instance, inflammatory processes involve the body's immune response to injury or infection, leading to symptoms such as redness, swelling, and pain. Infectious disease processes are caused by pathogenic microorganisms, resulting in conditions like pneumonia or sepsis. Neoplastic processes pertain to abnormal cell growth, which can be benign or malignant, as seen in tumors. Degenerative processes involve the gradual deterioration of function or structure, often observed in conditions like osteoarthritis. Lastly, metabolic processes encompass disorders that disrupt normal biochemical pathways, such as diabetes. Understanding these processes is crucial for surgical technologists to anticipate and assist in surgical interventions effectively.

3.1.4.3 Malignancies:

Malignancies refer to cancerous growths that arise from the uncontrolled division of abnormal cells. These tumors can invade surrounding tissues and metastasize to distant organs through the lymphatic system or bloodstream. Malignancies are classified into various types, including carcinomas (originating from epithelial cells), sarcomas (from connective tissues), leukemias (blood-forming tissues), and lymphomas (immune system tissues). The pathophysiology of malignancies involves genetic mutations, environmental factors, and lifestyle choices, leading to alterations in cellular regulation. Surgical technologists play a crucial role in the surgical management of malignancies, assisting in procedures such as tumor resections, biopsies, and palliative surgeries. Understanding the characteristics and behaviors of different malignancies is essential for surgical technologists, as it informs the surgical approach, instrumentation, and patient care strategies. Early detection and intervention are vital for improving patient outcomes and survival rates in individuals diagnosed with malignancies.

3.1.4.4 Traumatic injuries:

Traumatic injuries refer to physical harm inflicted on the body due to external forces, which can result from accidents, falls, violence, or other sudden events. These injuries can vary in severity, ranging from minor cuts and bruises to life-threatening conditions such as fractures, internal bleeding, or organ damage. Common types of traumatic injuries include contusions, lacerations, fractures, dislocations, and concussions.

The management of traumatic injuries often requires immediate medical attention to stabilize the patient, prevent further injury, and initiate appropriate surgical interventions if necessary. Surgical technologists play a crucial role in the operating room by preparing the sterile field, assisting the surgical team, and ensuring that all necessary instruments and supplies are available. Understanding the nature of traumatic injuries is essential for surgical technologists, as it enables them to anticipate the needs of the surgical team and contribute to effective patient care during trauma surgeries.

3.2 Microbiology:

Microbiology is the branch of science that studies microorganisms, which are microscopic entities that can exist as single cells or cell clusters. This field encompasses various types of organisms, including bacteria, viruses, fungi, protozoa, and algae. Microbiology is crucial in understanding the role of these organisms in health, disease, and the environment. In the context of surgical technology, it is essential to comprehend how microorganisms can cause infections and influence surgical outcomes. The principles of microbiology guide the development of aseptic techniques, sterilization methods, and infection control practices in the operating room. Knowledge of microbiology allows surgical technologists to recognize the potential pathogens present in surgical settings, understand their transmission routes, and implement appropriate measures to minimize the risk of surgical site infections. Thus, a solid foundation in microbiology is vital for ensuring patient safety and promoting successful surgical interventions.

3.2.1 Apply principles of surgical microbiology to operative practice:

This category emphasizes the critical role of microbiology in surgical settings, focusing on the prevention and management of infections. It involves understanding the types of microorganisms—bacteria, viruses, fungi, and parasites—that can cause surgical site infections (SSIs) and their mechanisms of pathogenesis. Surgical technologists must apply microbiological principles to ensure aseptic techniques are maintained throughout the surgical process, from preoperative preparation to postoperative care. This includes the proper sterilization of instruments, the use of appropriate antiseptics, and the implementation of infection control measures. Knowledge of microbial resistance patterns and the appropriate use of prophylactic antibiotics is essential for minimizing infection risks. By integrating microbiological principles into operative practice, surgical technologists contribute to patient safety, enhance surgical outcomes, and reduce the incidence of healthcare-associated infections, thereby promoting a sterile and safe surgical environment.

3.2.1.1   Classification and pathogenesis of microorganisms:

Microorganisms are classified into several categories, primarily bacteria, viruses, fungi, and protozoa, based on their cellular structure, reproduction methods, and metabolic processes. Bacteria can be further divided into gram-positive and gram-negative based on their cell wall composition, while viruses are classified by their nucleic acid type (DNA or RNA) and structure. Fungi are categorized as yeasts or molds, and protozoa are classified by their motility and life cycle stages.

Pathogenesis refers to the mechanisms by which microorganisms cause disease. This involves several steps, including adherence to host tissues, invasion of host defenses, and the production of toxins or enzymes that damage host cells. Understanding the classification and pathogenesis of microorganisms is crucial for surgical technologists, as it informs infection control practices, selection of appropriate antimicrobial agents, and the implementation of aseptic techniques during surgical procedures to minimize the risk of postoperative infections.

3.2.1.1.1   Cultures:

Cultures refer to the laboratory process of growing microorganisms from a sample to identify the specific pathogens present. This process is crucial in surgical microbiology as it helps determine the causative agents of infections, guiding appropriate antibiotic therapy. Samples can be obtained from various sources, including blood, urine, wound exudates, and body fluids. Once collected, these samples are inoculated onto culture media that provide the necessary nutrients for microbial growth.

The cultures are then incubated under controlled conditions to promote growth, which can take anywhere from hours to days, depending on the organism. After incubation, colonies are examined for characteristics such as morphology and color, and further tests are conducted to identify the microorganisms. Understanding culture results is essential for surgical technologists, as it informs the surgical team about potential infections and the need for aseptic techniques to prevent complications during operative procedures.

3.2.1.2   Infection control procedures:

Infection control procedures are systematic practices designed to prevent the transmission of infectious agents in healthcare settings, particularly during surgical procedures. These protocols encompass a range of strategies aimed at minimizing the risk of infection to patients, healthcare workers, and the environment. Key components include proper hand hygiene, the use of personal protective equipment (PPE), sterilization of surgical instruments, and the implementation of aseptic techniques.

Infection control also involves environmental cleaning, waste management, and surveillance of infection rates to identify and mitigate potential outbreaks. Surgical technologists play a vital role in adhering to these procedures, ensuring that the surgical field remains sterile and that all instruments and supplies are appropriately processed. By rigorously following infection control protocols, surgical teams can significantly reduce the incidence of surgical site infections (SSIs) and enhance patient safety and outcomes.

3.2.1.2.1   Aseptic technique:

Aseptic technique refers to a set of specific practices and procedures performed under carefully controlled conditions to minimize contamination by pathogens. This technique is crucial in the surgical environment to prevent infections during invasive procedures. It involves the use of sterile instruments, drapes, and supplies, as well as the application of hand hygiene protocols, such as thorough handwashing and the use of antiseptic solutions.

Surgical technologists must maintain a sterile field, ensuring that all items within this area remain free from microorganisms. This includes proper gowning, gloving, and the use of barriers to protect both the patient and surgical team. Additionally, aseptic technique encompasses the careful handling of instruments and materials to avoid cross-contamination. Adherence to these principles is essential for patient safety, promoting optimal surgical outcomes, and reducing the risk of postoperative infections.

3.2.1.3   Principles of tissue handling:

The principles of tissue handling refer to the techniques and practices employed to manage, manipulate, and protect tissues during surgical procedures. Proper tissue handling is crucial to minimize trauma, preserve blood supply, and promote optimal healing. Key principles include gentle manipulation to avoid unnecessary damage, maintaining moisture to prevent desiccation, and using appropriate instruments designed for specific tissue types. Surgical technologists must be aware of the anatomical structures and their functions to avoid compromising tissue integrity. Additionally, adhering to aseptic techniques is essential to prevent infection. Understanding the biological response of tissues to surgical intervention informs the choice of techniques and instruments, ensuring that the surgical field remains conducive to healing. Effective communication with the surgical team enhances coordination, allowing for timely and appropriate tissue handling throughout the procedure. Mastery of these principles is vital for achieving successful surgical outcomes and patient recovery.

3.2.1.3.1 Halsted principles:

The Halsted principles, formulated by Dr. William Halsted, are foundational guidelines for surgical technique and tissue handling that aim to minimize trauma and promote optimal healing. These principles include:

1. Gentle handling of tissues: Surgeons should manipulate tissues with care to preserve their integrity and function, reducing the risk of ischemia and necrosis.

2. Control of hemostasis: Effective management of bleeding is crucial. Surgeons must employ techniques to ensure that blood vessels are adequately ligated or cauterized to prevent excessive blood loss.

3. Preservation of blood supply: Maintaining the vascular supply to tissues is vital for healing. Surgeons should avoid unnecessary dissection that could compromise blood flow.

4. Minimizing tension on tissues: Proper suturing techniques should be employed to avoid excessive tension, which can lead to tissue ischemia and delayed healing.

These principles guide surgical technologists in assisting with procedures that prioritize patient safety and recovery.

3.2.1.3.2 Tissue manipulation methods:

Tissue manipulation methods refer to the techniques employed by surgical technologists and surgeons to handle, reposition, and protect tissues during surgical procedures. These methods are crucial for minimizing trauma to the tissues, ensuring optimal exposure of the surgical site, and facilitating effective surgical intervention. Common techniques include the use of forceps, retractors, and sponges to grasp and hold tissues, allowing for clear visibility and access. Additionally, gentle traction and counter-traction are applied to maintain tissue integrity while avoiding excessive pressure that could lead to ischemia or necrosis. Understanding the anatomy and physiology of the tissues involved is essential for selecting appropriate manipulation methods. Proper tissue handling not only enhances surgical outcomes but also reduces the risk of complications such as infection and delayed healing. Mastery of these techniques is vital for surgical technologists to support the surgical team effectively and ensure patient safety.

3.2.1.3.3 Traction/counter traction:

Traction refers to the application of a force to stretch or pull tissues in a specific direction, facilitating better visualization and access to the surgical site. It is essential in procedures where anatomical structures need to be moved aside to expose underlying tissues or organs. Counter traction is the opposing force applied to stabilize the tissue being manipulated, ensuring that the area remains in the desired position without causing damage. This technique is critical in maintaining the integrity of surrounding structures while allowing the surgeon to operate effectively. Proper use of traction and counter traction minimizes tissue trauma, reduces bleeding, and enhances surgical efficiency. Surgical technologists must understand the principles of these techniques, as they play a vital role in positioning instruments and assisting the surgical team in achieving optimal exposure during procedures.

3.2.1.4 Stages of, and factors influencing wound healing:

Wound healing is a complex biological process that occurs in four overlapping stages: hemostasis, inflammation, proliferation, and remodeling. Hemostasis involves the immediate response to injury, where blood vessels constrict and platelets aggregate to form a clot. Inflammation follows, characterized by increased blood flow and immune cell infiltration to prevent infection. The proliferation stage sees the formation of granulation tissue, re-epithelialization, and angiogenesis, promoting tissue regeneration. Finally, remodeling occurs, where collagen is reorganized and strengthened, leading to scar maturation.

Factors influencing wound healing include the patient's age, nutritional status, underlying health conditions (such as diabetes), oxygenation, and the presence of infection. Additionally, external factors like wound care practices, moisture balance, and the use of dressings can significantly impact healing outcomes. Understanding these stages and factors is crucial for surgical technologists to optimize patient care and facilitate effective wound management.

3.2.1.4.1 Condition of patient:

The condition of the patient significantly influences the wound healing process. Factors such as age, nutritional status, underlying medical conditions, and the presence of infections can affect the body's ability to heal. For instance, elderly patients may experience slower healing due to decreased cellular regeneration and compromised immune responses. Nutritional deficiencies, particularly in proteins, vitamins A and C, and zinc, can impair collagen synthesis and epithelialization, essential components of wound healing. Chronic conditions like diabetes mellitus can lead to poor circulation and neuropathy, further complicating the healing process. Additionally, the presence of infections can lead to increased inflammation and tissue damage, delaying recovery. Understanding these factors allows surgical technologists to anticipate potential complications and collaborate with the surgical team to implement appropriate interventions, ultimately enhancing patient outcomes and promoting effective healing.

3.2.1.4.2 Wound type:

Wound types are categorized based on their characteristics, mechanisms of injury, and healing processes. The primary classifications include acute and chronic wounds. Acute wounds typically result from trauma, surgery, or other sudden injuries and generally heal within a predictable timeframe. Examples include surgical incisions, abrasions, and lacerations. Chronic wounds, on the other hand, do not follow the normal healing trajectory and persist for an extended period, often due to underlying conditions such as diabetes or venous insufficiency. They include pressure ulcers, diabetic foot ulcers, and venous stasis ulcers. Additionally, wounds can be classified as clean, contaminated, or infected, depending on the presence of microorganisms. Understanding the type of wound is crucial for determining the appropriate treatment and intervention strategies, as each type has unique healing requirements and potential complications that must be managed effectively to promote optimal recovery.

3.2.1.5   Surgical wound classification:
Surgical wound classification is a systematic method used to categorize surgical wounds based on their degree of contamination and the risk of infection. There are four primary classifications:

1. Clean (Class I): These wounds are created under sterile conditions, with no inflammation present, and no entry into the respiratory, gastrointestinal, or genitourinary tracts. The risk of infection is low.

2. Clean-Contaminated (Class II): These wounds involve surgical procedures that enter the respiratory, gastrointestinal, or genitourinary tracts under controlled conditions, with minimal spillage. The risk of infection is moderate.

3. Contaminated (Class III): These wounds occur when there is a breach in sterile technique or when there is a presence of acute inflammation. The risk of infection is high.

4. Dirty or Infected (Class IV): These wounds are associated with existing infection or necrosis, indicating a high level of contamination and a significant risk of postoperative infection.

Understanding these classifications is crucial for surgical technologists in ensuring proper wound management and infection control protocols.

3.2.2 Identify and address factors that can influence an infectious process:
Infectious processes are influenced by various factors that can either promote or inhibit the spread of pathogens. Key factors include the mode of transmission, the virulence of the microorganism, the host's immune response, and environmental conditions.

Transmission can occur through direct contact, airborne particles, or contaminated surfaces. The virulence, or the ability of a pathogen to cause disease, is affected by its genetic makeup and mechanisms of resistance. The host's immune response plays a critical role; individuals with compromised immunity are more susceptible to infections.

Environmental factors such as temperature, humidity, and cleanliness also significantly impact the survival and proliferation of pathogens. Surgical technologists must identify these factors in the surgical setting, implementing strict aseptic techniques, sterilization protocols, and proper waste disposal to mitigate the risk of infection and ensure patient safety.

3.3   Surgical Pharmacology:
Surgical pharmacology is the branch of pharmacology that focuses on the study and application of drugs used in surgical settings. It encompasses the understanding of various medications, including anesthetics, analgesics, antibiotics, and other therapeutic agents, and their effects on patients undergoing surgical procedures. This field is crucial for surgical technologists, as it involves knowledge of drug classifications, mechanisms of action, dosages, routes of administration, and potential side effects.

Surgical pharmacology also includes the safe handling, preparation, and administration of medications in the operating room, ensuring compliance with legal and ethical standards. Understanding pharmacokinetics and pharmacodynamics is essential, as these principles guide the timing and selection of drugs to optimize patient outcomes. Ultimately, surgical pharmacology is integral to enhancing patient safety, managing pain, preventing infections, and facilitating effective surgical interventions.

3.3.1 Apply principles of surgical pharmacology to operative practice:
Surgical pharmacology involves the study of drugs and their effects on the surgical patient, emphasizing the safe and effective use of medications in the perioperative environment. Applying these principles to operative practice requires a thorough understanding of pharmacokinetics (how drugs are absorbed, distributed, metabolized, and excreted) and pharmacodynamics (the effects of drugs on the body). Surgical technologists must be knowledgeable about various classifications of medications, including anesthetics, analgesics, antibiotics, and anticoagulants, and their specific roles during surgery. This includes recognizing indications, contraindications, potential side effects, and interactions with other medications. Additionally, surgical technologists must ensure proper storage, preparation, and administration of medications, adhering to established protocols to maintain patient safety. By integrating surgical pharmacology principles into practice, surgical technologists contribute to optimal patient outcomes and enhance the overall efficiency of the surgical team.

3.3.1.1   Anesthesia related agents and medications:
Anesthesia related agents and medications are pharmacological substances used to induce a state of controlled unconsciousness, analgesia, and muscle relaxation during surgical procedures. These agents can be classified into three main categories: general anesthetics, regional anesthetics, and local anesthetics. General anesthetics, such as propofol and sevoflurane, are administered to render the patient completely unconscious and are typically delivered via inhalation or intravenous routes. Regional anesthetics, like epidurals and spinal blocks, target specific areas of the

body to provide pain relief while maintaining consciousness. Local anesthetics, such as lidocaine, are used for minor procedures to numb a small area. Understanding the pharmacodynamics and pharmacokinetics of these agents is crucial for surgical technologists, as they must assist in the safe administration and monitoring of anesthesia, ensuring patient safety and comfort throughout the surgical experience.

3.3.1.2 Blood and fluid replacement:

Blood and fluid replacement refers to the administration of intravenous fluids and blood products to restore or maintain adequate circulating volume and tissue perfusion during surgical procedures. This practice is critical in managing patients who experience significant blood loss, dehydration, or electrolyte imbalances.

In the operating room, surgical technologists must understand the types of fluids used, including crystalloids (e.g., normal saline, lactated Ringer's solution) and colloids (e.g., albumin, hydroxyethyl starch), as well as blood components such as red blood cells, platelets, and plasma.

The surgical team must monitor vital signs and laboratory values to guide fluid resuscitation and ensure the patient's hemodynamic stability. Proper blood and fluid replacement is essential to prevent complications such as hypovolemic shock, organ dysfunction, and delayed recovery. Knowledge of indications, contraindications, and potential reactions to transfusions is vital for safe surgical practice.

3.3.1.3 Complications from drug interactions:

Drug interactions occur when the effects of one medication are altered by the presence of another medication, food, or substance. These interactions can lead to adverse effects, reduced therapeutic efficacy, or increased toxicity. In the surgical setting, complications from drug interactions are particularly critical, as they can affect patient outcomes during and after surgery. For instance, anticoagulants may interact with certain anesthetics, increasing the risk of bleeding. Additionally, some antibiotics can diminish the effectiveness of oral contraceptives, leading to unintended pregnancies. It is essential for surgical technologists to be aware of potential drug interactions to assist in medication management and ensure patient safety. Proper communication with the surgical team regarding a patient's medication history is vital, as it allows for the identification of possible interactions and the implementation of appropriate precautions to mitigate risks during surgical procedures.

3.3.1.3.1 Malignant hyperthermia:

Malignant hyperthermia (MH) is a rare but life-threatening condition triggered by certain anesthetic agents, particularly volatile anesthetics and succinylcholine. It is characterized by a hypermetabolic response to these agents, leading to a rapid increase in calcium release from the sarcoplasmic reticulum of skeletal muscle cells. This results in muscle rigidity, increased carbon dioxide production, elevated body temperature, and metabolic acidosis. The condition is often genetic, linked to mutations in the ryanodine receptor (RYR1) gene, which plays a critical role in calcium regulation within muscle cells. Early recognition and immediate intervention are crucial; treatment typically involves the administration of dantrolene, which acts to reduce calcium release and restore normal muscle function. Surgical technologists must be aware of the signs of MH, as prompt action can significantly improve patient outcomes and prevent severe complications or death during surgical procedures.

3.3.1.4 Methods of anesthesia administration:

Anesthesia administration refers to the techniques used to deliver anesthetic agents to patients to induce a state of controlled unconsciousness, analgesia, or muscle relaxation during surgical procedures. The primary methods include inhalation, intravenous (IV), regional, and local anesthesia. Inhalation anesthesia involves the administration of anesthetic gases or vapors through a breathing mask or endotracheal tube, allowing for rapid onset and easy control of the anesthetic depth. Intravenous anesthesia involves the injection of anesthetic drugs directly into the bloodstream, providing quick effects and precise dosage control. Regional anesthesia blocks sensation in specific body areas through nerve blocks or spinal/epidural techniques, while local anesthesia numbs a small, targeted area. Each method has distinct indications, advantages, and considerations, and the choice depends on the type of surgery, patient health, and desired outcomes. Understanding these methods is crucial for surgical technologists to ensure patient safety and optimal surgical conditions.

3.3.1.4.1 General:

General anesthesia is a medically induced state of unconsciousness characterized by the absence of sensation and awareness. It is achieved through the administration of anesthetic agents, which can be delivered via inhalation or intravenous routes. The primary goal of general anesthesia is to provide analgesia, amnesia, and muscle relaxation, allowing for surgical procedures to be performed without discomfort to the patient.

During the administration of general anesthesia, the anesthetist closely monitors vital signs, including heart rate, blood pressure, and oxygen saturation, to ensure patient safety. Induction agents, such as propofol or thiopental, are typically used to initiate anesthesia, followed by maintenance agents, such as sevoflurane or isoflurane, to sustain the anesthetic state throughout the procedure. Recovery from general anesthesia involves the gradual return of consciousness and physiological functions, with patients often requiring monitoring in a post-anesthesia care unit (PACU) until stable.

3.3.1.4.2   Local:

Local anesthesia refers to the administration of anesthetic agents to a specific area of the body, resulting in a temporary loss of sensation in that localized region while allowing the patient to remain fully conscious. This method is commonly used for minor surgical procedures, such as skin biopsies, dental work, or small excisions, where the surgical site can be isolated from the surrounding tissues. Local anesthetics, such as lidocaine or bupivacaine, are typically injected directly into the tissue or applied topically. The onset of action is rapid, often within minutes, and the effects can last from one to several hours, depending on the agent used and the dosage administered. Local anesthesia is advantageous as it minimizes systemic effects, reduces recovery time, and allows for quicker patient discharge. It is essential for surgical technologists to understand the indications, contraindications, and potential complications associated with local anesthesia to ensure patient safety.

3.3.1.4.3   Block:

A block, also known as a regional anesthesia block, is a method of anesthesia that involves the injection of anesthetic agents near a cluster of nerves to block sensation in a specific area of the body. This technique is commonly used for surgeries on the limbs, abdomen, or pelvis, allowing for pain relief without the need for general anesthesia. The most common types of blocks include spinal blocks, epidural blocks, and peripheral nerve blocks.

During a block procedure, the anesthesiologist or nurse anesthetist identifies the target nerves using anatomical landmarks or imaging techniques. After administering the local anesthetic, the patient remains conscious and can often cooperate during the procedure while experiencing minimal discomfort. The advantages of using a block include reduced systemic medication exposure, faster recovery times, and the ability to provide postoperative pain control. Understanding the indications, contraindications, and potential complications of blocks is essential for surgical technologists.

3.3.1.5   Types, uses, action, and interactions of drugs and solution:

Drugs and solutions used in surgical settings can be categorized into several types, including anesthetics, analgesics, antibiotics, and antiseptics. Anesthetics induce loss of sensation or consciousness, while analgesics provide pain relief. Antibiotics prevent or treat infections, and antiseptics reduce microbial load on skin or surfaces. The action of these drugs refers to their mechanism of action, such as blocking nerve signals or inhibiting bacterial growth. Understanding drug interactions is crucial, as certain combinations can enhance or diminish therapeutic effects or increase toxicity. For example, mixing certain anesthetics with sedatives can lead to respiratory depression. Surgical technologists must be knowledgeable about these factors to ensure patient safety and effective outcomes during surgical procedures. Proper administration and monitoring of these drugs and solutions are essential in maintaining the patient's physiological stability throughout the surgical process.

3.3.1.5.1   Hemostatic agents:

Hemostatic agents are substances used to promote hemostasis, the process of stopping bleeding during surgical procedures. These agents can be classified into several categories, including mechanical, chemical, and biological hemostatic agents. Mechanical agents, such as gauze and sponges, provide physical barriers to bleeding. Chemical agents, like tranexamic acid and topical thrombin, facilitate clot formation by enhancing the coagulation cascade. Biological agents, such as fibrin sealants, utilize components derived from human or animal sources to promote clotting.

The choice of hemostatic agent depends on factors such as the type of surgery, the location of the bleeding, and the patient's individual characteristics. Proper application and understanding of these agents are crucial for surgical technologists, as they play a vital role in minimizing blood loss and ensuring patient safety during operative procedures.

3.3.1.5.2   Antibiotics:

Antibiotics are a class of antimicrobial agents specifically designed to combat bacterial infections by inhibiting bacterial growth or killing bacteria outright. They function through various mechanisms, including disrupting cell wall synthesis, inhibiting protein synthesis, or interfering with nucleic acid metabolism. Commonly used antibiotics include penicillins, cephalosporins, macrolides, and tetracyclines, each with specific indications based on the type of bacteria and infection severity.

In surgical settings, antibiotics are crucial for prophylaxis to prevent postoperative infections, particularly in procedures involving implants or where the risk of infection is heightened. It is essential to understand the spectrum of activity, potential side effects, and interactions with other medications. Additionally, awareness of antibiotic resistance is vital, as misuse can lead to resistant strains, complicating treatment options. Proper selection and administration of antibiotics are critical responsibilities for surgical technologists to ensure patient safety and optimal surgical outcomes.

3.3.1.5.3   IV solutions:

Intravenous (IV) solutions are sterile liquids administered directly into the bloodstream via an intravenous line. They are essential for maintaining fluid balance, delivering medications, providing nutrition, and correcting electrolyte imbalances in patients. IV solutions can be classified into crystalloid and colloid solutions. Crystalloids, such as normal saline and lactated Ringer's solution, contain small molecules that can easily pass through cell membranes, making them suitable for hydration and electrolyte replenishment. Colloids, like dextran and hydroxyethyl starch, contain larger molecules that remain in the vascular space, helping to expand blood volume and maintain blood pressure. The choice of IV solution depends on the patient's condition, the desired therapeutic effect, and potential interactions with other medications. Proper administration and monitoring of IV solutions are critical to prevent complications such as fluid overload, infection, or adverse reactions, highlighting the surgical technologist's role in patient safety during surgical procedures.

3.3.1.6 <u>Weights, measures, and conversions:</u>

Weights, measures, and conversions refer to the standardized systems used to quantify and express the mass, volume, and dimensions of surgical instruments, supplies, and medications. In the surgical environment, precise measurements are crucial for ensuring patient safety and effective outcomes. The metric system is predominantly used in healthcare, where grams (g) and milliliters (mL) are standard units for weight and volume, respectively. Understanding conversions between metric and imperial systems is essential, particularly when dealing with medications or materials that may be labeled in different units. For example, converting ounces to milliliters or pounds to kilograms is often necessary. Surgical technologists must be proficient in these conversions to accurately prepare and administer medications, calculate dosages, and ensure the correct amount of sterile supplies is utilized during procedures. Mastery of weights, measures, and conversions is vital for maintaining a safe and efficient surgical environment.

3.3.2 <u>Maintain awareness of maximum dosage:</u>

Maintaining awareness of maximum dosage refers to the critical responsibility of surgical technologists to understand and monitor the maximum allowable amounts of medications administered to patients during surgical procedures. This knowledge is essential to prevent potential adverse effects, including toxicity or overdose, which can lead to severe complications or even death. Surgical technologists must be familiar with various medications, including anesthetics, antibiotics, and analgesics, and their respective maximum dosages based on patient factors such as age, weight, and medical history. This awareness extends to recognizing the importance of double-checking dosages with the surgical team, especially when multiple medications are involved. By maintaining vigilance regarding maximum dosages, surgical technologists contribute to patient safety, ensuring that the surgical environment is both effective and secure. This practice underscores the importance of teamwork and communication within the surgical team, ultimately enhancing patient outcomes.

CST
Practice
Questions
[SET 1]

Question 1: Which of the following is the most appropriate method for verifying patient identity before surgery?
A) Asking the patient to state their name and date of birth
B) Checking the patient's wristband only
C) Confirming the patient's identity with a family member
D) Reviewing the patient's chart without patient interaction

Question 2: What is the primary purpose of performing a preoperative skin antisepsis?
A) To moisturize the skin
B) To reduce the risk of surgical site infections
C) To enhance the absorption of anesthesia
D) To identify any skin allergies

Question 3: During the preoperative preparation for a surgical procedure, the surgical team decides to use a waterless hand antiseptic. Which of the following steps is crucial when using a waterless hand antiseptic to ensure proper hand hygiene?
A) Apply the antiseptic to dry hands and rub until dry.
B) Rinse hands with water before applying the antiseptic.
C) Apply the antiseptic and rinse with water after 30 seconds.
D) Apply the antiseptic to wet hands and rub until dry.

Question 4: Sarah, a surgical technologist, is preparing for a total knee arthroplasty. The surgeon mentions the possibility of using computer-assisted navigation. What additional equipment should Sarah ensure is available?
A) Tourniquet system
B) Computer navigation system
C) Arthroscopy tower
D) Electrocautery unit

Question 5: Emily, a 45-year-old patient, is undergoing spinal fusion surgery. The surgeon decides to use a synthetic tissue graft. What is a key consideration when using synthetic tissue grafts in this type of procedure?
A) Ensuring the graft is radiopaque for imaging purposes
B) Matching the graft's mechanical properties to the host tissue
C) Selecting a graft that promotes rapid vascularization
D) Choosing a graft with antibacterial properties

Question 6: During a laparoscopic cholecystectomy on a patient named Mr. Smith, the surgeon requests an instrument to grasp and manipulate the gallbladder. Which instrument should the surgical technologist provide?
A) Metzenbaum scissors
B) Kocher clamp
C) Maryland dissector
D) Babcock forceps

Question 7: During a spinal fusion surgery, the surgical technologist is asked to prepare an autograft bone for implantation. What is the first step the technologist should take to ensure the graft is viable?
A) Soak the bone graft in saline solution.
B) Pass the bone graft directly to the surgeon.
C) Irrigate the bone graft with antibiotic solution.
D) Ensure the bone graft is kept moist with a sterile sponge.

Question 8: In the context of administrative duties, which task is a surgical technologist least likely to perform?
A) Scheduling surgeries
B) Sterilizing surgical instruments
C) Maintaining patient records
D) Ordering surgical supplies

Question 9: During a surgical procedure, the surgical technologist notices that the sponge count is incorrect. What is the most appropriate immediate action?
A) Continue with the procedure and inform the surgeon at the end.
B) Stop the procedure and perform an immediate recount.
C) Ignore the discrepancy and assume it is a counting error.
D) Inform the circulating nurse and surgeon immediately.

Question 10: Which of the following practices is most effective in ensuring cost containment in the surgical setting?
A) Reusing single-use items whenever possible
B) Implementing a just-in-time inventory system
C) Stockpiling supplies to avoid shortages
D) Allowing surgeons to use any preferred brand of surgical instruments

Question 11: After completing a cholecystectomy on Mr. Smith, the surgical technologist is responsible for removing the drapes and other equipment. During this process, what is the correct procedure for handling the suction tubing?
A) Leave the suction tubing attached to the suction canister.
B) Disconnect the suction tubing and discard it immediately.
C) Disconnect the suction tubing, cap the ends, and dispose of it in a biohazard bag.
D) Disconnect the suction tubing and place it on the sterile field.

Question 12: What is the primary function of the cerebellum in the human brain?
A) Regulation of emotions
B) Coordination of voluntary movements

C) Production of cerebrospinal fluid
D) Processing of visual information

Question 13: During a surgical procedure, the autoclave used for sterilizing instruments malfunctions. As a Certified Surgical Technologist, what is the most appropriate immediate action to ensure patient safety?
A) Continue using the instruments that were previously sterilized.
B) Manually clean the instruments with antiseptic solution.
C) Use a backup autoclave to re-sterilize the instruments.
D) Delay the surgery until the autoclave is repaired.

Question 14: What is the correct sequence for gowning and gloving a sterile team member?
A) Don gloves first, then gown
B) Don gown first, then gloves
C) Don mask first, then gown, then gloves
D) Don cap first, then gloves, then gown

Question 15: During the preoperative assessment of Mr. Smith, a 65-year-old patient scheduled for a total hip replacement, the surgical technologist notices that Mr. Smith has not removed his hearing aids. What is the most appropriate action for the surgical technologist to take?
A) Allow Mr. Smith to keep his hearing aids in place for the surgery.
B) Remove the hearing aids and place them in a labeled container for safekeeping.
C) Inform the anesthesiologist and proceed with the surgery.
D) Ask Mr. Smith to remove his hearing aids and give them to a family member.

Question 16: Which type of malignancy is characterized by the presence of Reed-Sternberg cells?
A) Non-Hodgkin lymphoma
B) Hodgkin lymphoma
C) Multiple myeloma
D) Acute myeloid leukemia

Question 17: Which of the following is the most appropriate method for removing excess blood from the operative site during surgery?
A) Using a sterile gauze pad
B) Applying a tourniquet
C) Utilizing a suction device
D) Allowing natural coagulation

Question 18: During a laparoscopic cholecystectomy, the surgeon asks the surgical technologist to identify the structure labeled "CBD" on the imaging screen. What does "CBD" stand for in this context?
A) Common Bile Duct
B) Cystic Bile Duct
C) Common Biliary Drain

D) Cystic Biliary Duct

Question 19: During a laparoscopic cholecystectomy on a 45-year-old patient named Mr. Smith, the surgeon accidentally punctures the cystic artery, leading to significant bleeding. What is the most appropriate action for the surgical technologist to take in this emergency?
A) Apply direct pressure to the bleeding site immediately.
B) Increase the insufflation pressure to reduce bleeding.
C) Hand the surgeon a hemostatic clamp and prepare suction.
D) Convert to an open procedure to control the bleeding.

Question 20: In a case where Mrs. Smith is undergoing an arteriovenous (AV) fistula creation for hemodialysis, which vessel is typically connected to the cephalic vein?
A) Brachial artery
B) Radial artery
C) Ulnar artery
D) Subclavian artery

Question 21: Which bone is primarily responsible for the formation of the elbow joint along with the humerus and the radius?
A) Scapula
B) Ulna
C) Clavicle
D) Femur

Question 22: Which hormone is primarily responsible for the regulation of the menstrual cycle in females?
A) Testosterone
B) Estrogen
C) Insulin
D) Cortisol

Question 23: What is the primary purpose of using cautery in postoperative procedures during the removal of drapes and other equipment from the patient?
A) To reduce the risk of infection
B) To ensure complete hemostasis
C) To minimize tissue adhesion
D) To enhance wound healing

Question 24: During the transfer of a patient from the operating table to the stretcher, what is the primary role of the Certified Surgical Technologist?
A) Direct the anesthesia provider to manage the patient's airway.
B) Coordinate the movement by counting aloud and guiding the team.
C) Hold the patient's head and neck to prevent injury.
D) Ensure all surgical instruments are accounted for.

Question 25: During a surgical procedure, Dr. Smith and Nurse Johnson have a disagreement about the correct instrument to use. As a Certified Surgical Technologist, how should you handle this situation to maintain a professional and efficient operating room environment?
A) Ignore the disagreement and continue with your tasks.
B) Side with Dr. Smith since he is the lead surgeon.
C) Suggest a brief pause to discuss the issue and reach a consensus.
D) Report the disagreement to the hospital administration immediately.

Question 26: Sarah, a surgical technologist, is preparing the Da Vinci system for a complex robotic-assisted hysterectomy. Which of the following steps is crucial for ensuring the robotic instruments are correctly draped?
A) Ensuring the robotic instruments are sterilized before the procedure.
B) Draping the robotic instruments after they are attached to the robotic arms.
C) Draping the robotic instruments before they are attached to the robotic arms.
D) Ensuring the robotic instruments are draped simultaneously with the robotic arms.

Question 27: What is the primary function of the sinoatrial (SA) node in the heart?
A) To pump blood to the lungs
B) To act as the heart's natural pacemaker
C) To receive deoxygenated blood from the body
D) To prevent backflow of blood into the atria

Question 28: During a surgical procedure, a fire breaks out in the operating room. What is the first action that the surgical technologist should take to ensure the safety of the patient and staff?
A) Call for help and alert the fire department.
B) Use a fire extinguisher to put out the fire.
C) Remove the patient from the immediate danger area.
D) Turn off all electrical equipment in the operating room.

Question 29: What is the most appropriate method for disposing of contaminated sharps after surgery in compliance with Standard Precautions?
A) Place them in a regular trash bin.
B) Place them in a puncture-resistant sharps container.
C) Place them in a biohazard bag.
D) Place them in an autoclave for sterilization.

Question 30: Mrs. Smith is scheduled for a laparoscopic cholecystectomy. During the preoperative phase, which document should be reviewed to ensure that all necessary preoperative instructions have been communicated and understood by the patient?

A) Preoperative teaching record
B) Operative report
C) Postoperative care plan
D) Discharge summary

Question 31: During the preoperative setup for an orthopedic surgery on a patient named Ms. Johnson, the surgical technologist notices that the suction unit is not providing adequate suction. What should be the first step in troubleshooting this issue?
A) Replace the suction canister.
B) Increase the suction pressure.
C) Inspect the suction tubing for kinks or blockages.
D) Switch to a different suction unit.

Question 32: During a laparoscopic cholecystectomy, which of the following steps should the surgical technologist anticipate immediately after the pneumoperitoneum is established?
A) Insertion of the laparoscope
B) Clipping of the cystic artery and duct
C) Dissection of the gallbladder from the liver bed
D) Closure of the port sites

Question 33: Mrs. Smith is scheduled for a pediatric surgery. The surgical technologist is responsible for preparing the operating room environment. What is the recommended temperature range for the operating room to ensure the pediatric patient's safety and comfort?
A) 60°F to 65°F
B) 68°F to 73°F
C) 70°F to 75°F
D) 75°F to 80°F

Question 34: During a laparoscopic cholecystectomy on a patient named Mr. Smith, which draping technique should be used to ensure the laparoscopic equipment remains sterile throughout the procedure?
A) Drape the patient first, then cover the laparoscopic equipment with a separate sterile drape.
B) Drape the laparoscopic equipment first, then drape the patient.
C) Drape the patient and the laparoscopic equipment simultaneously using a single sterile drape.
D) Use a sterile cover only for the laparoscopic equipment, leaving the patient undraped.

Question 35: What is the primary reason for verifying the availability of surgical equipment before a procedure?
A) To ensure the surgical team is familiar with the equipment
B) To prevent delays during the surgery
C) To comply with hospital policy
D) To maintain the cleanliness of the operating room

Question 36: During an intraoperative procedure using a computer navigation system, the surgical

technologist notices a discrepancy between the system's guidance and the actual anatomical structures. What should be the immediate course of action?
A) Continue the surgery and adjust manually
B) Recalibrate the navigation system
C) Restart the computer navigation system
D) Ignore the discrepancy if it is minor

Question 37: Which of the following is a critical step to ensure the safety and effectiveness of phacoemulsification during cataract surgery?
A) Using a high-frequency laser
B) Maintaining the correct intraocular pressure
C) Applying topical antibiotics preoperatively
D) Performing a corneal transplant

Question 38: During the preoperative preparation for Mr. Johnson, a 65-year-old patient scheduled for hip replacement surgery, which of the following patient safety devices is most crucial to apply to prevent deep vein thrombosis (DVT)?
A) Sequential compression device (SCD)
B) Pulse oximeter
C) Foley catheter
D) Nasal cannula

Question 39: Which of the following is the most reliable method to test the sharpness of surgical scissors?
A) Cutting through a piece of gauze
B) Visual inspection under a magnifying glass
C) Running a finger along the blade
D) Using a sharpness testing device

Question 40: Which of the following actions is essential to maintain aseptic technique when donning sterile gloves?
A) Touching the outside of the glove with bare hands.
B) Using the closed gloving technique.
C) Adjusting the glove fit by touching the sterile gown.
D) Donning gloves before the sterile gown.

Question 41: Which of the following is a common cause of fires in the operating room?
A) Use of non-sterile instruments
B) Electrical equipment malfunction
C) Inadequate hand hygiene
D) Poor lighting conditions

Question 42: During an orthopedic surgery on Mrs. Johnson, the power drill suddenly stops working. As the Certified Surgical Technologist, what should you do first to troubleshoot this equipment malfunction?
A) Check the battery or power supply.
B) Replace the drill with a new one.
C) Inform the surgeon immediately.
D) Sterilize a backup drill.

Question 43: Which of the following thermal technologies is most commonly used for tissue
dissection and coagulation during laparoscopic surgery?
A) Cryotherapy
B) Ultrasonic scalpel
C) Laser ablation
D) Radiofrequency ablation

Question 44: During an orthopedic surgery, the surgical technologist is responsible for monitoring the use of irrigation solutions. What is the most important factor to consider when managing these solutions?
A) The temperature of the irrigation solution.
B) The color of the irrigation solution.
C) The volume of irrigation solution used.
D) The type of irrigation solution being used.

Question 45: During surgery, which of the following is the most critical indicator of significant blood loss that requires immediate intervention?
A) Decreased urine output
B) Increased respiratory rate
C) Drop in blood pressure
D) Elevated heart rate

Question 46: In preparing Ms. Smith, a 45-year-old patient for a knee arthroscopy, what is the correct tension for the safety strap to ensure both safety and comfort?
A) Tight enough to leave an indentation on the skin
B) Loose enough to fit a hand underneath easily
C) Snug, allowing minimal movement but not causing discomfort
D) Not applied, as it is unnecessary for this procedure

Question 47: During the preoperative preparation for Mr. Johnson's knee replacement surgery, the surgical team is about to perform the Universal Protocol (Time Out). Which of the following steps is NOT part of the Time Out procedure?
A) Confirming the patient's identity using two identifiers
B) Verifying the surgical site and procedure
C) Reviewing the patient's allergies and medical history
D) Ensuring the surgical instruments are sterile

Question 48: When should contaminated sharps be disposed of in a sharps container after surgery?
A) Immediately after use.
B) At the end of the surgical procedure.
C) When the sharps container is full.
D) Before the patient leaves the operating room.

Question 49: During a post-operative debrief, Dr. Johnson mentions that he prefers a different suture material for closing incisions. What should the Certified Surgical Technologist do to ensure this preference is consistently followed in future surgeries?

A) Make a mental note and remember to use the new suture material.
B) Update Dr. Johnson's preference card to reflect the new suture material.
C) Inform the circulating nurse to remind the team during the next surgery.
D) Use the new suture material only if Dr. Johnson specifically asks for it.

Question 50: During an intraoperative procedure, the surgeon instructs you to assist in applying a splint to Ms. Smith's lower leg. What is the primary purpose of applying padding before the splint?
A) To provide additional support to the limb.
B) To prevent skin irritation and pressure sores.
C) To make the splint easier to remove.
D) To ensure the splint adheres to the skin.

Question 51: During a laparoscopic cholecystectomy, the surgeon asks you to connect and activate a Jackson-Pratt (JP) drain to a suction apparatus. What is the correct sequence of steps to ensure proper function?
A) Connect the drain to the suction tubing, activate the suction, then compress the bulb.
B) Compress the bulb, connect the drain to the suction tubing, then activate the suction.
C) Connect the drain to the suction tubing, compress the bulb, then activate the suction.
D) Activate the suction, compress the bulb, then connect the drain to the suction tubing.

Question 52: During a laparoscopic cholecystectomy, what is the primary responsibility of the surgical technologist when the surgeon is dissecting the cystic duct and artery?
A) Adjusting the insufflation pressure
B) Retracting the liver for better visualization
C) Passing the appropriate instruments to the surgeon
D) Monitoring the patient's vital signs

Question 53: When preparing suture material for a surgical procedure, which of the following steps is essential to ensure sterility?
A) Open the suture packet with bare hands.
B) Use sterile gloves to handle the suture material.
C) Place the suture material on a non-sterile surface.
D) Cut the suture material with non-sterile scissors.

Question 54: Sarah, a 45-year-old patient, is being prepared for a laparoscopic cholecystectomy. Which monitoring device should be applied to continuously measure her cardiac electrical activity during the procedure?
A) Capnography
B) Electrocardiogram (ECG) leads
C) Pulse oximeter
D) Blood pressure cuff

Question 55: During a tympanoplasty procedure on Mr. Johnson, the surgeon needs to graft tissue to repair the tympanic membrane. Which of the following structures is most commonly used for this graft?
A) Nasal septum
B) Temporalis fascia
C) Buccal mucosa
D) Palatal mucosa

Question 56: During a laparoscopic cholecystectomy on a patient named John, the surgeon requests a Maryland dissector. Which of the following actions should the surgical technologist take to ensure the instrument is passed correctly?
A) Pass the instrument with the tips pointed downwards.
B) Pass the instrument with the tips pointed upwards.
C) Pass the instrument with the tips in a neutral position.
D) Pass the instrument with the tips facing the surgeon.

Question 57: Which of the following steps is most crucial in preventing cross-contamination during the room clean-up process after a surgical procedure?
A) Disposing of all sharps immediately
B) Wiping down the surgical lights
C) Using a high-level disinfectant on all surfaces
D) Removing all linens and waste first

Question 58: During an orthopedic surgery on a patient named Mrs. Johnson, the anesthesiologist requests an infusion of 1 gram of cefazolin. As the surgical technologist, what should you do next?
A) Prepare the cefazolin and administer it immediately.
B) Verify the medication and dosage with the circulating nurse before preparing it.
C) Ask the surgeon to confirm the request before proceeding.
D) Wait until the end of the surgery to administer the cefazolin.

Question 59: What is the primary reason for monitoring the amount of solution used during an intraoperative procedure?
A) To ensure the surgical team has enough supplies
B) To prevent contamination of the sterile field
C) To maintain accurate fluid balance for the patient
D) To comply with hospital inventory protocols

Question 60: During a laparoscopic cholecystectomy on a patient named Mr. Johnson, the surgeon requests the use of a thermal device to achieve hemostasis. Which device should the surgical technologist prepare?
A) Harmonic Scalpel
B) Bipolar Forceps
C) Monopolar Electrosurgery
D) Cryotherapy Probe

Question 61: Which of the following best describes a comminuted fracture?
A) A fracture where the bone is broken into multiple pieces
B) A fracture where the bone is partially bent
C) A fracture where the bone is broken straight across
D) A fracture where the bone is broken in a spiral pattern

Question 62: In a spinal fusion surgery for a patient named Sarah, the surgical technologist is preparing a synthetic tissue graft. What is the primary consideration to ensure the graft's effectiveness?
A) The graft's tensile strength.
B) The graft's immunogenicity.
C) The graft's size and shape compatibility.
D) The graft's color and texture.

Question 63: After a successful laparoscopic cholecystectomy on Mr. Johnson, the surgical technologist is responsible for removing the drapes and other equipment from the patient. Which of the following steps should be performed first?
A) Remove the surgical drapes from the patient.
B) Disconnect the insufflation tubing from the trocar.
C) Remove the trocars from the patient's abdomen.
D) Turn off the electrosurgical unit.

Question 64: Which hemostatic agent is most appropriate for controlling capillary bleeding in a highly vascular area during surgery?
A) Bone wax
B) Fibrin sealant
C) Tourniquet
D) Electrocautery

Question 65: Which of the following is the most appropriate method for handling surgical instruments during the removal of drapes postoperatively?
A) Place all instruments on the patient's chest
B) Hand instruments directly to the circulating nurse
C) Leave instruments on the drapes until they are removed
D) Place instruments back in the instrument tray immediately

Question 66: During a phacoemulsification procedure on Mr. Johnson, the surgeon encounters a dense cataract. Which of the following settings should the surgical technologist adjust to optimize the ultrasound power for effective emulsification?
A) Increase the aspiration flow rate
B) Decrease the ultrasound power
C) Increase the ultrasound power
D) Decrease the irrigation flow rate

Question 67: What is the primary purpose of performing a leak test on a laparoscopic insufflator before surgery?
A) To ensure the insufflator is properly calibrated for gas flow
B) To verify the insufflator's pressure settings
C) To check for any gas leakage in the tubing and connections
D) To confirm the insufflator's power supply is functioning

Question 68: What is the most effective active listening technique to ensure understanding during a preoperative team briefing?
A) Nodding occasionally
B) Paraphrasing the speaker's points
C) Maintaining eye contact
D) Taking notes

Question 69: During the intraoperative phase of phacoemulsification on Ms. Thompson, the surgeon notices a surge in the anterior chamber. What immediate action should the surgical technologist take to stabilize the chamber?
A) Increase the irrigation flow rate
B) Decrease the aspiration flow rate
C) Increase the ultrasound power
D) Decrease the irrigation flow rate

Question 70: During the preoperative preparation for a laparoscopic cholecystectomy on Mr. Smith, where is the most appropriate placement for the bovie pad to ensure patient safety?
A) Over a bony prominence
B) On the upper arm
C) On the thigh
D) On the abdomen

Question 71: What is the first step a Certified Surgical Technologist should take when an autoclave fails to reach the required temperature for sterilization?
A) Replace the autoclave's heating element.
B) Check the water level in the autoclave reservoir.
C) Restart the autoclave cycle.
D) Contact the biomedical engineering department immediately.

Question 72: Which stage of grief, according to Kübler-Ross, is characterized by the patient refusing to accept the reality of their terminal diagnosis?
A) Anger
B) Depression
C) Denial
D) Bargaining

Question 73: What is the primary purpose of a surgeon's preference card in a surgical setting?
A) To list the surgical instruments and supplies preferred by the surgeon
B) To document the patient's medical history and allergies

C) To outline the postoperative care plan for the patient
D) To provide a detailed billing summary for the surgery

Question 74: Which of the following steps is essential during a medical hand wash to ensure proper asepsis?
A) Using a nail brush for 30 seconds
B) Rinsing hands with hot water
C) Keeping hands lower than elbows during rinsing
D) Cleaning under fingernails

Question 75: During a laparoscopic cholecystectomy on a patient named Sarah, the surgeon decides to use intraoperative ultrasound to assess the biliary anatomy. Which ultrasound probe is most suitable for this purpose?
A) Phased array probe
B) Linear array probe
C) Curvilinear array probe
D) Endocavitary probe

Question 76: Ms. Smith is scheduled for a total hip replacement. Which positioning device should be used to ensure proper alignment and stabilization of the operative leg during the procedure?
A) Wilson frame
B) Hip positioner
C) Knee crutches
D) Mayfield headrest

Question 77: Sarah, a patient undergoing a liver resection, requires intraoperative ultrasound to locate a lesion. What is the most critical factor for ensuring optimal ultrasound imaging during this procedure?
A) The patient's body mass index (BMI).
B) The type of ultrasound probe used.
C) The experience of the surgical technologist.
D) The amount of saline used for acoustic coupling.

Question 78: What is the primary purpose of ensuring the bovie pad is securely attached to the patient before starting an electrosurgical procedure?
A) To prevent the patient from moving
B) To ensure the patient remains sterile
C) To provide a return path for the electrical current
D) To monitor the patient's heart rate

Question 79: During the preoperative preparation for Mr. Johnson's laparoscopic cholecystectomy, the surgical technologist needs to verify the availability of essential equipment. Which of the following is the most critical piece of equipment to ensure is available and functioning properly?
A) Electrosurgical unit
B) Suction apparatus
C) Laparoscopic camera system
D) Surgical lights

Question 80: Which cranial nerve is responsible for the sense of smell?
A) Optic Nerve (II)
B) Oculomotor Nerve (III)
C) Olfactory Nerve (I)
D) Trigeminal Nerve (V)

Question 81: During preoperative preparation, which device is essential for monitoring a patient's end-tidal CO2 levels?
A) Pulse oximeter
B) Capnograph
C) Electrocardiogram (ECG)
D) Thermometer

Question 82: Ms. Smith, a patient scheduled for an elective knee replacement, expresses confusion about the risks associated with the procedure. What is the best course of action for the surgical technologist?
A) Explain the risks and benefits of the procedure to the patient.
B) Ask the patient to sign the consent form regardless of her confusion.
C) Inform the surgeon or nurse to re-explain the procedure to the patient.
D) Ignore the patient's concerns and proceed with the preoperative preparations.

Question 83: What does dark red or maroon blood suggest during an intraoperative procedure?
A) Arterial bleeding
B) Venous bleeding
C) Capillary bleeding
D) Hemolysis

Question 84: During a preoperative assessment, the surgical technologist needs to ensure x-ray safety for a patient named Mr. Smith, who is scheduled for a hip replacement surgery. Which of the following measures is the most appropriate to minimize Mr. Smith's exposure to x-rays during the procedure?
A) Positioning the x-ray machine as close to the patient as possible
B) Using lead aprons and thyroid shields on the patient
C) Increasing the x-ray exposure time to capture clearer images
D) Allowing the patient to hold the x-ray film to reduce movement

Question 85: Which of the following is the most appropriate initial management for a patient with a suspected cervical spine injury from a traumatic accident?
A) Immediate removal of the cervical collar
B) Application of a thoracic brace
C) Immobilization with a cervical collar
D) Administration of intravenous fluids

Question 86: During a total knee arthroplasty on a

patient named Mrs. Johnson, the surgeon instructs you to prepare the dressing for the wound site. Which of the following is the most appropriate type of dressing to use to minimize the risk of infection?
A) Gauze dressing without any antiseptic.
B) Transparent film dressing.
C) Hydrocolloid dressing.
D) Sterile, non-adherent dressing with an antiseptic layer.

Question 87: 5 Which of the following microorganisms is most commonly associated with surgical site infections (SSIs)?
A) Escherichia coli
B) Staphylococcus aureus
C) Pseudomonas aeruginosa
D) Candida albicans

Question 88: What is the most effective immediate action to take if a fire breaks out in the operating room?
A) Evacuate the patient immediately
B) Use a fire extinguisher to put out the fire
C) Shut off the gas supply
D) Call for help and wait for instructions

Question 89: Which of the following is the most critical piece of information to verify on the preoperative checklist before the patient is taken to the operating room?
A) Patient's insurance details
B) Patient's consent form
C) Patient's dietary restrictions
D) Patient's family contact information

Question 90: A patient presents with a widespread rash and fever three days after surgery. Which of the following should be the primary concern?
A) Allergic reaction to latex
B) Surgical site infection
C) Drug-induced hypersensitivity
D) Contact dermatitis from adhesive dressings

Question 91: Which of the following is the most appropriate action for a surgical technologist to take when a patient expresses anxiety about their upcoming surgery?
A) Ignore the patient's concerns and focus on preparing the surgical instruments.
B) Reassure the patient by providing accurate information about the procedure.
C) Tell the patient that their anxiety is normal and will go away on its own.
D) Suggest the patient speak to their family members about their concerns.

Question 92: A patient named Sarah is undergoing surgery for breast cancer. The surgeon plans to perform a sentinel lymph node biopsy to check for metastasis. Which lymph nodes are most likely to be the sentinel nodes in this case?
A) Axillary lymph nodes
B) Inguinal lymph nodes
C) Cervical lymph nodes
D) Mesenteric lymph nodes

Question 93: Mrs. Johnson is scheduled for an elective cholecystectomy. Her preoperative laboratory results indicate a hemoglobin level of 8.5 g/dL. What should be the surgical technologist's primary concern regarding this lab result?
A) The patient might have an increased risk of infection.
B) The patient might have an increased risk of bleeding.
C) The patient might have an increased risk of poor oxygenation during surgery.
D) The patient might have an increased risk of electrolyte imbalance.

Question 94: When preparing a wound site for dressing, which of the following steps is essential to maintain sterility?
A) Using non-sterile gloves to handle the dressing
B) Cleaning the wound with sterile saline solution
C) Applying the dressing with bare hands
D) Using the same dressing for multiple wounds

Question 95: During a lung resection surgery on Mrs. Smith, the surgeon needs to avoid damaging the phrenic nerve. Which anatomical landmark should the surgical technologist use to locate the phrenic nerve?
A) Anterior to the hilum of the lung
B) Posterior to the hilum of the lung
C) Lateral to the trachea
D) Medial to the esophagus

Question 96: When restocking supplies in the operating room, what is the best practice to ensure sterility and readiness for the next procedure?
A) Placing new supplies in the front of the storage area
B) Checking expiration dates and rotating stock
C) Storing supplies in their original packaging
D) Ensuring all supplies are within easy reach

Question 97: Ms. Johnson is undergoing an exploratory laparotomy to investigate abdominal pain. The surgeon needs an incision that allows wide access to the entire abdominal cavity. Which incision should the surgeon choose?
A) Pfannenstiel incision
B) McBurney incision
C) Midline incision
D) Kocher incision

Question 98: What is the primary mechanism by which a harmonic scalpel achieves hemostasis during surgery?

A) Electrical cauterization
B) Ultrasonic vibrations
C) Laser energy
D) Radiofrequency waves

Question 99: What is the primary purpose of using computer navigation systems during orthopedic surgery?
A) To reduce the need for surgical instruments
B) To enhance the accuracy of implant placement
C) To shorten the duration of the surgery
D) To eliminate the need for imaging techniques

Question 100: During the postoperative phase, the surgical technologist is tasked with removing drapes and other equipment from the patient. What is the correct procedure for handling nondisposable instruments?
A) Place nondisposable instruments in a basin of sterile water.
B) Disassemble and soak nondisposable instruments in enzymatic cleaner.
C) Immediately place nondisposable instruments in a sterilization container.
D) Hand nondisposable instruments to the scrub nurse for immediate reuse.

Question 101: Which of the following is a critical step in the preoperative preparation of a surgical microscope?
A) Calibrating the microscope's magnification settings
B) Ensuring the microscope is connected to the anesthesia machine
C) Sterilizing the microscope's entire body
D) Placing the microscope in the sterile field

Question 102: During a cataract surgery on Mrs. Smith, the surgeon asks the surgical technologist to identify the fluid-filled space between the cornea and the iris. What is the correct identification?
A) Vitreous chamber
B) Anterior chamber
C) Posterior chamber
D) Aqueous humor

Question 103: Which of the following is a key principle in ensuring electrical safety in the operating room?
A) Using extension cords to connect multiple devices
B) Ensuring all equipment is properly grounded
C) Overloading circuits to maximize efficiency
D) Using non-conductive materials for all surfaces

Question 104: When removing equipment from the patient postoperatively, what is the primary consideration?
A) Speed of removal
B) Maintaining sterility
C) Patient comfort
D) Minimizing noise

Question 105: During the preoperative preparation for a knee replacement surgery, the surgical technologist, Alex, notices a small tear in the sterile package of surgical instruments. What should Alex do next?
A) Use the instruments as long as they appear clean
B) Reseal the package with sterile tape and proceed
C) Discard the package and obtain a new sterile set
D) Continue with the surgery and inform the surgeon later

Question 106: Which of the following is the most critical safety measure to implement when using a laser in the operating room?
A) Ensuring the patient is draped with non-reflective materials
B) Wearing standard surgical masks
C) Using smoke evacuators
D) Applying wet towels around the surgical site

Question 107: During the preoperative preparation for a laparoscopic cholecystectomy on a patient named Mr. Smith, the surgical technologist is responsible for ensuring the suction system is properly set up. Which of the following steps is crucial to verify the functionality of the suction system?
A) Ensure the suction canister is empty.
B) Check that the suction tubing is securely connected.
C) Verify the suction pressure is set to 200 mmHg.
D) Confirm the suction system is plugged into the electrical outlet.

Question 108: Which classification of surgical instrument is a Kocher clamp?
A) Cutting and dissecting
B) Clamping and occluding
C) Grasping and holding
D) Retracting and exposing

Question 109: What is the primary reason for accurately reporting the amount of medication and solution used during a surgical procedure?
A) To ensure the patient receives the correct dosage postoperatively
B) To maintain an accurate inventory of medical supplies
C) To provide precise information for the patient's medical record
D) To comply with hospital administrative policies

Question 110: What is the primary reason for using a fenestrated drape when preparing specialty equipment for a surgical procedure?
A) To allow for multiple instruments to be passed through the drape.
B) To provide a sterile barrier while allowing access to the surgical site.
C) To cover the entire surgical field with one drape.
D) To minimize the use of additional drapes during the procedure.

Question 111: Sarah, a surgical technologist, is preparing for an upcoming surgery and notices that the inventory of surgical gloves is low. What should she do to ensure proper cost containment?
A) Ignore the low inventory and proceed with the surgery.
B) Order a large quantity of gloves to avoid future shortages.
C) Report the low inventory to the supply manager and request a restock based on usage trends.
D) Borrow gloves from another department without informing anyone.

Question 112: Which of the following is the most effective method for reducing surgical smoke in the operating room?
A) Using high-efficiency particulate air (HEPA) filters
B) Wearing high-filtration surgical masks
C) Utilizing a smoke evacuation system
D) Increasing room ventilation

Question 113: In the context of intraoperative procedures, what is a significant safety concern when using an argon laser?
A) Potential for deep tissue burns.
B) Risk of retinal damage to the surgical team.
C) High incidence of postoperative infections.
D) Excessive smoke production during use.

Question 114: Mr. Johnson is scheduled for a laparoscopic cholecystectomy. During the preoperative phase, the surgical technologist notices that the informed consent form is missing the surgeon's signature. What should the surgical technologist do next?
A) Proceed with the surgery as the patient has signed the consent form.
B) Inform the circulating nurse to get the surgeon's signature before proceeding.
C) Ask the patient to sign the consent form again.
D) Ignore the missing signature as it is not crucial.

Question 115: Which artery is primarily responsible for supplying blood to the lower extremities?
A) Brachial artery
B) Femoral artery
C) Carotid artery
D) Radial artery

Question 116: During the postoperative phase, the surgical technologist must ensure that all instruments used during Mrs. Johnson's appendectomy are accounted for. Which of the following steps is most crucial in this process?
A) Counting the instruments before removing the drapes.
B) Counting the instruments after removing the drapes.
C) Counting the instruments after the patient has been transferred to the recovery room.
D) Counting the instruments while the patient is being extubated.

Question 117: During the postoperative phase after an appendectomy on Ms. Smith, the surgical technologist must remove the drapes and equipment. What is the correct sequence for removing the drapes?
A) Remove the drapes starting from the head of the patient.
B) Remove the drapes starting from the feet of the patient.
C) Remove the drapes starting from the sides of the patient.
D) Remove the drapes starting from the surgical site outward.

Question 118: Sarah, a 35-year-old patient, is undergoing a hysterectomy. During the procedure, the surgeon needs to avoid damaging the structure that transports eggs from the ovaries to the uterus. Which structure is the surgeon referring to?
A) Ureter
B) Fallopian tube
C) Round ligament
D) Broad ligament

Question 119: During a surgical procedure, the patient experiences a sudden drop in blood pressure and heart rate. What is the first action the surgical technologist should take?
A) Administer epinephrine.
B) Notify the surgeon immediately.
C) Increase the IV fluid rate.
D) Begin chest compressions.

Question 120: What is the primary function of the glomerulus in the kidney?
A) Filtration of blood
B) Reabsorption of water
C) Secretion of hormones
D) Concentration of urine

Question 121: Dr. Smith has updated his preference card to include a new suture material for abdominal surgeries. As a Certified Surgical Technologist, what is the most appropriate action to ensure this change is reflected in future procedures?
A) Verbally inform the surgical team of the change before each surgery.
B) Update the preference card in the computer system immediately.
C) Write a note on the physical preference card and update it later.
D) Wait until the end of the week to make all updates at once.

Question 122: What is the primary reason for verifying the correct type and size of implantable

items with the surgeon before the procedure begins?
A) To ensure the implant matches the patient's insurance coverage
B) To confirm the implant is available in the sterile field
C) To prevent surgical complications and ensure proper fit
D) To reduce the overall cost of the surgery

Question 123: During a neurosurgical procedure on Mr. Johnson, the surgical technologist is responsible for setting up the operating microscope. Which of the following steps is crucial to ensure proper focus and clarity of the microscope?
A) Adjusting the microscope's light intensity
B) Balancing the microscope's weight distribution
C) Calibrating the microscope's ocular lenses
D) Ensuring the microscope's objective lens is clean

Question 124: During the preoperative preparation for a surgery on patient Mr. Johnson, the surgical technologist notices a tear in the sterile glove after assisting with gowning. What should be the immediate next step?
A) Continue with the procedure and replace the glove later.
B) Replace the glove immediately without notifying anyone.
C) Notify the surgical team and replace the glove immediately.
D) Ignore the tear if it is small and proceed with the surgery.

Question 125: During an orthopedic surgery on Mr. Johnson, the surgeon excises a bone fragment and asks for it to be sent for microbiological culture. How should the Certified Surgical Technologist handle this specimen?
A) Place the specimen in formalin and label it with the patient's name and date of birth.
B) Place the specimen in a sterile container without any preservative and label it with the patient's name, date of birth, and "Microbiological Culture."
C) Place the specimen in a sterile container with saline and label it with the patient's name, date of birth, and "Histopathology."
D) Wrap the specimen in a sterile gauze soaked in saline and label it with the patient's name and date of birth.

Question 126: After a successful laparoscopic cholecystectomy on Mr. Johnson, the surgical technologist is tasked with removing the drapes and other equipment. During this process, what is the most crucial step to ensure safety when dealing with the cautery device?
A) Turn off the cautery device and unplug it before removing the drapes.
B) Remove the drapes first, then turn off the cautery device.

C) Leave the cautery device on standby mode while removing the drapes.
D) Ask the surgeon to remove the drapes while the cautery device is still on.

Question 127: After a cholecystectomy, Mr. Johnson reports severe abdominal pain, a fever of 102°F, and yellowing of the skin. As a Certified Surgical Technologist, what is the most appropriate action to take?
A) Reassure the patient that these symptoms are normal post-surgery.
B) Administer over-the-counter pain medication and monitor.
C) Report the symptoms immediately to the surgeon.
D) Suggest the patient to increase fluid intake and rest.

Question 128: What is the primary benefit of utilizing online continuing education platforms for Certified Surgical Technologists?
A) Limited access to course materials
B) Inconsistent course quality
C) Flexibility in learning schedule
D) High costs compared to traditional methods

Question 129: Which of the following practices is most effective in ensuring cost containment in the surgical setting?
A) Reusing single-use items after sterilization
B) Implementing a standardized inventory management system
C) Ordering supplies in bulk without considering usage rates
D) Using the most expensive surgical instruments available

Question 130: What is the primary purpose of using a surgical skin antiseptic prior to an incision?
A) To reduce the risk of postoperative infection
B) To remove all resident bacteria from the skin
C) To sterilize the surgical instruments
D) To provide a sterile field for the surgical team

Question 131: Which of the following is the most appropriate suction tip to use during a tonsillectomy procedure to ensure effective removal of blood and debris?
A) Poole suction tip
B) Yankauer suction tip
C) Frazier suction tip
D) Rosen suction tip

Question 132: After a successful appendectomy on Mr. Johnson, the surgical technologist is responsible for removing the drapes and other equipment. What is the first step in this process?
A) Remove the surgical instruments from the sterile field.
B) Disconnect the suction and electrosurgical units.
C) Remove the drapes by pulling them towards the

patient's head.

D) Ensure all counts are correct and accounted for.

Question 133: What is the primary advantage of using an ultrasonic scalpel over traditional electrocautery for hemostasis in surgery?
A) Lower risk of thermal injury to surrounding tissues
B) Higher coagulation temperatures
C) Easier to use
D) More cost-effective

Question 134: Which of the following is the most appropriate step to take before using a pneumatic power drill in surgery?
A) Lubricate the drill with oil
B) Check the air hose for leaks
C) Sterilize the drill using an autoclave
D) Ensure the drill is fully charged

Question 135: During a laparoscopic procedure, which mechanical device is often utilized to control bleeding from small vessels?
A) Laparoscopic stapler
B) Harmonic scalpel
C) Laparoscopic clip applier
D) Bipolar forceps

Question 136: During a surgical procedure, the surgeon asks you to assist in applying a cast to Mr. Johnson's fractured forearm. What is the first step you should take to ensure proper application?
A) Apply padding directly to the skin.
B) Immerse the casting material in water.
C) Position the limb in the desired alignment.
D) Cut the casting material to the appropriate length.

Question 137: Which of the following is a primary reason for using helium in laser technology during intraoperative procedures?
A) Helium is highly reactive and enhances laser precision.
B) Helium is a noble gas that helps stabilize the laser beam.
C) Helium is heavier than air and prevents laser scattering.
D) Helium is used to cool the laser equipment due to its high thermal conductivity.

Question 138: What is the most effective method for ensuring accurate interdepartmental communication regarding surgical schedules?
A) Verbal communication during morning briefings
B) Written memos distributed to all departments
C) Real-time updates through a centralized computer system
D) Weekly departmental meetings

Question 139: During a total hip replacement surgery on a patient named Mrs. Johnson, you notice a small tear in your sterile gown sleeve. What is the most appropriate action to follow

standard and universal precautions?
A) Continue the procedure and cover the tear with a sterile drape.
B) Notify the surgeon and replace the gown immediately.
C) Ask the circulating nurse to tape over the tear.
D) Continue the procedure and replace the gown after the surgery.

Question 140: During a total knee arthroplasty, the surgical technologist is responsible for ensuring the power equipment is functioning correctly. Which of the following steps should be performed first when assembling the power equipment?
A) Check the battery charge level.
B) Attach the appropriate blade or bit.
C) Verify the sterilization indicator.
D) Test the equipment for proper operation.

Question 141: Which of the following is the most effective way for a Certified Surgical Technologist to keep track of their continuing education credits using computer technology?
A) Using a paper-based logbook
B) Relying on email notifications from professional organizations
C) Utilizing a dedicated continuing education tracking software
D) Keeping a mental note of completed courses

Question 142: Which of the following is a key administrative duty of a CST in the operating room?
A) Scheduling surgeries
B) Documenting surgical counts
C) Managing patient records
D) Supervising the surgical team

Question 143: During a surgical procedure, a chemical spill occurs in the operating room. What is the first action a Certified Surgical Technologist (CST) should take to ensure safety?
A) Immediately start cleaning up the spill.
B) Evacuate the operating room.
C) Notify the surgical team and follow the facility's spill protocol.
D) Continue with the procedure and address the spill later.

Question 144: Which of the following actions should be taken immediately after a sharps container becomes three-quarters full?
A) Compress the contents to make more room.
B) Continue using the container until it is completely full.
C) Seal the container and replace it with a new one.
D) Transfer the sharps to a larger container.

Question 145: What is the most effective method for a surgical technologist to prevent the transmission of bloodborne pathogens during surgery?

A) Wearing a surgical mask
B) Double-gloving
C) Using a face shield
D) Handwashing before and after the procedure

Question 146: During a preoperative preparation, Sarah, a Certified Surgical Technologist, needs to perform a surgical scrub before assisting in a cardiac surgery. Which of the following steps is crucial to ensure proper aseptic technique?
A) Scrubbing from the elbow to the fingertips
B) Using a nail cleaner under running water before starting the scrub
C) Drying hands and arms with a reusable towel
D) Scrubbing for a minimum of 1 minute

Question 147: Which of the following is the primary reason for wearing a surgical mask during preoperative preparation?
A) To protect the surgical team from splashes
B) To prevent the spread of airborne pathogens from the surgical team to the patient
C) To keep the surgical team warm
D) To enhance communication within the surgical team

Question 148: Sarah, a surgical technologist, is preparing a pneumatic drill for use in a craniotomy. Which of the following actions is most critical to ensure the drill operates safely and effectively during the procedure?
A) Ensure the drill is properly lubricated.

B) Confirm the air pressure settings are within the recommended range.
C) Check the drill for visible signs of wear and tear.
D) Attach the drill to the air supply line.

Question 149: Which of the following is the most critical step in verifying the availability of surgical equipment before a procedure?
A) Checking the inventory list
B) Confirming equipment functionality
C) Ensuring sterility of instruments
D) Reviewing the surgeon's preference card

Question 150: During an orthopedic surgery, the surgical technologist notices a significant amount of smoke being generated by the electrocautery device. What is the best practice to minimize the potential hazards of surgical smoke?
A) Use high-efficiency particulate air (HEPA) filters in the operating room
B) Ensure all team members wear standard surgical masks
C) Utilize local exhaust ventilation (LEV) systems
D) Increase the room's air exchange rate

ANSWER WITH DETAILED EXPLANATION SET [1]

Question 1: Correct Answer: B) To break up and emulsify the cataractous lens
Rationale: The primary function of ultrasound technology in phacoemulsification is to break up and emulsify the cataractous lens, allowing for its removal. Option A is incorrect as visualization is achieved through a microscope. Option C is incorrect because irrigation is performed using a balanced salt solution. Option D is incorrect as suturing is not related to the ultrasound technology used in phacoemulsification.

Question 2: Correct Answer: D) Polydioxanone (PDS)
Rationale: Dr. Smith's preference card specifically lists Polydioxanone (PDS) for closing abdominal incisions due to its long-term tensile strength and minimal tissue reaction. Silk (A) is not suitable for abdominal incisions due to its high tissue reactivity. Polypropylene (B) is often used for vascular anastomoses but not typically for abdominal closures. Chromic gut (C) is absorbable but lacks the long-term strength required for abdominal incisions. Therefore, PDS is the correct choice.

Question 3: Correct Answer: B) Sterilization and rigorous screening of the donor tissue.
Rationale: The crucial step in minimizing the risk of disease transmission in allografts is the sterilization and rigorous screening of the donor tissue. Option A is incorrect because immediate implantation without processing would increase the risk of disease transmission. Option C, while important, is not specific to allograft preparation. Option D is incorrect because the donor being a close relative does not necessarily reduce the risk of disease transmission; the focus should be on the thorough screening and sterilization process.

Question 4: Correct Answer: B) To identify the root cause and prevent future occurrences
Rationale: The primary purpose of addressing an unexpected delay due to equipment malfunction during a postoperative debrief is to identify the root cause and prevent future occurrences. This helps improve patient safety and surgical efficiency. Option A is incorrect as assigning blame is not constructive. Option C, while important, is not the primary purpose of the debrief. Option D is irrelevant to the main goal of the debrief.

Question 5: Correct Answer: C) Pfannenstiel incision
Rationale: The Pfannenstiel incision is most commonly used for cesarean sections due to its cosmetic benefits and reduced risk of hernia. The midline incision (A) is used for general abdominal surgeries, McBurney's incision (B) is used for appendectomies, and the subcostal incision (D) is used for gallbladder surgeries. The Pfannenstiel incision offers better healing and less postoperative pain, making it the preferred choice for cesarean sections.

Question 6: Correct Answer: B) Addressing the conflict directly and facilitating open communication
Rationale: Addressing the conflict directly and facilitating open communication is the most effective strategy. This approach encourages transparency and mutual understanding, which are crucial for resolving conflicts. Ignoring the conflict (Option A) can lead to unresolved issues, while allowing the team leader to make a unilateral decision (Option C) may not address underlying problems. Blaming external factors (Option D) avoids responsibility and does not resolve the core issue.

Question 7: Correct Answer: C) Immediately update the computer system with the correct instrument.
Rationale: Immediately updating the computer system (C) ensures that future procedures have the correct instrument listed, minimizing the risk of errors. Informing Dr. Jones (A) is important but not sufficient alone. A mental note (B) is unreliable, and using the outdated instrument (D) compromises patient safety and procedural efficiency.

Question 8: Correct Answer: C) Ensure the drapes are placed with the adhesive edges facing towards the surgical site.
Rationale: The adhesive edges of the drapes should face towards the surgical site to secure the drapes and maintain sterility. Option A is incorrect as the adhesive edges should not face away. Option B is incorrect because multiple drapes are typically used for precision. Option D is partially correct but does not address the adhesive edge placement, which is crucial for maintaining a sterile field.

Question 9: Correct Answer: C) Sternum
Rationale: The sternum is part of the axial skeleton, which includes the skull, vertebral column, and rib cage. The scapula, humerus, and clavicle are part of the appendicular skeleton, which includes the limbs and girdles. The axial skeleton provides central support and protection for vital organs, while the appendicular skeleton facilitates movement and interaction with the environment.

Question 10: Correct Answer: A) Squeezing the drain bulb and then connecting it to the suction apparatus
Rationale: Squeezing the drain bulb before connecting it to the suction apparatus creates a vacuum necessary for optimal drainage. Connecting the drain first (B) or activating the suction apparatus before attaching the drain (D) would not establish the required negative pressure. Filling the drain bulb with saline (C) is incorrect and could lead to improper function and potential contamination.

Question 11: Correct Answer: B) Keeping the graft moist with saline
Rationale: Keeping the graft moist with saline is crucial to maintain its cellular viability and structural integrity. Sterilizing with high heat (A) and exposing to ultraviolet light (C) can damage the graft's cellular components. Freezing the graft (D) is used for preservation but must be done under specific conditions to avoid damaging the graft's viability. Therefore, maintaining moisture with saline is essential.

Question 12: Correct Answer: C) Vestibulocochlear

nerve (VIII)

Rationale: The vestibulocochlear nerve (VIII) is responsible for transmitting sensory information from the inner ear to the brain, including both auditory and balance information. The facial nerve (VII) (A) controls muscles of facial expression, the trigeminal nerve (V) (B) is involved in facial sensation and mastication, and the glossopharyngeal nerve (IX) (D) is involved in taste and other functions but not in transmitting auditory information.

Question 13: Correct Answer: B) Notify the surgeon immediately.

Rationale: The most appropriate initial action is to notify the surgeon immediately, as a rapidly expanding hematoma can indicate active bleeding that requires prompt surgical intervention. Applying a cold compress (A) or elevating the limb (C) may be supportive measures but do not address the underlying cause. Administering pain medication (D) does not address the potential need for urgent surgical management.

Question 14: Correct Answer: C) To verify the correct patient, procedure, and site

Rationale: The primary purpose of the Universal Protocol (Time Out) is to verify the correct patient, procedure, and site to prevent wrong-site, wrong-procedure, and wrong-patient surgeries. While confirming insurance information, ensuring instrument sterility, and reviewing credentials are important, they are not the primary focus of the Time Out. The Time Out is a critical safety step to ensure the surgical team is aligned and aware of the specifics of the surgery, thereby minimizing the risk of errors.

Question 15: Correct Answer: C) Notify the surgeon immediately.

Rationale: A sudden increase in dark, bloody drainage from a surgical drain can indicate a developing hematoma or active bleeding. The correct action is to notify the surgeon immediately for prompt evaluation and intervention. Increasing the frequency of monitoring (A) or documenting and continuing to monitor (D) are insufficient responses, and replacing the drain (B) is not appropriate without surgical consultation.

Question 16: Correct Answer: B) Prepare and pass a hemostatic clip applier.

Rationale: The immediate action to control bleeding from the cystic artery is to prepare and pass a hemostatic clip applier to the surgeon. This allows the surgeon to quickly clamp the artery and stop the bleeding. Suctioning (A) and irrigation (D) may help clear the view but do not control the bleeding. Increasing insufflation pressure (C) is not a standard method for controlling arterial bleeding and can cause other complications.

Question 17: Correct Answer: B) Use wet towels to protect surrounding tissues.

Rationale: Using wet towels to protect surrounding tissues is a critical precaution to prevent unintended thermal injury from the CO_2 beam coagulator. Option A is incorrect as maximum power increases the risk of tissue damage. Option C is incorrect because prolonged exposure can cause excessive thermal damage. Option D is incorrect because smoke evacuators are essential to maintain a clear surgical field and reduce inhalation of harmful fumes.

Question 18: Correct Answer: B) Assist Dr. Smith with gowning first, then open the sterile glove package.

Rationale: The correct sequence is to assist with gowning first to maintain sterility, followed by opening the sterile glove package. This ensures that the gown remains sterile while the gloves are being donned. Options A and D are incorrect because they disrupt the sterile field by handling gloves before the gown. Option C is partially correct but does not follow the proper sequence, risking contamination.

Question 19: Correct Answer: A) Pass the instrument with the handles first.

Rationale: The correct way to pass Metzenbaum scissors is with the handles first to allow the surgeon to grasp the instrument securely and immediately use it. Passing with the tips first (B) can be unsafe and inefficient. Passing with the tips pointing towards (C) or away from (D) the technologist can lead to accidental injury or contamination, making these options incorrect.

Question 20: Correct Answer: C) Vagus nerve (CN X)

Rationale: The vagus nerve (CN X) is responsible for the majority of parasympathetic outflow to the thoracic and abdominal organs. It innervates the heart, lungs, and digestive tract, playing a crucial role in autonomic control. The optic nerve (CN II) is related to vision, the trigeminal nerve (CN V) is involved in facial sensation and mastication, and the hypoglossal nerve (CN XII) controls tongue movements. Thus, CN X is the correct answer.

Question 21: Correct Answer: A) McBurney's point

Rationale: McBurney's point is the anatomical landmark used to locate the appendix, situated one-third the distance from the anterior superior iliac spine to the umbilicus. Murphy's point is related to gallbladder disease, Hesselbach's triangle is associated with inguinal hernias, and the Triangle of Calot is used in biliary surgery. Correct identification ensures accurate and efficient surgical procedures.

Question 22: Correct Answer: C) Non-woven fabric wraps

Rationale: Non-woven fabric wraps are ideal for steam sterilization as they allow steam penetration and maintain sterility. Aluminum foil (A) and wax paper (D) do not permit steam penetration, while plastic bags (B) can melt or impede sterilization. Non-woven fabric wraps provide the necessary barrier and permeability for effective sterilization.

Question 23: Correct Answer: B) Place the instrument in a flash sterilizer for a short cycle.

Rationale: The correct procedure for sterilizing an instrument for immediate use is to use a flash sterilizer, which ensures the instrument is properly sterilized in a short amount of time. Option A is incorrect because wiping does not sterilize the instrument. Option C is incorrect as soaking in disinfectant does not achieve sterilization. Option D is incorrect because spraying with antiseptic does not ensure complete sterilization.

Question 24: Correct Answer: B) Prone

Rationale: The prone position is commonly used for lumbar laminectomy as it provides optimal access to the spine. The supine position (A) is not suitable for posterior spinal surgeries. The lithotomy position (C) is used for gynecological and urological procedures. The lateral position (D) may be used for certain spinal surgeries but is not the standard for lumbar laminectomy.

Question 25: Correct Answer: D) Provide her with information on the hospital's confidentiality policies.

Rationale: Providing Mrs. Johnson with information on the hospital's confidentiality policies (Option D) ensures transparency and adherence to ethical and legal standards. Simply assuring her (Option A) without details may not fully address her concerns. Option B is incorrect as it misrepresents the access control of medical records. Telling her not to worry (Option C) dismisses her valid concerns and does not provide the necessary information.

Question 26: Correct Answer: A) Use a new set of sterile instruments for handling the graft.

Rationale: The most critical step to prevent contamination is using a new set of sterile instruments for handling the graft. This minimizes the risk of introducing pathogens. Option B is incorrect because rinsing with sterile water does not ensure sterility. Option C is incorrect because gloved hands alone do not guarantee sterility. Option D is important but secondary to using sterile instruments.

Question 27: Correct Answer: D) Hand nondisposable items directly to the circulating nurse.

Rationale: Nondisposable items should be handed directly to the circulating nurse to ensure they are accounted for and properly processed. Option A is incorrect because nondisposable items should not be placed in biohazard bags. Option B is incorrect as cleaning and disinfecting should occur after removal from the sterile field. Option C is incorrect because placing items on another sterile table is unnecessary and does not ensure proper handling.

Question 28: Correct Answer: C) Irrigate the area with saline to visualize the source of bleeding.

Rationale: Irrigating the area with saline helps clear the blood, allowing the surgeon to visualize the source of bleeding and apply appropriate hemostatic measures. Handing a hemostat (A) or using suction (B) without clear visualization may not effectively control the bleeding. Placing a sponge stick (D) is impractical in a laparoscopic procedure and may obscure the view.

Question 29: Correct Answer: A) To sterilize instruments for immediate use

Rationale: The primary purpose of a short cycle in sterilization is to sterilize instruments for immediate use. This cycle is designed for quick turnaround, ensuring that instruments are ready for use in a short amount of time. Options B, C, and D are incorrect as they either generalize the purpose (B), incorrectly state the method (C), or misinterpret the capacity (D) of the short cycle.

Question 30: Correct Answer: A) It provides real-time imaging of soft tissues.

Rationale: Intraoperative ultrasound is primarily advantageous because it provides real-time imaging of soft tissues, which aids in precise surgical navigation and decision-making. Option B is incorrect as the use of contrast agents depends on the specific procedure. Option C is partially correct but not the primary advantage. Option D is incorrect as intraoperative ultrasound can actually help reduce surgical time by providing immediate feedback.

Question 31: Correct Answer: B) Helium prevents oxidation of the laser components.

Rationale: Helium is used to purge the laser pathway to prevent oxidation of the laser components, ensuring the equipment functions optimally. Option A is incorrect as helium does not affect the laser's energy output. Option C is incorrect because helium does not reduce electrical interference. Option D is incorrect since helium's primary role is not to provide a sterile environment but to prevent oxidation.

Question 32: Correct Answer: B) Turn off the suction device, then remove the suction tubing.

Rationale: Turning off the suction device first ensures that no negative pressure is applied when removing the tubing, preventing tissue damage. Removing the tubing first (Option A) or checking the canister (Option C) before turning off the device could cause harm. Removing drapes (Option D) is unrelated to the immediate safety concern of suction.

Question 33: Correct Answer: B) Polydioxanone (PDS)

Rationale: Polydioxanone (PDS) is a synthetic absorbable suture that provides extended wound support, making it ideal for closing deep fascia layers. Polyglactin 910 (Vicryl) is absorbable but loses tensile strength faster than PDS. Silk is non-absorbable and can cause tissue reaction, and Chromic gut is absorbable but has a shorter absorption period, making them less suitable for deep fascia closure.

Question 34: Correct Answer: B) Duodenum

Rationale: The duodenum, the first part of the small intestine, is primarily responsible for nutrient absorption. The stomach mainly aids in the mechanical and chemical breakdown of food, the colon primarily absorbs water and electrolytes, and the esophagus serves as a conduit for food from the mouth to the stomach. Hence, the duodenum is the correct answer as it plays a crucial role in the absorption of nutrients.

Question 35: Correct Answer: B) Produces new skin cells

Rationale: The stratum basale is the deepest layer of the epidermis and is responsible for producing new skin cells, which is crucial for the healing process. Option A is incorrect because providing a barrier to infection is a function of the entire epidermis. Option C is incorrect as nutrient supply is mainly a function of the dermis. Option D is incorrect because regulating body temperature is a function of sweat glands and blood vessels in the dermis, not the stratum basale.

Question 36: Correct Answer: B) Venous bleeding
Rationale: Dark red blood typically indicates venous bleeding, as venous blood is deoxygenated and appears darker. Arterial bleeding (A) is usually bright red due to high oxygen content. Capillary bleeding (C) is generally slower and less voluminous, and oxygenated blood (D) would also be bright red. Recognizing the color can help in identifying the source and managing the bleeding appropriately.

Question 37: Correct Answer: B) Laparoscope
Rationale: The laparoscope is essential for a laparoscopic cholecystectomy as it allows visualization of the abdominal cavity. A bone saw (A) is used in orthopedic surgeries, a craniotomy set (C) is used for neurosurgical procedures, and a tourniquet (D) is used to control bleeding in extremity surgeries. Ensuring the correct instruments are available is crucial for the success of the procedure and patient safety.

Question 38: Correct Answer: B) Hydroxyapatite
Rationale: Hydroxyapatite is a common material used in synthetic tissue grafts due to its biocompatibility and osteoconductive properties. Collagen (A) is a natural protein, not synthetic. Autogenous bone (C) and allograft tissue (D) are not synthetic materials; they are harvested from the patient or donors, respectively. Therefore, Hydroxyapatite (B) is the correct answer as it is a synthetic material commonly used in grafts.

Question 39: Correct Answer: C) Platelet count
Rationale: Reviewing the platelet count is crucial before surgery to ensure proper coagulation status. Platelets play a key role in blood clotting, and an abnormal count can lead to excessive bleeding or clotting issues during surgery. While hemoglobin level (B) is important for oxygen transport, blood glucose level (A) for metabolic control, and serum creatinine level (D) for kidney function, they do not directly indicate coagulation status.

Question 40: Correct Answer: B) Supervising and providing feedback on the trainee's performance
Rationale: The primary responsibility of a preceptor is to supervise and provide feedback on the trainee's performance. This helps ensure that the trainee develops the necessary skills and knowledge. Option A is incorrect because the preceptor should not perform all tasks themselves. Option C is incorrect as it neglects the importance of oversight. Option D is partially correct but does not encompass the full scope of the preceptor's responsibilities.

Question 41: Correct Answer: D) By holding the needle holder at the handle
Rationale: Holding the needle holder at the handle ensures control and safety when passing it to the surgeon. Holding it at the tip (A) or the hinge (C) can compromise sterility and control. Placing it on the sterile field (B) can cause delays and is not the standard practice for passing instruments.

Question 42: Correct Answer: C) Coordinating with the surgical team for shift coverage
Rationale: A key administrative duty of a surgical technologist related to personnel management is coordinating with the surgical team for shift coverage. This ensures that there is adequate staffing for surgical procedures. Scheduling surgeries (A) is typically the responsibility of the surgical scheduler, ensuring compliance with safety protocols (B) is a broader responsibility, and maintaining patient records (D) is primarily the duty of medical records personnel.

Question 43: Correct Answer: B) Use a barcode scanner to scan each instrument and automatically update the EHR.
Rationale: Using a barcode scanner ensures accurate and immediate documentation of instruments in the EHR, reducing the risk of errors. Manually writing details (A) and updating from memory (D) can lead to inaccuracies. Verbally informing the circulating nurse (C) can result in miscommunication. The barcode scanner method is efficient and minimizes human error.

Question 44: Correct Answer: C) Check the distal pulses and notify the surgeon.
Rationale: Checking the distal pulses and notifying the surgeon is crucial to assess for potential vascular compromise or compartment syndrome. Elevating the leg (A) or applying a warm compress (B) could mask symptoms and delay proper diagnosis. Administering anticoagulants (D) without further assessment could be dangerous if there is a vascular injury.

Question 45: Correct Answer: C) Maintaining fluid balance and immune defense
Rationale: The primary function of the lymphatic system is to maintain fluid balance by returning interstitial fluid to the bloodstream and to provide immune defense by filtering pathogens and presenting them to lymphocytes. Unlike option A, which describes the circulatory system's role, option B which pertains to the bone marrow, and option D which relates to the liver, option C accurately captures the lymphatic system's essential roles.

Question 46: Correct Answer: B) Seal the drapes in a biohazard bag.
Rationale: The first step in disposing of contaminated drapes is to seal them in a biohazard bag to prevent the spread of infectious materials. Placing them in a regular trash bin (Option A) or rinsing with water (Option C) does not contain the contamination. Folding the drapes (Option D) is unnecessary and does not address contamination control.

Question 47: Correct Answer: A) To prevent contamination of sterile fields
Rationale: Securing cords and tubing to the drapes is crucial to prevent contamination of sterile fields. This practice ensures that the sterile environment is maintained throughout the procedure. While options B, C, and D are important considerations, they do not address the primary concern of maintaining a sterile field, which is essential for preventing infections and ensuring patient safety.

Question 48: Correct Answer: B) Adjust the focus on the endoscope
Rationale: The most appropriate first step when the image is blurry is to adjust the focus on the

endoscope. Increasing the brightness of the monitor (Option A) will not correct the blurriness. Replacing the light source (Option C) is unnecessary if the light is functioning. Checking the insufflation pressure (Option D) is irrelevant to image clarity. Adjusting the focus directly addresses the issue of a blurry image.

Question 49: Correct Answer: C) Cystic duct
Rationale: The cystic duct must be carefully identified and preserved during a laparoscopic cholecystectomy to prevent bile leakage and ensure proper removal of the gallbladder. The hepatic artery and portal vein are nearby but not directly involved in this procedure. The common bile duct should also be preserved, but the cystic duct is specifically ligated and cut during the surgery.

Question 50: Correct Answer: B) Use a nail cleaner to clean under the nails.
Rationale: Using a nail cleaner to clean under the nails is essential to remove debris and reduce microbial load, ensuring the effectiveness of the surgical scrub. Option A is incorrect because hot water can irritate the skin. Option C is incorrect as drying should be done after rinsing, not scrubbing. Option D is incorrect because applying lotion can compromise sterility.

Question 51: Correct Answer: A) Checking the expiration dates of sterile supplies
Rationale: Checking the expiration dates of sterile supplies is essential to ensure that all materials used during surgery are safe and effective. While reviewing the patient's medical history (B) and confirming the surgeon's preferences (C) are important preoperative tasks, they do not directly relate to verifying equipment availability. Ensuring proper ventilation (D) is crucial for maintaining a sterile environment but is not part of the equipment verification process.

Question 52: Correct Answer: A) Electrosurgical unit
Rationale: The electrosurgical unit is a nondisposable item that requires special handling during postoperative procedures to prevent damage and ensure its longevity. Unlike surgical drapes, gloves, and sponges, which are disposable, the electrosurgical unit is a reusable piece of equipment. Proper care and handling are essential to maintain its functionality and safety for future surgical procedures.

Question 53: Correct Answer: B) To understand the communication breakdown and improve protocols
Rationale: The focus during the debrief should be to understand the communication breakdown and improve protocols to prevent similar issues in the future. This enhances patient care and teamwork. Option A is incorrect as reprimanding is not productive. Option C is important but not the primary focus of the debrief. Option D is not relevant to the main goal of improving communication and protocols.

Question 54: Correct Answer: D) Shaking the package to hear for loose contents
Rationale: Shaking the package to hear for loose contents is not a reliable method to confirm sterility. Reliable methods include checking the sterilization indicator, inspecting for moisture or dampness, and ensuring the package is properly sealed. Shaking the package does not provide any information about the sterility and could potentially damage the contents, making it an inappropriate method for confirming package integrity.

Question 55: Correct Answer: C) Iris
Rationale: The iris is the part of the eye that controls the diameter and size of the pupil, thereby regulating the amount of light that reaches the retina. The cornea and lens focus light onto the retina, but they do not control light entry. The sclera is the white part of the eye and does not play a role in light regulation. Thus, the iris is the correct answer.

Question 56: Correct Answer: A) Arm Boards
Rationale: Arm boards are essential for positioning the patient's arms securely during a laparoscopic cholecystectomy, preventing nerve damage and ensuring proper positioning. Stirrups are used for gynecological procedures, chest rolls are for prone positions, and a headrest is for head and neck support. Therefore, arm boards are the correct choice for this procedure.

Question 57: Correct Answer: B) Notify the surgeon and anesthesiologist.
Rationale: The first action is to notify the surgeon and anesthesiologist, as they are responsible for diagnosing and managing intraoperative emergencies. Administering epinephrine (A) and increasing IV fluid rate (C) are actions that require medical orders. Chest compressions (D) are only necessary if the patient is in cardiac arrest, which is not indicated by a sudden drop in blood pressure alone.

Question 58: Correct Answer: B) Notify the surgeon immediately.
Rationale: The presence of a firm, swollen area near the incision site may indicate a hematoma, which can lead to complications if not addressed promptly. Notifying the surgeon immediately ensures that the situation is assessed and managed appropriately. Applying a warm compress (A) or administering pain medication (C) may mask symptoms, and encouraging ambulation (D) could exacerbate the condition. Immediate notification is critical for proper intervention.

Question 59: Correct Answer: C) Padding all bony prominences
Rationale: Padding all bony prominences is essential to prevent pressure sores and nerve damage. While placing a pillow under the abdomen (A) and turning the head (B) are important for comfort and airway management, they do not address the primary concern of pressure injury. Securing the arms above the head (D) can lead to brachial plexus injury and is not recommended.

Question 60: Correct Answer: B) Increased intracranial pressure
Rationale: Insufflation of the abdomen with carbon dioxide during laparoscopic procedures can lead to increased intra-abdominal pressure, which in turn can increase intracranial pressure. This is due to the reduced venous return from the brain. Options A) and C) are incorrect as insufflation typically leads to

increased heart and respiratory rates due to hypercapnia. Option D) is incorrect because increased intra-abdominal pressure actually decreases venous return.

Question 61: Correct Answer: C) Medication-induced rash

Rationale: Medication-induced rash is a common postoperative complication, often resulting from antibiotics or other medications administered during or after surgery. Unlike surgical site infection, which would present with localized symptoms, or deep vein thrombosis, which involves swelling and pain in the limbs, a medication-induced rash is more likely to appear on the chest and arms. Allergic reactions to anesthesia typically manifest immediately post-surgery, not two days later.

Question 62: Correct Answer: A) To maintain sterility and prevent contamination

Rationale: Draping the Da Vinci robotic system is crucial to maintain a sterile field and prevent contamination during surgery. This is essential for patient safety and infection control. While protecting the robotic arms (B) and enhancing visibility (C) are important, they are secondary to sterility. Proper calibration (D) is necessary but unrelated to draping.

Question 63: Correct Answer: B) Post the laser warning sign immediately and then proceed.

Rationale: The correct action is to post the laser warning sign immediately and then proceed. This ensures that all personnel are aware of the laser in use, preventing accidental exposure. Continuing the procedure and informing the supervisor later (Option A) or asking the circulating nurse (Option C) could delay the necessary warning. Ignoring the missing sign (Option D) is a breach of safety protocols and could endanger others.

Question 64: Correct Answer: B) Ensuring the ratchet mechanism is functional

Rationale: The primary consideration when assembling self-retaining retractors is ensuring the ratchet mechanism is functional. This ensures that the retractor can hold tissues apart without manual effort. While sterilization (C) is crucial for infection control, and sharp blades (A) and lightweight design (D) may be beneficial, they are not the primary concern for functionality during assembly. The ratchet mechanism's functionality directly impacts the retractor's effectiveness in maintaining exposure.

Question 65: Correct Answer: B) Application of a hemostatic clip

Rationale: The application of a hemostatic clip is most appropriate for controlling bleeding from a small vessel during laparoscopic procedures. Manual pressure with a gauze pad (A) is impractical in a laparoscopic setting. A tourniquet (C) is not suitable for this type of surgery. Topical hemostatic agents (D) are useful but not as effective as clips for direct vessel control.

Question 66: Correct Answer: A) Double-bagging the waste in biohazard bags.

Rationale: Double-bagging contaminated waste in biohazard bags ensures an additional layer of protection against leaks and spills, maintaining compliance with Standard Precautions. Labeling with the patient's name (Option B) is not required and breaches confidentiality. Immediate incineration (Option C) is not always feasible. Transporting in a regular cart (Option D) does not provide adequate containment.

Question 67: Correct Answer: A) Epidermis

Rationale: The epidermis is the outermost layer of the skin and serves as the primary barrier against pathogens and environmental damage. The dermis, hypodermis, and subcutaneous tissue are deeper layers that provide structural support, insulation, and cushioning but do not serve as the primary barrier. The epidermis contains specialized cells like keratinocytes that produce keratin, a protein that reinforces this barrier function.

Question 68: Correct Answer: B) Offer reassurance and notify the attending physician about her symptoms.

Rationale: The correct action is to offer reassurance and notify the attending physician about the patient's symptoms. This ensures that Mrs. Smith's pain and anxiety are managed appropriately by the medical team. Option A is incorrect as surgical technologists are not authorized to administer medication. Option C is inappropriate as it neglects the patient's immediate need for pain relief. Option D, while well-meaning, does not address the underlying issue of severe pain.

Question 69: Correct Answer: B) Following standardized surgical procedures and protocols

Rationale: Following standardized surgical procedures and protocols ensures consistency, reduces waste, and optimizes resource use, contributing to cost containment. Using the most expensive supplies (A) does not guarantee better outcomes and increases costs. Frequently changing suppliers (C) can disrupt supply chains and reduce reliability. Encouraging excessive use of drapes and gowns (D) leads to unnecessary expenses and waste.

Question 70: Correct Answer: B) To reduce the risk of postoperative wound infections

Rationale: The primary purpose of administering preoperative antibiotics is to reduce the risk of postoperative wound infections by eliminating potential pathogens. Treating existing infections (A) is not the primary goal in a preoperative context. Enhancing anesthesia (C) and managing pain (D) are not related to the prophylactic use of antibiotics.

Question 71: Correct Answer: C) Check the integrity of the stapler and ensure it is functioning correctly.

Rationale: The first step is to check the integrity and functionality of the stapler to prevent any malfunctions during surgery. Loading the stapler (A) and handing it directly to the surgeon (B) should only be done after ensuring it is functional. Re-sterilizing the stapler (D) is unnecessary if it has already been sterilized according to protocol.

Question 72: Correct Answer: A) Biceps brachii

Rationale: The biceps brachii is primarily responsible for flexion of the forearm at the elbow. The triceps brachii is responsible for extension of the forearm, the deltoid is involved in shoulder abduction, and the latissimus dorsi is involved in shoulder adduction and extension. Identifying the biceps brachii as the correct muscle ensures proper understanding of muscle functions in surgical procedures.

Question 73: Correct Answer: C) The patient is experiencing hypoxia.

Rationale: Dark and sluggish blood typically indicates hypoxia, where there is a lack of oxygen in the blood. Hypovolemia (A) would result in decreased blood volume, not necessarily dark blood. High oxygen saturation (B) would result in bright red blood. Normal blood pH (D) does not affect the color of the blood in this manner.

Question 74: Correct Answer: B) Remove the drapes slowly and carefully, ensuring all instruments are accounted for

Rationale: The correct procedure is to remove the drapes slowly and carefully to ensure that all instruments are accounted for and to avoid any injury to the patient. Option A is incorrect as pulling the drapes quickly can cause discomfort and potential injury. Option C is incorrect because cutting the drapes can be hazardous and is not standard practice. Option D is incorrect as shaking the drapes can dislodge instruments, posing a risk to the patient and staff.

Question 75: Correct Answer: B) Verifying the surgeon's current preferences with the surgeon directly.

Rationale: Verifying the surgeon's current preferences with the surgeon directly ensures that the preference card reflects the most accurate and up-to-date information. This step is crucial for maintaining efficiency and reducing the risk of errors during surgery. Updating based on trends (A) or adding potentially useful items (C) may not align with the surgeon's specific needs. Removing unused items (D) without confirmation could lead to the omission of necessary tools.

Question 76: Correct Answer: A) To monitor urine output during surgery

Rationale: The main reason for using a Foley catheter during a cystectomy is to monitor urine output during surgery. This helps assess kidney function and fluid balance. Option B is incorrect because anesthesia is not delivered this way, option C is incorrect as Foley catheters do not prevent blood clots, and option D is incorrect because bladder pressure measurement is not the catheter's primary function. Monitoring urine output is crucial for patient safety during the procedure.

Question 77: Correct Answer: B) Confirm the DNR order with the patient and document it in the preoperative checklist.

Rationale: The surgical technologist should confirm the DNR order with the patient and document it in the preoperative checklist. This ensures that all team members are aware of the patient's wishes. Temporarily suspending the DNR order (Option A) or ignoring it (Option C) goes against the patient's rights. Informing the anesthesia team to disregard the DNR

order (Option D) is inappropriate and could lead to ethical and legal issues.

Question 78: Correct Answer: C) The type of tissue being retracted

Rationale: The primary consideration when selecting a retractor is the type of tissue being retracted. This ensures minimal tissue damage and optimal exposure. While the size of the incision (A), the surgeon's preference (B), and the patient's age (D) are important, they are secondary to understanding the tissue characteristics. Using the correct retractor for the tissue type ensures better surgical outcomes and reduces complications.

Question 79: Correct Answer: A) To ensure the surgical team is familiar with the surgeon's preferred instruments and supplies

Rationale: Reviewing the surgeon's preference card is crucial for ensuring that the surgical team is aware of the specific instruments, supplies, and techniques preferred by the surgeon. This preparation helps in minimizing delays and enhancing the efficiency of the procedure. Options B, C, and D, while important, do not directly relate to the primary purpose of the preference card, which is to streamline the intraoperative process by catering to the surgeon's specific needs.

Question 80: Correct Answer: B) To reflect changes in the surgeon's technique or preferences

Rationale: The primary reason for revising a surgeon's preference card is to reflect changes in the surgeon's technique or preferences. This ensures that the surgical team is prepared with the correct instruments and supplies, leading to a more efficient and effective surgery. Options A, C, and D are plausible but incorrect; while they may be secondary benefits, the main focus is on accommodating the surgeon's specific needs and preferences.

Question 81: Correct Answer: B) Verifying the medication label with the surgeon's order

Rationale: Verifying the medication label with the surgeon's order is crucial to ensure the correct medication is administered. While checking the expiration date (A), storing the medication correctly (C), and recording the administration (D) are important, they do not directly prevent the administration of the wrong medication. Verification ensures patient safety by confirming the correct drug, dosage, and route.

Question 82: Correct Answer: C) Dispose of the sharps in a puncture-resistant container.

Rationale: The correct action is to dispose of the sharps in a puncture-resistant container to prevent needlestick injuries and contamination. Placing sharps in a regular trash bin (Option A) poses a risk of injury and contamination. Recapping needles (Option B) is discouraged due to the risk of needlestick injuries. Soaking sharps in disinfectant (Option D) does not eliminate the physical hazard they pose.

Question 83: Correct Answer: C) Appendicitis

Rationale: Appendicitis is the inflammation of the appendix, often requiring surgical removal known as an appendectomy. Cholecystitis is the inflammation of the gallbladder, diverticulitis involves inflammation of the diverticula in the colon, and pancreatitis is the inflammation of the pancreas. Therefore, appendicitis is the correct answer as it specifically involves the appendix and often necessitates surgical intervention.

Question 84: Correct Answer: C) Autoclaving instruments

Rationale: Autoclaving instruments is the most effective method to ensure sterility as it uses high-pressure steam to eliminate all microorganisms. Wiping with alcohol (Option A) and rinsing with sterile water (Option D) do not provide complete sterilization. Soaking in saline solution (Option B) can actually promote corrosion and does not sterilize the instruments. Therefore, autoclaving is the gold standard for sterilizing surgical instruments.

Question 85: Correct Answer: B) Cystic duct

Rationale: The cystic duct must be correctly identified and clipped to safely remove the gallbladder during a laparoscopic cholecystectomy. The common hepatic duct (A) and common bile duct (C) are major bile ducts that should not be clipped. The right hepatic duct (D) drains bile from the right lobe of the liver and is not involved in gallbladder removal. Misidentifying these structures can lead to severe complications.

Question 86: Correct Answer: B) Diaphragm

Rationale: The diaphragm is the primary muscle responsible for inspiration, contracting to create a vacuum that allows air to enter the lungs. Intercostal muscles assist in respiration but are secondary to the diaphragm. The pectoralis major and latissimus dorsi are involved in movements of the upper limb and trunk but do not play a primary role in respiration. Therefore, the correct answer is B) Diaphragm.

Question 87: Correct Answer: B) Mayo scissors

Rationale: Mayo scissors are specifically designed for cutting through tougher tissues and materials, making them ideal for safely removing drapes without causing damage to the surgical site. Metzenbaum scissors are too delicate for this task, hemostats are used for clamping blood vessels, and Adson forceps are used for grasping tissue, not cutting. Mayo scissors provide the necessary strength and precision needed for this postoperative procedure.

Question 88: Correct Answer: B) Use a smoke evacuator to remove the smoke from the surgical site.

Rationale: The correct action is to use a smoke evacuator to remove the smoke from the surgical site. This ensures the safety of both the patient and the surgical team by preventing inhalation of potentially harmful particles. Increasing the laser power (Option A) could exacerbate the issue, applying saline (Option C) is not a standard response to smoke, and ignoring the smoke (Option D) is unsafe and unprofessional.

Question 89: Correct Answer: A) Drape the C-arm with a sterile cover before positioning it over the patient.

Rationale: Draping the C-arm with a sterile cover before positioning it over the patient ensures the equipment does not contaminate the sterile field. Option B risks contamination during positioning. Option C is insufficient as it does not fully protect the sterile field. Option D fails to maintain sterility of the equipment, which is essential for preventing infection.

Question 90: Correct Answer: C) Electronic Health Records (EHR)

Rationale: Electronic Health Records (EHR) ensure accurate and consistent communication by providing a centralized, real-time, and accessible platform for patient information. Unlike verbal communication (A) and written notes (B), which are prone to errors and misinterpretation, EHRs maintain a detailed and permanent record. Informal meetings (D) lack the structured documentation necessary for reliable communication. Therefore, EHRs are the most effective method for ensuring accurate interdepartmental communication.

Question 91: Correct Answer: C) Isopropyl alcohol

Rationale: Isopropyl alcohol is a key component in waterless surgical scrubs due to its rapid and effective antimicrobial properties. Chlorhexidine gluconate (A) is used in traditional scrubs but not typically in waterless formulations. Hydrogen peroxide (B) and sodium hypochlorite (D) are not commonly used in waterless surgical scrubs due to their potential for irritation and less rapid action compared to isopropyl alcohol.

Question 92: Correct Answer: D) Mask, goggles, gown, gloves

Rationale: The correct sequence for donning PPE is mask first, followed by goggles, then the gown, and finally gloves. This order ensures that the most critical areas (face and eyes) are protected first, minimizing contamination risk. Options A and C incorrectly place the gown before the mask and goggles, which could lead to contamination. Option B correctly starts with the mask but incorrectly sequences the gown before the goggles.

Question 93: Correct Answer: B) Speak up immediately and suggest a review of each team member's responsibilities.

Rationale: Speaking up immediately and suggesting a review ensures that everyone is clear on their roles before the procedure begins, promoting effective group dynamics. Waiting (A) or assuming (C) could lead to confusion and errors, while discussing privately (D) might not address the immediate need for clarity. This proactive approach fosters better communication and teamwork.

Question 94: Correct Answer: D) Evaluating the patient's airway and potential for difficult intubation

Rationale: Evaluating the patient's airway and potential for difficult intubation is crucial due to the increased risk of airway management issues in bariatric patients. While understanding the procedure, nutritional status, and psychological readiness are important, they do not directly address the immediate perioperative risk of airway complications. This assessment helps prevent serious intraoperative issues and ensures patient safety.

Question 95: Correct Answer: C) A cloth soaked in a hospital-approved disinfectant.

Rationale: Using a cloth soaked in a hospital-approved disinfectant ensures that all surfaces are properly disinfected, reducing the risk of infection. A dry cloth (Option A) only removes dust but does not disinfect. Sterile water (Option B) and saline solution (Option D) do not contain disinfecting agents, making them ineffective for proper disinfection.

Question 96: Correct Answer: C) Tachycardia
Rationale: During significant blood loss, the body compensates by increasing the heart rate (tachycardia) to maintain cardiac output and blood pressure. Option A) is incorrect as urine output typically decreases to conserve fluid. Option B) is incorrect because vasodilation would lower blood pressure further. Option D) is incorrect because decreased cardiac output would not help in maintaining blood pressure; it would worsen the hypotension.

Question 97: Correct Answer: D) Disconnect the cautery device from the power source and place it in a designated safe area.
Rationale: The correct procedure is to disconnect the cautery device from the power source and place it in a designated safe area to prevent any accidental burns or electrical hazards. Option A is incorrect as wrapping it in a sterile drape does not address the power source. Option B is partially correct but does not include disconnection. Option C is irrelevant to safety. Disconnecting and safely storing the device is essential for postoperative safety.

Question 98: Correct Answer: C) Padding bony prominences to prevent pressure sores.
Rationale: Padding bony prominences is essential to prevent pressure sores and ensure patient comfort. Option A is incorrect because the wrist should be in a functional position, not full extension. Option B is incorrect as the splint should extend beyond the fracture site to immobilize the joint above and below. Option D is incorrect as some splint materials are not rigid immediately and need time to set.

Question 99: Correct Answer: C) Open cholecystectomy set
Rationale: The open cholecystectomy set should be prioritized because it is essential for converting to an open procedure if complications arise during the laparoscopic cholecystectomy. The C-arm fluoroscope and harmonic scalpel are useful but not critical for this specific scenario. The cryotherapy unit is unrelated to the procedure. The open cholecystectomy set ensures readiness for a safe and effective conversion if needed.

Question 100: Correct Answer: C) Decreased urine output
Rationale: Decreased urine output is a critical sign of significant intraoperative blood loss, indicating reduced renal perfusion due to hypovolemia. Increased blood pressure (A) and decreased heart rate (B) are not typical responses to blood loss; rather, blood pressure usually drops, and heart rate increases. Elevated body temperature (D) is not directly related to blood loss. Monitoring urine output helps in assessing the patient's volume status and guiding fluid resuscitation.

Question 101: Correct Answer: A) It provides a real-time, dynamic view of the biliary anatomy.
Rationale: The primary advantage of using intraoperative ultrasound during a laparoscopic cholecystectomy is that it provides a real-time, dynamic view of the biliary anatomy, which helps in accurately identifying structures such as the common bile duct. While options B and C are partially correct, they do not address the primary advantage. Option D is incorrect because the use of ultrasound may not necessarily reduce the overall time of the surgery.

Question 102: Correct Answer: B) It enhances the surgeon's ability to visualize soft tissue structures in real-time.
Rationale: Intraoperative ultrasound technology provides real-time imaging, which significantly enhances the surgeon's ability to visualize soft tissue structures during surgery. This advantage is crucial for precise surgical interventions. While reducing postoperative imaging (A), decreasing surgery duration (C), and eliminating other imaging modalities (D) are potential benefits, they are not the primary advantages. Real-time visualization is the most critical feature that directly impacts surgical accuracy and outcomes.

Question 103: Correct Answer: B) Diaphragm
Rationale: The diaphragm is the primary muscle responsible for inhalation. When it contracts, it flattens and increases the thoracic cavity's volume, allowing air to be drawn into the lungs. While intercostal muscles assist in expanding the chest cavity, they are secondary to the diaphragm. Abdominal muscles are more involved in forced exhalation, and the pectoralis major primarily functions in arm movement. Thus, the diaphragm is the correct answer due to its primary role in inhalation.

Question 104: Correct Answer: C) Muscle rigidity
Rationale: Muscle rigidity is a hallmark sign of malignant hyperthermia, a life-threatening condition triggered by certain anesthetic agents. It is often accompanied by a rapid increase in body temperature, tachycardia, and hypercapnia. Bradycardia, hypotension, and hypothermia are not typically associated with malignant hyperthermia and may result from other intraoperative complications. Recognizing muscle rigidity promptly allows for immediate treatment with dantrolene and supportive measures, improving patient outcomes.

Question 105: Correct Answer: B) Allowing the child to bring a favorite toy or blanket
Rationale: Allowing the child to bring a favorite toy or blanket helps comfort and reduce anxiety. Sedatives (A) are not the first line of management and may not be suitable for all children. Isolation (C) can increase anxiety, and discussing detailed surgical risks (D) can overwhelm and frighten the child. A familiar object provides emotional security and eases the preoperative experience.

Question 106: Correct Answer: A) Immediately inform the surgeon and wait for further instructions.
Rationale: Informing the surgeon and waiting for further instructions ensures that any adjustments are made safely and effectively, maintaining the integrity

of the surgical field. Option B is incorrect as repositioning without informing the surgeon can disrupt the procedure. Option C is incorrect as replacing the retractor may not be necessary. Option D is incorrect because tightening without informing the surgeon can cause unintended tissue damage.

Question 107: Correct Answer: D) Verify the count of nondisposable items with the circulating nurse.

Rationale: Verifying the count of nondisposable items with the circulating nurse ensures that all items are accounted for and none are left inside the patient or misplaced. Counting instruments before removing drapes (A) is important but not the final verification step. Placing items in a single bin (B) is not best practice due to potential damage. Documenting use (C) is important but secondary to verifying counts.

Question 108: Correct Answer: B) Inform the surgeon immediately and assist in changing the glove.

Rationale: The correct action is to inform the surgeon immediately and assist in changing the glove to maintain aseptic technique. Ignoring the tear (Option A) or covering it with a sterile adhesive bandage (Option C) does not ensure sterility. Asking the circulating nurse (Option D) delays the immediate action needed. Promptly changing the glove prevents contamination and maintains the sterile field.

Question 109: Correct Answer: B) Address the conflict immediately in a calm and respectful manner

Rationale: Addressing the conflict immediately in a calm and respectful manner ensures that the issue does not escalate and disrupt the procedure. Ignoring the conflict (Option A) or allowing team members to resolve it on their own (Option D) can lead to further tension. Reporting the conflict after the procedure (Option C) does not provide an immediate solution, which is crucial in a surgical setting.

Question 110: Correct Answer: B) Serum creatinine level

Rationale: Serum creatinine level is essential to evaluate renal function before surgery, as impaired kidney function can affect the metabolism and excretion of anesthetic agents, leading to potential complications. While white blood cell count (A) can indicate infection, hematocrit level (C) reflects blood volume and oxygen-carrying capacity, and prothrombin time (D) assesses clotting ability, they do not specifically evaluate renal function.

Question 111: Correct Answer: C) Use the hospital's EHR system to access the records directly.

Rationale: Using the hospital's EHR system to access the records directly is the most efficient and immediate method, ensuring that Alex has the necessary information without delay. Calling or emailing the medical records department (Options A and B) may cause unnecessary delays, and waiting until the end of the procedure (Option D) could compromise patient care. Direct access through the EHR system facilitates timely and accurate interdepartmental communication. ---

Question 112: Correct Answer: B) Use of electrocautery

Rationale: Electrocautery is most appropriate for achieving hemostasis in highly vascular areas as it uses electrical current to coagulate blood vessels, providing immediate and effective control of bleeding. A tourniquet (A) is used for limb surgeries to control blood flow, a pressure dressing (C) is more suitable for postoperative care, and hemostatic agents (D) are adjuncts rather than primary methods.

Question 113: Correct Answer: B) Clean the wound site with sterile saline solution.

Rationale: The first step in preparing a wound site for dressing application is to clean the wound with a sterile saline solution. This helps to remove any debris and reduce the risk of infection. Option A is incorrect as applying a dressing without cleaning can lead to infection. Option C is incorrect because non-sterile gauze can introduce contaminants. Option D is incorrect because cleaning should precede any application of ointments to ensure the wound is free from contaminants.

Question 114: Correct Answer: A) Iliac crest

Rationale: The iliac crest is a reliable landmark for locating the L4 vertebra, as it is generally at the level of the L4-L5 intervertebral disc. The sacral promontory is too inferior, the spinous process of T12 is too superior, and the inferior angle of the scapula is unrelated to lumbar vertebrae. Accurate identification of the L4 vertebra is essential for precise instrumentation in spinal fusion procedures.

Question 115: Correct Answer: B) Verifying the patient's anatomical landmarks after draping

Rationale: Verifying the patient's anatomical landmarks after draping is crucial for accurate data input into the computer navigation system. This step ensures that the system's data aligns correctly with the patient's anatomy, which is essential for precise surgical guidance. While calibrating the system (A) and ensuring sterile instruments (D) are important, they do not directly impact the accuracy of the navigation data. Entering demographic data (C) is necessary but not as critical as verifying anatomical landmarks for surgical precision.

Question 116: Correct Answer: B) Use a flash sterilizer with a cycle of 3 minutes at 270°F.

Rationale: Flash sterilization, also known as immediate-use steam sterilization, is the most appropriate method for sterilizing instruments quickly. Option A is incorrect because alcohol is not a reliable sterilant for surgical instruments. Option C is incorrect as rinsing with sterile saline does not sterilize the instrument. Option D is incorrect because chemical sterilants require longer exposure times and are not suitable for immediate use.

Question 117: Correct Answer: C) Placing in an enzymatic cleaner

Rationale: Placing surgical instruments in an enzymatic cleaner immediately after use is the most effective method for decontamination. Enzymatic cleaners break down organic material such as blood and tissue, which helps prevent the formation of biofilms. Soaking in saline solution (A) and rinsing with tap water (B) are not effective in breaking down organic material, and wiping with a sterile cloth (D) does not adequately remove contaminants.

Question 118: Correct Answer: B) Transport John on a stretcher with side rails up and ensure he is covered with a blanket.

Rationale: Transporting John on a stretcher with side rails up and ensuring he is covered with a blanket ensures his safety and comfort. Allowing him to walk (Option A) or sit in a wheelchair (Option C) increases the risk of falls or injury. Asking him to wait (Option D) is not appropriate as it delays the surgical schedule and does not address the need for safe transport.

Question 119: Correct Answer: A) To enhance visualization by creating a pneumoperitoneum

Rationale: Insufflation during laparoscopic surgery involves introducing gas (usually CO_2) into the abdominal cavity to create a pneumoperitoneum. This lifts the abdominal wall away from the internal organs, enhancing visualization and providing space for surgical instruments. Sterilizing instruments (B) and providing oxygen to the patient (C) are unrelated to insufflation, while reducing infection risk (D) is not a direct function of insufflation.

Question 120: Correct Answer: B) It uses ultrasonic vibrations to cut and coagulate tissue simultaneously.

Rationale: The harmonic scalpel uses ultrasonic vibrations to cut and coagulate tissue at the same time, which minimizes bleeding and reduces the need for additional hemostatic measures. Option A is incorrect because the harmonic scalpel is typically effective on vessels up to 5mm, not 7mm. Option C, while partially correct, is not the primary advantage. Option D is incorrect as the harmonic scalpel is generally more expensive than traditional electrosurgical devices.

Question 121: Correct Answer: C) Sudden onset of severe pain unrelieved by medication

Rationale: Sudden onset of severe pain unrelieved by medication is an abnormal postoperative finding that could indicate complications such as infection, hemorrhage, or deep vein thrombosis, and should be reported immediately. Slight redness, small amounts of serous drainage, and mild swelling are common and generally expected postoperative findings. These do not typically indicate serious complications unless they worsen significantly.

Question 122: Correct Answer: B) Thrombin

Rationale: Thrombin is a potent hemostatic agent that directly converts fibrinogen to fibrin, promoting clot formation. Epinephrine is primarily used for vasoconstriction, Lidocaine is an anesthetic, and Heparin is an anticoagulant. Therefore, Thrombin is the most effective chemical agent for achieving hemostasis during surgery.

Question 123: Correct Answer: D) The patient's understanding of the surgeon's credentials

Rationale: Informed consent requires the patient's understanding of the procedure, voluntary agreement, and signature on the consent form. The surgeon's credentials are not a necessary component of informed consent. While knowing the surgeon's qualifications may reassure the patient, it is not required for the legal and ethical process of informed consent.

Question 124: Correct Answer: A) Notify the surgeon immediately.

Rationale: Notifying the surgeon immediately is crucial for a rapidly expanding hematoma, as it may indicate a serious underlying issue requiring surgical intervention. Increasing IV fluids (B) does not address the source of bleeding. Warm compresses (C) could exacerbate bleeding. Repositioning the patient (D) does not address the hematoma. Prompt communication with the surgeon ensures timely management and intervention.

Question 125: Correct Answer: C) Deltoid

Rationale: The deltoid muscle is primarily responsible for the abduction of the arm at the shoulder joint. The biceps brachii flexes the elbow, the trapezius elevates and rotates the scapula, and the latissimus dorsi extends and adducts the arm. Therefore, only the deltoid muscle is involved in arm abduction, making it the correct choice.

Question 126: Correct Answer: B) Double-check the implant type with the surgical team during the time-out procedure.

Rationale: The best practice is to double-check the implant type with the surgical team during the time-out procedure. This ensures that everyone is in agreement and reduces the risk of errors. Option A is incorrect as the preoperative plan may change. Option C is incorrect because weight and height alone are not sufficient criteria. Option D is incorrect because the most commonly used screws may not be appropriate for every patient.

Question 127: Correct Answer: B) Place the specimen in a sterile container without any preservative and label it with the patient's name, date of birth, and "Frozen Section."

Rationale: For a frozen section, the specimen should be placed in a sterile container without any preservative to avoid altering the tissue. Labeling must include the patient's name, date of birth, and the specific instruction "Frozen Section." Incorrect options either involve preservatives (A, D) or lack the necessary labeling (C), which could compromise the diagnostic process.

Question 128: Correct Answer: B) Open the first flap of the sterile package away from the body.

Rationale: Alex should open the first flap of the sterile package away from the body to prevent contamination from the body or clothing. Option A is incorrect because opening towards the body can cause contamination. Option C is incorrect as touching the inside of the sterile package with bare hands compromises sterility. Option D is incorrect because placing the sterile package on a non-sterile surface before opening can lead to contamination.

Question 129: Correct Answer: B) Double-bag the contaminated materials in biohazard bags and seal them.

Rationale: Double-bagging and sealing contaminated materials in biohazard bags ensures that infectious materials are contained and handled according to Standard Precautions, minimizing the risk of exposure. Option A is incorrect as regular trash bins do not provide the necessary containment. Option C is incorrect because rinsing contaminated drapes can spread pathogens. Option D is incorrect as sharps containers are specifically for sharp objects, not general contaminated waste.

Question 130: Correct Answer: A) Verify the allograft's expiration date.

Rationale: Verifying the allograft's expiration date is essential to ensure its viability and safety for use in surgery. Immersing in iodine solution (B) is not standard practice and can damage the tissue. Cutting the allograft immediately after removal from the freezer (C) can lead to structural damage. Storing in a dry environment (D) is incorrect as it should be kept in a controlled, sterile environment.

Question 131: Correct Answer: B) Check the circuit breaker and reset it if necessary.

Rationale: The most appropriate next step is to check the circuit breaker and reset it if necessary, as it may have tripped due to an overload or fault. Replacing the grounding pad (Option A) is unnecessary if it is already properly placed. Increasing the power setting (Option C) could be dangerous without addressing the root cause. Using a different outlet (Option D) might not solve the underlying electrical issue and could pose additional risks.

Question 132: Correct Answer: A) To create an anastomosis

Rationale: Linear staplers are primarily used to create anastomoses in gastrointestinal surgery, ensuring a secure and consistent connection between two sections of the bowel. While ligating blood vessels (B), closing skin incisions (C), and performing tissue biopsies (D) are important surgical tasks, they are not the primary functions of a linear stapler. Linear staplers provide a quick and reliable method for joining tissues, which is crucial in gastrointestinal procedures.

Question 133: Correct Answer: C) To enhance the contrast of tissues

Rationale: Adjusting the color temperature of surgical lights enhances the contrast of tissues, making it easier for surgeons to differentiate between various anatomical structures. Matching ambient lighting (A) and conserving energy (D) are not primary concerns in the operating room. While reducing eye strain (B) is important, it is a secondary benefit compared to the critical need for improved tissue contrast.

Question 134: Correct Answer: C) Assigning unique identification numbers to each patient

Rationale: Assigning unique identification numbers to each patient is the best practice for maintaining confidentiality. This method prevents unauthorized access to personal information. Using patient names (Option A) and discussing details with colleagues (Option D) can breach confidentiality. Storing data on a shared network drive (Option B) may expose sensitive information to unauthorized users.

Question 135: Correct Answer: B) To assist in patient triage and transportation

Rationale: The primary role of a CST during a hospital-wide disaster drill is to assist in patient triage and transportation. This ensures that patients are quickly and efficiently moved to appropriate care areas. Options A, C, and D are incorrect because CSTs do not perform surgeries independently, manage hospital communications, or oversee the entire disaster response plan. Their role is more focused on supporting surgical and patient care activities during emergencies.

Question 136: Correct Answer: B) To reduce the x-ray beam size and limit exposure

Rationale: The primary reason for using a collimator is to reduce the x-ray beam size and limit exposure. Enhancing image clarity (A) and increasing radiation dose (C) are not the main purposes of a collimator. Stabilizing the x-ray machine (D) is unrelated to the function of a collimator. By limiting the beam size, collimators help protect both the patient and surgical team from unnecessary radiation exposure.

Question 137: Correct Answer: C) Arterial bleeding

Rationale: Bright red, pulsatile bleeding is characteristic of arterial bleeding due to the high oxygen content and pressure in arteries. Venous bleeding (A) is darker and not pulsatile. Capillary bleeding (B) is slow and oozing, and lymphatic fluid (D) is typically clear or slightly yellow. Recognizing these characteristics is crucial for appropriate intraoperative management.

Question 138: Correct Answer: C) Acknowledge the patient's feelings and notify the surgical team.

Rationale: The correct response is to acknowledge the patient's feelings and notify the surgical team. This approach ensures the patient's emotional needs are addressed and allows the surgical team to provide appropriate support. Reassuring the patient (A) may seem comforting but does not address underlying concerns. Ignoring the comment (B) is inappropriate and neglects the patient's emotional state. Telling the patient that fear is normal (D) is dismissive and does not provide a solution.

Question 139: Correct Answer: B) Use a sterile adhesive drape to secure the tubing to the drapes.

Rationale: Using a sterile adhesive drape to secure the tubing to the drapes maintains the sterile field and prevents contamination. Taping the tubing to the patient's skin (A) risks compromising sterility. Allowing the tubing to hang freely (C) increases the risk of contamination and tripping hazards. Placing the tubing on the instrument tray (D) can clutter the tray and is not a secure method.

Question 140: Correct Answer: C) Distended abdomen

Rationale: A distended abdomen is a key sign of internal bleeding, indicating that blood may be accumulating in the abdominal cavity. Elevated blood pressure (A) and increased urine output (D) are not typical signs of internal bleeding. Decreased heart rate (B) is less common and not as directly indicative of internal bleeding as a distended abdomen. Recognizing this sign promptly can lead to quicker intervention and improved patient outcomes.

Question 141: Correct Answer: C) Remove the

drapes from the patient

Rationale: The first action should be to remove the burning drapes from the patient to prevent injury. While calling for help (A) and using a fire extinguisher (B) are important, they are secondary to ensuring the patient's immediate safety. Turning off the oxygen supply (D) is also crucial but should follow the removal of the burning material to prevent further harm.

Question 142: Correct Answer: C) To prevent deep vein thrombosis (DVT)

Rationale: The primary purpose of applying sequential compression devices (SCDs) is to prevent deep vein thrombosis (DVT) by promoting blood circulation in the lower extremities. This is crucial in surgical patients who are at increased risk of blood clots due to prolonged immobility. Options A, B, and D are incorrect because SCDs are not primarily used for preventing infections, enhancing wound healing, or reducing postoperative pain, though improved circulation can have secondary benefits.

Question 143: Correct Answer: B) Inform the anesthesiologist immediately.

Rationale: A sudden drop in blood pressure is a critical event that requires immediate attention from the anesthesiologist to assess and manage the cause. Increasing IV fluids (Option A) or adjusting the patient's position (Option C) may be necessary but only after consulting the anesthesiologist. Checking the surgical site (Option D) is important but secondary to informing the anesthesiologist.

Question 144: Correct Answer: C) Metzenbaum Scissors

Rationale: Metzenbaum Scissors are primarily used for cutting delicate tissue during surgery. Mayo Scissors are used for cutting heavier tissues, Allis Forceps are used for grasping and holding tissues, and Babcock Forceps are used for grasping delicate tissues without causing trauma. Metzenbaum Scissors have a longer handle-to-blade ratio, making them ideal for precise cutting of delicate tissues, which is not the intended use of the other instruments listed.

Question 145: Correct Answer: A) To drain bile and prevent bile leakage

Rationale: The primary purpose of a T-tube in a laparoscopic cholecystectomy is to drain bile and prevent bile leakage. Unlike option B, which is incorrect because irrigation is not the T-tube's function, option C is incorrect because medications are not administered this way, and option D is incorrect because it does not measure intra-abdominal pressure. The T-tube ensures proper bile drainage post-surgery, preventing complications.

Question 146: Correct Answer: B) Selecting the appropriate cuff size based on the limb circumference

Rationale: Selecting the appropriate cuff size based on the limb circumference is crucial to ensure effective and safe use of a pneumatic tourniquet. Option A is incorrect as the tourniquet should be applied proximal to the surgical site, not directly over it. Option C is incorrect because the pressure should be individualized, not maximized. Option D is incorrect as prolonged application without breaks can lead to tissue damage and other complications.

Question 147: Correct Answer: C) Linear array ultrasound

Rationale: Linear array ultrasound is ideal for visualizing superficial structures, such as veins, and is commonly used to confirm central venous catheter placement. TEE (A) is used for cardiac imaging, Doppler ultrasound (B) measures blood flow but is not specific for catheter placement, and curvilinear array ultrasound (D) is used for deeper structures, making them less suitable for this task.

Question 148: Correct Answer: B) Cochlea

Rationale: The cochlea is the spiral-shaped organ in the inner ear that contains hair cells. These hair cells convert sound waves into electrical signals, which are then transmitted to the brain via the auditory nerve. The tympanic membrane (A) vibrates in response to sound waves but does not convert them into electrical signals. The Eustachian tube (C) equalizes pressure in the middle ear, and the semicircular canals (D) are involved in balance, not hearing.

Question 149: Correct Answer: B) Use a draw sheet to assist in moving the patient.

Rationale: Using a draw sheet to assist in moving the patient is essential to ensure a smooth and safe transfer. It helps distribute the patient's weight evenly and reduces the risk of injury to both the patient and the staff. Option A is incorrect because the stretcher should be at the same height or slightly lower, but this alone does not ensure safety. Option C is incorrect as the patient should not assist due to the risk of injury. Option D is incorrect because monitoring equipment should only be disconnected when absolutely necessary and after ensuring the patient is stable.

Question 150: Correct Answer: A) Use latex-free gloves and equipment throughout the procedure.

Rationale: The correct action is to use latex-free gloves and equipment throughout the procedure to prevent an allergic reaction. Administering an antihistamine (Option B) is not a preventive measure for latex allergy. Scheduling in a latex-free operating room (Option C) is ideal but not always feasible. Informing the team (Option D) is important but insufficient without using latex-free equipment.

CST Exam Practice Questions [SET 2]

Question 1: Which of the following is the most appropriate method for verifying patient identity before surgery?
A) Asking the patient to state their name and date of birth
B) Checking the patient's wristband only
C) Confirming the patient's identity with a family member
D) Reviewing the patient's chart without patient interaction

Question 2: What is the primary purpose of performing a preoperative skin antisepsis?
A) To moisturize the skin
B) To reduce the risk of surgical site infections
C) To enhance the absorption of anesthesia
D) To identify any skin allergies

Question 3: During the preoperative preparation for a surgical procedure, the surgical team decides to use a waterless hand antiseptic. Which of the following steps is crucial when using a waterless hand antiseptic to ensure proper hand hygiene?
A) Apply the antiseptic to dry hands and rub until dry.
B) Rinse hands with water before applying the antiseptic.
C) Apply the antiseptic and rinse with water after 30 seconds.
D) Apply the antiseptic to wet hands and rub until dry.

Question 4: Sarah, a surgical technologist, is preparing for a total knee arthroplasty. The surgeon mentions the possibility of using computer-assisted navigation. What additional equipment should Sarah ensure is available?
A) Tourniquet system
B) Computer navigation system
C) Arthroscopy tower
D) Electrocautery unit

Question 5: Emily, a 45-year-old patient, is undergoing spinal fusion surgery. The surgeon decides to use a synthetic tissue graft. What is a key consideration when using synthetic tissue grafts in this type of procedure?
A) Ensuring the graft is radiopaque for imaging purposes
B) Matching the graft's mechanical properties to the host tissue
C) Selecting a graft that promotes rapid vascularization
D) Choosing a graft with antibacterial properties

Question 6: During a laparoscopic cholecystectomy on a patient named Mr. Smith, the surgeon requests an instrument to grasp and manipulate the gallbladder. Which instrument should the surgical technologist provide?
A) Metzenbaum scissors
B) Kocher clamp
C) Maryland dissector
D) Babcock forceps

Question 7: During a spinal fusion surgery, the surgical technologist is asked to prepare an autograft bone for implantation. What is the first step the technologist should take to ensure the graft is viable?
A) Soak the bone graft in saline solution.
B) Pass the bone graft directly to the surgeon.
C) Irrigate the bone graft with antibiotic solution.
D) Ensure the bone graft is kept moist with a sterile sponge.

Question 8: In the context of administrative duties, which task is a surgical technologist least likely to perform?
A) Scheduling surgeries
B) Sterilizing surgical instruments
C) Maintaining patient records
D) Ordering surgical supplies

Question 9: During a surgical procedure, the surgical technologist notices that the sponge count is incorrect. What is the most appropriate immediate action?
A) Continue with the procedure and inform the surgeon at the end.
B) Stop the procedure and perform an immediate recount.
C) Ignore the discrepancy and assume it is a counting error.
D) Inform the circulating nurse and surgeon immediately.

Question 10: Which of the following practices is most effective in ensuring cost containment in the surgical setting?
A) Reusing single-use items whenever possible
B) Implementing a just-in-time inventory system
C) Stockpiling supplies to avoid shortages
D) Allowing surgeons to use any preferred brand of surgical instruments

Question 11: After completing a cholecystectomy on Mr. Smith, the surgical technologist is responsible for removing the drapes and other equipment. During this process, what is the correct procedure for handling the suction tubing?
A) Leave the suction tubing attached to the suction canister.
B) Disconnect the suction tubing and discard it immediately.
C) Disconnect the suction tubing, cap the ends, and dispose of it in a biohazard bag.
D) Disconnect the suction tubing and place it on the

sterile field.

Question 12: What is the primary function of the cerebellum in the human brain?
A) Regulation of emotions
B) Coordination of voluntary movements
C) Production of cerebrospinal fluid
D) Processing of visual information

Question 13: During a surgical procedure, the autoclave used for sterilizing instruments malfunctions. As a Certified Surgical Technologist, what is the most appropriate immediate action to ensure patient safety?
A) Continue using the instruments that were previously sterilized.
B) Manually clean the instruments with antiseptic solution.
C) Use a backup autoclave to re-sterilize the instruments.
D) Delay the surgery until the autoclave is repaired.

Question 14: What is the correct sequence for gowning and gloving a sterile team member?
A) Don gloves first, then gown
B) Don gown first, then gloves
C) Don mask first, then gown, then gloves
D) Don cap first, then gloves, then gown

Question 15: During the preoperative assessment of Mr. Smith, a 65-year-old patient scheduled for a total hip replacement, the surgical technologist notices that Mr. Smith has not removed his hearing aids. What is the most appropriate action for the surgical technologist to take?
A) Allow Mr. Smith to keep his hearing aids in place for the surgery.
B) Remove the hearing aids and place them in a labeled container for safekeeping.
C) Inform the anesthesiologist and proceed with the surgery.
D) Ask Mr. Smith to remove his hearing aids and give them to a family member.

Question 16: Which type of malignancy is characterized by the presence of Reed-Sternberg cells?
A) Non-Hodgkin lymphoma
B) Hodgkin lymphoma
C) Multiple myeloma
D) Acute myeloid leukemia

Question 17: Which of the following is the most appropriate method for removing excess blood from the operative site during surgery?
A) Using a sterile gauze pad
B) Applying a tourniquet
C) Utilizing a suction device
D) Allowing natural coagulation

Question 18: During a laparoscopic cholecystectomy, the surgeon asks the surgical technologist to identify the structure labeled "CBD" on the imaging screen. What does "CBD" stand for in this context?
A) Common Bile Duct
B) Cystic Bile Duct
C) Common Biliary Drain
D) Cystic Biliary Duct

Question 19: During a laparoscopic cholecystectomy on a 45-year-old patient named Mr. Smith, the surgeon accidentally punctures the cystic artery, leading to significant bleeding. What is the most appropriate action for the surgical technologist to take in this emergency?
A) Apply direct pressure to the bleeding site immediately.
B) Increase the insufflation pressure to reduce bleeding.
C) Hand the surgeon a hemostatic clamp and prepare suction.
D) Convert to an open procedure to control the bleeding.

Question 20: In a case where Mrs. Smith is undergoing an arteriovenous (AV) fistula creation for hemodialysis, which vessel is typically connected to the cephalic vein?
A) Brachial artery
B) Radial artery
C) Ulnar artery
D) Subclavian artery

Question 21: Which bone is primarily responsible for the formation of the elbow joint along with the humerus and the radius?
A) Scapula
B) Ulna
C) Clavicle
D) Femur

Question 22: Which hormone is primarily responsible for the regulation of the menstrual cycle in females?
A) Testosterone
B) Estrogen
C) Insulin
D) Cortisol

Question 23: What is the primary purpose of using cautery in postoperative procedures during the removal of drapes and other equipment from the patient?
A) To reduce the risk of infection
B) To ensure complete hemostasis
C) To minimize tissue adhesion
D) To enhance wound healing

Question 24: During the transfer of a patient from the operating table to the stretcher, what is the primary role of the Certified Surgical Technologist?
A) Direct the anesthesia provider to manage the

patient's airway.
B) Coordinate the movement by counting aloud and guiding the team.
C) Hold the patient's head and neck to prevent injury.
D) Ensure all surgical instruments are accounted for.

Question 25: During a surgical procedure, Dr. Smith and Nurse Johnson have a disagreement about the correct instrument to use. As a Certified Surgical Technologist, how should you handle this situation to maintain a professional and efficient operating room environment?
A) Ignore the disagreement and continue with your tasks.
B) Side with Dr. Smith since he is the lead surgeon.
C) Suggest a brief pause to discuss the issue and reach a consensus.
D) Report the disagreement to the hospital administration immediately.

Question 26: Sarah, a surgical technologist, is preparing the Da Vinci system for a complex robotic-assisted hysterectomy. Which of the following steps is crucial for ensuring the robotic instruments are correctly draped?
A) Ensuring the robotic instruments are sterilized before the procedure.
B) Draping the robotic instruments after they are attached to the robotic arms.
C) Draping the robotic instruments before they are attached to the robotic arms.
D) Ensuring the robotic instruments are draped simultaneously with the robotic arms.

Question 27: What is the primary function of the sinoatrial (SA) node in the heart?
A) To pump blood to the lungs
B) To act as the heart's natural pacemaker
C) To receive deoxygenated blood from the body
D) To prevent backflow of blood into the atria

Question 28: During a surgical procedure, a fire breaks out in the operating room. What is the first action that the surgical technologist should take to ensure the safety of the patient and staff?
A) Call for help and alert the fire department.
B) Use a fire extinguisher to put out the fire.
C) Remove the patient from the immediate danger area.
D) Turn off all electrical equipment in the operating room.

Question 29: What is the most appropriate method for disposing of contaminated sharps after surgery in compliance with Standard Precautions?
A) Place them in a regular trash bin.
B) Place them in a puncture-resistant sharps container.
C) Place them in a biohazard bag.
D) Place them in an autoclave for sterilization.

Question 30: Mrs. Smith is scheduled for a laparoscopic cholecystectomy. During the preoperative phase, which document should be reviewed to ensure that all necessary preoperative instructions have been communicated and understood by the patient?
A) Preoperative teaching record
B) Operative report
C) Postoperative care plan
D) Discharge summary

Question 31: During the preoperative setup for an orthopedic surgery on a patient named Ms. Johnson, the surgical technologist notices that the suction unit is not providing adequate suction. What should be the first step in troubleshooting this issue?
A) Replace the suction canister.
B) Increase the suction pressure.
C) Inspect the suction tubing for kinks or blockages.
D) Switch to a different suction unit.

Question 32: During a laparoscopic cholecystectomy, which of the following steps should the surgical technologist anticipate immediately after the pneumoperitoneum is established?
A) Insertion of the laparoscope
B) Clipping of the cystic artery and duct
C) Dissection of the gallbladder from the liver bed
D) Closure of the port sites

Question 33: Mrs. Smith is scheduled for a pediatric surgery. The surgical technologist is responsible for preparing the operating room environment. What is the recommended temperature range for the operating room to ensure the pediatric patient's safety and comfort?
A) 60°F to 65°F
B) 68°F to 73°F
C) 70°F to 75°F
D) 75°F to 80°F

Question 34: During a laparoscopic cholecystectomy on a patient named Mr. Smith, which draping technique should be used to ensure the laparoscopic equipment remains sterile throughout the procedure?
A) Drape the patient first, then cover the laparoscopic equipment with a separate sterile drape.
B) Drape the laparoscopic equipment first, then drape the patient.
C) Drape the patient and the laparoscopic equipment simultaneously using a single sterile drape.
D) Use a sterile cover only for the laparoscopic equipment, leaving the patient undraped.

Question 35: What is the primary reason for verifying the availability of surgical equipment before a procedure?
A) To ensure the surgical team is familiar with the equipment

B) To prevent delays during the surgery
C) To comply with hospital policy
D) To maintain the cleanliness of the operating room

Question 36: During an intraoperative procedure using a computer navigation system, the surgical technologist notices a discrepancy between the system's guidance and the actual anatomical structures. What should be the immediate course of action?
A) Continue the surgery and adjust manually
B) Recalibrate the navigation system
C) Restart the computer navigation system
D) Ignore the discrepancy if it is minor

Question 37: Which of the following is a critical step to ensure the safety and effectiveness of phacoemulsification during cataract surgery?
A) Using a high-frequency laser
B) Maintaining the correct intraocular pressure
C) Applying topical antibiotics preoperatively
D) Performing a corneal transplant

Question 38: During the preoperative preparation for Mr. Johnson, a 65-year-old patient scheduled for hip replacement surgery, which of the following patient safety devices is most crucial to apply to prevent deep vein thrombosis (DVT)?
A) Sequential compression device (SCD)
B) Pulse oximeter
C) Foley catheter
D) Nasal cannula

Question 39: Which of the following is the most reliable method to test the sharpness of surgical scissors?
A) Cutting through a piece of gauze
B) Visual inspection under a magnifying glass
C) Running a finger along the blade
D) Using a sharpness testing device

Question 40: Which of the following actions is essential to maintain aseptic technique when donning sterile gloves?
A) Touching the outside of the glove with bare hands.
B) Using the closed gloving technique.
C) Adjusting the glove fit by touching the sterile gown.
D) Donning gloves before the sterile gown.

Question 41: Which of the following is a common cause of fires in the operating room?
A) Use of non-sterile instruments
B) Electrical equipment malfunction
C) Inadequate hand hygiene
D) Poor lighting conditions

Question 42: During an orthopedic surgery on Mrs. Johnson, the power drill suddenly stops working. As the Certified Surgical Technologist, what should you do first to troubleshoot this equipment malfunction?
A) Check the battery or power supply.

B) Replace the drill with a new one.
C) Inform the surgeon immediately.
D) Sterilize a backup drill.

Question 43: Which of the following thermal technologies is most commonly used for tissue dissection and coagulation during laparoscopic surgery?
A) Cryotherapy
B) Ultrasonic scalpel
C) Laser ablation
D) Radiofrequency ablation

Question 44: During an orthopedic surgery, the surgical technologist is responsible for monitoring the use of irrigation solutions. What is the most important factor to consider when managing these solutions?
A) The temperature of the irrigation solution.
B) The color of the irrigation solution.
C) The volume of irrigation solution used.
D) The type of irrigation solution being used.

Question 45: During surgery, which of the following is the most critical indicator of significant blood loss that requires immediate intervention?
A) Decreased urine output
B) Increased respiratory rate
C) Drop in blood pressure
D) Elevated heart rate

Question 46: In preparing Ms. Smith, a 45-year-old patient for a knee arthroscopy, what is the correct tension for the safety strap to ensure both safety and comfort?
A) Tight enough to leave an indentation on the skin
B) Loose enough to fit a hand underneath easily
C) Snug, allowing minimal movement but not causing discomfort
D) Not applied, as it is unnecessary for this procedure

Question 47: During the preoperative preparation for Mr. Johnson's knee replacement surgery, the surgical team is about to perform the Universal Protocol (Time Out). Which of the following steps is NOT part of the Time Out procedure?
A) Confirming the patient's identity using two identifiers
B) Verifying the surgical site and procedure
C) Reviewing the patient's allergies and medical history
D) Ensuring the surgical instruments are sterile

Question 48: When should contaminated sharps be disposed of in a sharps container after surgery?
A) Immediately after use.
B) At the end of the surgical procedure.
C) When the sharps container is full.
D) Before the patient leaves the operating room.

Question 49: During a post-operative debrief, Dr. Johnson mentions that he prefers a different suture material for closing incisions. What should the Certified Surgical Technologist do to ensure this preference is consistently followed in future surgeries?

A) Make a mental note and remember to use the new suture material.
B) Update Dr. Johnson's preference card to reflect the new suture material.
C) Inform the circulating nurse to remind the team during the next surgery.
D) Use the new suture material only if Dr. Johnson specifically asks for it.

Question 50: During an intraoperative procedure, the surgeon instructs you to assist in applying a splint to Ms. Smith's lower leg. What is the primary purpose of applying padding before the splint?

A) To provide additional support to the limb.
B) To prevent skin irritation and pressure sores.
C) To make the splint easier to remove.
D) To ensure the splint adheres to the skin.

Question 51: During a laparoscopic cholecystectomy, the surgeon asks you to connect and activate a Jackson-Pratt (JP) drain to a suction apparatus. What is the correct sequence of steps to ensure proper function?

A) Connect the drain to the suction tubing, activate the suction, then compress the bulb.
B) Compress the bulb, connect the drain to the suction tubing, then activate the suction.
C) Connect the drain to the suction tubing, compress the bulb, then activate the suction.
D) Activate the suction, compress the bulb, then connect the drain to the suction tubing.

Question 52: During a laparoscopic cholecystectomy, what is the primary responsibility of the surgical technologist when the surgeon is dissecting the cystic duct and artery?

A) Adjusting the insufflation pressure
B) Retracting the liver for better visualization
C) Passing the appropriate instruments to the surgeon
D) Monitoring the patient's vital signs

Question 53: When preparing suture material for a surgical procedure, which of the following steps is essential to ensure sterility?

A) Open the suture packet with bare hands.
B) Use sterile gloves to handle the suture material.
C) Place the suture material on a non-sterile surface.
D) Cut the suture material with non-sterile scissors.

Question 54: Sarah, a 45-year-old patient, is being prepared for a laparoscopic cholecystectomy. Which monitoring device should be applied to continuously measure her cardiac electrical activity during the procedure?

A) Capnography
B) Electrocardiogram (ECG) leads
C) Pulse oximeter
D) Blood pressure cuff

Question 55: During a tympanoplasty procedure on Mr. Johnson, the surgeon needs to graft tissue to repair the tympanic membrane. Which of the following structures is most commonly used for this graft?

A) Nasal septum
B) Temporalis fascia
C) Buccal mucosa
D) Palatal mucosa

Question 56: During a laparoscopic cholecystectomy on a patient named John, the surgeon requests a Maryland dissector. Which of the following actions should the surgical technologist take to ensure the instrument is passed correctly?

A) Pass the instrument with the tips pointed downwards.
B) Pass the instrument with the tips pointed upwards.
C) Pass the instrument with the tips in a neutral position.
D) Pass the instrument with the tips facing the surgeon.

Question 57: Which of the following steps is most crucial in preventing cross-contamination during the room clean-up process after a surgical procedure?

A) Disposing of all sharps immediately
B) Wiping down the surgical lights
C) Using a high-level disinfectant on all surfaces
D) Removing all linens and waste first

Question 58: During an orthopedic surgery on a patient named Mrs. Johnson, the anesthesiologist requests an infusion of 1 gram of cefazolin. As the surgical technologist, what should you do next?

A) Prepare the cefazolin and administer it immediately.
B) Verify the medication and dosage with the circulating nurse before preparing it.
C) Ask the surgeon to confirm the request before proceeding.
D) Wait until the end of the surgery to administer the cefazolin.

Question 59: What is the primary reason for monitoring the amount of solution used during an intraoperative procedure?

A) To ensure the surgical team has enough supplies
B) To prevent contamination of the sterile field
C) To maintain accurate fluid balance for the patient
D) To comply with hospital inventory protocols

Question 60: During a laparoscopic cholecystectomy on a patient named Mr. Johnson, the surgeon requests the use of a thermal device

to achieve hemostasis. Which device should the surgical technologist prepare?
A) Harmonic Scalpel
B) Bipolar Forceps
C) Monopolar Electrosurgery
D) Cryotherapy Probe

Question 61: Which of the following best describes a comminuted fracture?
A) A fracture where the bone is broken into multiple pieces
B) A fracture where the bone is partially bent
C) A fracture where the bone is broken straight across
D) A fracture where the bone is broken in a spiral pattern

Question 62: In a spinal fusion surgery for a patient named Sarah, the surgical technologist is preparing a synthetic tissue graft. What is the primary consideration to ensure the graft's effectiveness?
A) The graft's tensile strength.
B) The graft's immunogenicity.
C) The graft's size and shape compatibility.
D) The graft's color and texture.

Question 63: After a successful laparoscopic cholecystectomy on Mr. Johnson, the surgical technologist is responsible for removing the drapes and other equipment from the patient. Which of the following steps should be performed first?
A) Remove the surgical drapes from the patient.
B) Disconnect the insufflation tubing from the trocar.
C) Remove the trocars from the patient's abdomen.
D) Turn off the electrosurgical unit.

Question 64: Which hemostatic agent is most appropriate for controlling capillary bleeding in a highly vascular area during surgery?
A) Bone wax
B) Fibrin sealant
C) Tourniquet
D) Electrocautery

Question 65: Which of the following is the most appropriate method for handling surgical instruments during the removal of drapes postoperatively?
A) Place all instruments on the patient's chest
B) Hand instruments directly to the circulating nurse
C) Leave instruments on the drapes until they are removed
D) Place instruments back in the instrument tray immediately

Question 66: During a phacoemulsification procedure on Mr. Johnson, the surgeon encounters a dense cataract. Which of the following settings should the surgical technologist adjust to optimize the ultrasound power for effective emulsification?

A) Increase the aspiration flow rate
B) Decrease the ultrasound power
C) Increase the ultrasound power
D) Decrease the irrigation flow rate

Question 67: What is the primary purpose of performing a leak test on a laparoscopic insufflator before surgery?
A) To ensure the insufflator is properly calibrated for gas flow
B) To verify the insufflator's pressure settings
C) To check for any gas leakage in the tubing and connections
D) To confirm the insufflator's power supply is functioning

Question 68: What is the most effective active listening technique to ensure understanding during a preoperative team briefing?
A) Nodding occasionally
B) Paraphrasing the speaker's points
C) Maintaining eye contact
D) Taking notes

Question 69: During the intraoperative phase of phacoemulsification on Ms. Thompson, the surgeon notices a surge in the anterior chamber. What immediate action should the surgical technologist take to stabilize the chamber?
A) Increase the irrigation flow rate
B) Decrease the aspiration flow rate
C) Increase the ultrasound power
D) Decrease the irrigation flow rate

Question 70: During the preoperative preparation for a laparoscopic cholecystectomy on Mr. Smith, where is the most appropriate placement for the bovie pad to ensure patient safety?
A) Over a bony prominence
B) On the upper arm
C) On the thigh
D) On the abdomen

Question 71: What is the first step a Certified Surgical Technologist should take when an autoclave fails to reach the required temperature for sterilization?
A) Replace the autoclave's heating element.
B) Check the water level in the autoclave reservoir.
C) Restart the autoclave cycle.
D) Contact the biomedical engineering department immediately.

Question 72: Which stage of grief, according to Kübler-Ross, is characterized by the patient refusing to accept the reality of their terminal diagnosis?
A) Anger
B) Depression
C) Denial
D) Bargaining

Question 73: What is the primary purpose of a surgeon's preference card in a surgical setting?
A) To list the surgical instruments and supplies preferred by the surgeon
B) To document the patient's medical history and allergies
C) To outline the postoperative care plan for the patient
D) To provide a detailed billing summary for the surgery

Question 74: Which of the following steps is essential during a medical hand wash to ensure proper asepsis?
A) Using a nail brush for 30 seconds
B) Rinsing hands with hot water
C) Keeping hands lower than elbows during rinsing
D) Cleaning under fingernails

Question 75: During a laparoscopic cholecystectomy on a patient named Sarah, the surgeon decides to use intraoperative ultrasound to assess the biliary anatomy. Which ultrasound probe is most suitable for this purpose?
A) Phased array probe
B) Linear array probe
C) Curvilinear array probe
D) Endocavitary probe

Question 76: Ms. Smith is scheduled for a total hip replacement. Which positioning device should be used to ensure proper alignment and stabilization of the operative leg during the procedure?
A) Wilson frame
B) Hip positioner
C) Knee crutches
D) Mayfield headrest

Question 77: Sarah, a patient undergoing a liver resection, requires intraoperative ultrasound to locate a lesion. What is the most critical factor for ensuring optimal ultrasound imaging during this procedure?
A) The patient's body mass index (BMI).
B) The type of ultrasound probe used.
C) The experience of the surgical technologist.
D) The amount of saline used for acoustic coupling.

Question 78: What is the primary purpose of ensuring the bovie pad is securely attached to the patient before starting an electrosurgical procedure?
A) To prevent the patient from moving
B) To ensure the patient remains sterile
C) To provide a return path for the electrical current
D) To monitor the patient's heart rate

Question 79: During the preoperative preparation for Mr. Johnson's laparoscopic cholecystectomy, the surgical technologist needs to verify the availability of essential equipment. Which of the following is the most critical piece of equipment

to ensure is available and functioning properly?
A) Electrosurgical unit
B) Suction apparatus
C) Laparoscopic camera system
D) Surgical lights

Question 80: Which cranial nerve is responsible for the sense of smell?
A) Optic Nerve (II)
B) Oculomotor Nerve (III)
C) Olfactory Nerve (I)
D) Trigeminal Nerve (V)

Question 81: During preoperative preparation, which device is essential for monitoring a patient's end-tidal CO2 levels?
A) Pulse oximeter
B) Capnograph
C) Electrocardiogram (ECG)
D) Thermometer

Question 82: Ms. Smith, a patient scheduled for an elective knee replacement, expresses confusion about the risks associated with the procedure. What is the best course of action for the surgical technologist?
A) Explain the risks and benefits of the procedure to the patient.
B) Ask the patient to sign the consent form regardless of her confusion.
C) Inform the surgeon or nurse to re-explain the procedure to the patient.
D) Ignore the patient's concerns and proceed with the preoperative preparations.

Question 83: What does dark red or maroon blood suggest during an intraoperative procedure?
A) Arterial bleeding
B) Venous bleeding
C) Capillary bleeding
D) Hemolysis

Question 84: During a preoperative assessment, the surgical technologist needs to ensure x-ray safety for a patient named Mr. Smith, who is scheduled for a hip replacement surgery. Which of the following measures is the most appropriate to minimize Mr. Smith's exposure to x-rays during the procedure?
A) Positioning the x-ray machine as close to the patient as possible
B) Using lead aprons and thyroid shields on the patient
C) Increasing the x-ray exposure time to capture clearer images
D) Allowing the patient to hold the x-ray film to reduce movement

Question 85: Which of the following is the most appropriate initial management for a patient with a suspected cervical spine injury from a traumatic accident?

A) Immediate removal of the cervical collar
B) Application of a thoracic brace
C) Immobilization with a cervical collar
D) Administration of intravenous fluids

Question 86: During a total knee arthroplasty on a patient named Mrs. Johnson, the surgeon instructs you to prepare the dressing for the wound site. Which of the following is the most appropriate type of dressing to use to minimize the risk of infection?
A) Gauze dressing without any antiseptic.
B) Transparent film dressing.
C) Hydrocolloid dressing.
D) Sterile, non-adherent dressing with an antiseptic layer.

Question 87: 5 Which of the following microorganisms is most commonly associated with surgical site infections (SSIs)?
A) Escherichia coli
B) Staphylococcus aureus
C) Pseudomonas aeruginosa
D) Candida albicans

Question 88: What is the most effective immediate action to take if a fire breaks out in the operating room?
A) Evacuate the patient immediately
B) Use a fire extinguisher to put out the fire
C) Shut off the gas supply
D) Call for help and wait for instructions

Question 89: Which of the following is the most critical piece of information to verify on the preoperative checklist before the patient is taken to the operating room?
A) Patient's insurance details
B) Patient's consent form
C) Patient's dietary restrictions
D) Patient's family contact information

Question 90: A patient presents with a widespread rash and fever three days after surgery. Which of the following should be the primary concern?
A) Allergic reaction to latex
B) Surgical site infection
C) Drug-induced hypersensitivity
D) Contact dermatitis from adhesive dressings

Question 91: Which of the following is the most appropriate action for a surgical technologist to take when a patient expresses anxiety about their upcoming surgery?
A) Ignore the patient's concerns and focus on preparing the surgical instruments.
B) Reassure the patient by providing accurate information about the procedure.
C) Tell the patient that their anxiety is normal and will go away on its own.
D) Suggest the patient speak to their family members about their concerns.

Question 92: A patient named Sarah is undergoing surgery for breast cancer. The surgeon plans to perform a sentinel lymph node biopsy to check for metastasis. Which lymph nodes are most likely to be the sentinel nodes in this case?
A) Axillary lymph nodes
B) Inguinal lymph nodes
C) Cervical lymph nodes
D) Mesenteric lymph nodes

Question 93: Mrs. Johnson is scheduled for an elective cholecystectomy. Her preoperative laboratory results indicate a hemoglobin level of 8.5 g/dL. What should be the surgical technologist's primary concern regarding this lab result?
A) The patient might have an increased risk of infection.
B) The patient might have an increased risk of bleeding.
C) The patient might have an increased risk of poor oxygenation during surgery.
D) The patient might have an increased risk of electrolyte imbalance.

Question 94: When preparing a wound site for dressing, which of the following steps is essential to maintain sterility?
A) Using non-sterile gloves to handle the dressing
B) Cleaning the wound with sterile saline solution
C) Applying the dressing with bare hands
D) Using the same dressing for multiple wounds

Question 95: During a lung resection surgery on Mrs. Smith, the surgeon needs to avoid damaging the phrenic nerve. Which anatomical landmark should the surgical technologist use to locate the phrenic nerve?
A) Anterior to the hilum of the lung
B) Posterior to the hilum of the lung
C) Lateral to the trachea
D) Medial to the esophagus

Question 96: When restocking supplies in the operating room, what is the best practice to ensure sterility and readiness for the next procedure?
A) Placing new supplies in the front of the storage area
B) Checking expiration dates and rotating stock
C) Storing supplies in their original packaging
D) Ensuring all supplies are within easy reach

Question 97: Ms. Johnson is undergoing an exploratory laparotomy to investigate abdominal pain. The surgeon needs an incision that allows wide access to the entire abdominal cavity. Which incision should the surgeon choose?
A) Pfannenstiel incision
B) McBurney incision

C) Midline incision
D) Kocher incision

Question 98: What is the primary mechanism by which a harmonic scalpel achieves hemostasis during surgery?
A) Electrical cauterization
B) Ultrasonic vibrations
C) Laser energy
D) Radiofrequency waves

Question 99: What is the primary purpose of using computer navigation systems during orthopedic surgery?
A) To reduce the need for surgical instruments
B) To enhance the accuracy of implant placement
C) To shorten the duration of the surgery
D) To eliminate the need for imaging techniques

Question 100: During the postoperative phase, the surgical technologist is tasked with removing drapes and other equipment from the patient. What is the correct procedure for handling nondisposable instruments?
A) Place nondisposable instruments in a basin of sterile water.
B) Disassemble and soak nondisposable instruments in enzymatic cleaner.
C) Immediately place nondisposable instruments in a sterilization container.
D) Hand nondisposable instruments to the scrub nurse for immediate reuse.

Question 101: Which of the following is a critical step in the preoperative preparation of a surgical microscope?
A) Calibrating the microscope's magnification settings
B) Ensuring the microscope is connected to the anesthesia machine
C) Sterilizing the microscope's entire body
D) Placing the microscope in the sterile field

Question 102: During a cataract surgery on Mrs. Smith, the surgeon asks the surgical technologist to identify the fluid-filled space between the cornea and the iris. What is the correct identification?
A) Vitreous chamber
B) Anterior chamber
C) Posterior chamber
D) Aqueous humor

Question 103: Which of the following is a key principle in ensuring electrical safety in the operating room?
A) Using extension cords to connect multiple devices
B) Ensuring all equipment is properly grounded
C) Overloading circuits to maximize efficiency
D) Using non-conductive materials for all surfaces

Question 104: When removing equipment from the patient postoperatively, what is the primary consideration?
A) Speed of removal
B) Maintaining sterility
C) Patient comfort
D) Minimizing noise

Question 105: During the preoperative preparation for a knee replacement surgery, the surgical technologist, Alex, notices a small tear in the sterile package of surgical instruments. What should Alex do next?
A) Use the instruments as long as they appear clean
B) Reseal the package with sterile tape and proceed
C) Discard the package and obtain a new sterile set
D) Continue with the surgery and inform the surgeon later

Question 106: Which of the following is the most critical safety measure to implement when using a laser in the operating room?
A) Ensuring the patient is draped with non-reflective materials
B) Wearing standard surgical masks
C) Using smoke evacuators
D) Applying wet towels around the surgical site

Question 107: During the preoperative preparation for a laparoscopic cholecystectomy on a patient named Mr. Smith, the surgical technologist is responsible for ensuring the suction system is properly set up. Which of the following steps is crucial to verify the functionality of the suction system?
A) Ensure the suction canister is empty.
B) Check that the suction tubing is securely connected.
C) Verify the suction pressure is set to 200 mmHg.
D) Confirm the suction system is plugged into the electrical outlet.

Question 108: Which classification of surgical instrument is a Kocher clamp?
A) Cutting and dissecting
B) Clamping and occluding
C) Grasping and holding
D) Retracting and exposing

Question 109: What is the primary reason for accurately reporting the amount of medication and solution used during a surgical procedure?
A) To ensure the patient receives the correct dosage postoperatively
B) To maintain an accurate inventory of medical supplies
C) To provide precise information for the patient's medical record
D) To comply with hospital administrative policies

Question 110: What is the primary reason for using a fenestrated drape when preparing specialty equipment for a surgical procedure?
A) To allow for multiple instruments to be passed

through the drape.
B) To provide a sterile barrier while allowing access to the surgical site.
C) To cover the entire surgical field with one drape.
D) To minimize the use of additional drapes during the procedure.

Question 111: Sarah, a surgical technologist, is preparing for an upcoming surgery and notices that the inventory of surgical gloves is low. What should she do to ensure proper cost containment?
A) Ignore the low inventory and proceed with the surgery.
B) Order a large quantity of gloves to avoid future shortages.
C) Report the low inventory to the supply manager and request a restock based on usage trends.
D) Borrow gloves from another department without informing anyone.

Question 112: Which of the following is the most effective method for reducing surgical smoke in the operating room?
A) Using high-efficiency particulate air (HEPA) filters
B) Wearing high-filtration surgical masks
C) Utilizing a smoke evacuation system
D) Increasing room ventilation

Question 113: In the context of intraoperative procedures, what is a significant safety concern when using an argon laser?
A) Potential for deep tissue burns.
B) Risk of retinal damage to the surgical team.
C) High incidence of postoperative infections.
D) Excessive smoke production during use.

Question 114: Mr. Johnson is scheduled for a laparoscopic cholecystectomy. During the preoperative phase, the surgical technologist notices that the informed consent form is missing the surgeon's signature. What should the surgical technologist do next?
A) Proceed with the surgery as the patient has signed the consent form.
B) Inform the circulating nurse to get the surgeon's signature before proceeding.
C) Ask the patient to sign the consent form again.
D) Ignore the missing signature as it is not crucial.

Question 115: Which artery is primarily responsible for supplying blood to the lower extremities?
A) Brachial artery
B) Femoral artery
C) Carotid artery
D) Radial artery

Question 116: During the postoperative phase, the surgical technologist must ensure that all instruments used during Mrs. Johnson's appendectomy are accounted for. Which of the
following steps is most crucial in this process?
A) Counting the instruments before removing the drapes.
B) Counting the instruments after removing the drapes.
C) Counting the instruments after the patient has been transferred to the recovery room.
D) Counting the instruments while the patient is being extubated.

Question 117: During the postoperative phase after an appendectomy on Ms. Smith, the surgical technologist must remove the drapes and equipment. What is the correct sequence for removing the drapes?
A) Remove the drapes starting from the head of the patient.
B) Remove the drapes starting from the feet of the patient.
C) Remove the drapes starting from the sides of the patient.
D) Remove the drapes starting from the surgical site outward.

Question 118: Sarah, a 35-year-old patient, is undergoing a hysterectomy. During the procedure, the surgeon needs to avoid damaging the structure that transports eggs from the ovaries to the uterus. Which structure is the surgeon referring to?
A) Ureter
B) Fallopian tube
C) Round ligament
D) Broad ligament

Question 119: During a surgical procedure, the patient experiences a sudden drop in blood pressure and heart rate. What is the first action the surgical technologist should take?
A) Administer epinephrine.
B) Notify the surgeon immediately.
C) Increase the IV fluid rate.
D) Begin chest compressions.

Question 120: What is the primary function of the glomerulus in the kidney?
A) Filtration of blood
B) Reabsorption of water
C) Secretion of hormones
D) Concentration of urine

Question 121: Dr. Smith has updated his preference card to include a new suture material for abdominal surgeries. As a Certified Surgical Technologist, what is the most appropriate action to ensure this change is reflected in future procedures?
A) Verbally inform the surgical team of the change before each surgery.
B) Update the preference card in the computer system immediately.
C) Write a note on the physical preference card and

update it later.
D) Wait until the end of the week to make all updates at once.

Question 122: What is the primary reason for verifying the correct type and size of implantable items with the surgeon before the procedure begins?
A) To ensure the implant matches the patient's insurance coverage
B) To confirm the implant is available in the sterile field
C) To prevent surgical complications and ensure proper fit
D) To reduce the overall cost of the surgery

Question 123: During a neurosurgical procedure on Mr. Johnson, the surgical technologist is responsible for setting up the operating microscope. Which of the following steps is crucial to ensure proper focus and clarity of the microscope?
A) Adjusting the microscope's light intensity
B) Balancing the microscope's weight distribution
C) Calibrating the microscope's ocular lenses
D) Ensuring the microscope's objective lens is clean

Question 124: During the preoperative preparation for a surgery on patient Mr. Johnson, the surgical technologist notices a tear in the sterile glove after assisting with gowning. What should be the immediate next step?
A) Continue with the procedure and replace the glove later.
B) Replace the glove immediately without notifying anyone.
C) Notify the surgical team and replace the glove immediately.
D) Ignore the tear if it is small and proceed with the surgery.

Question 125: During an orthopedic surgery on Mr. Johnson, the surgeon excises a bone fragment and asks for it to be sent for microbiological culture. How should the Certified Surgical Technologist handle this specimen?
A) Place the specimen in formalin and label it with the patient's name and date of birth.
B) Place the specimen in a sterile container without any preservative and label it with the patient's name, date of birth, and "Microbiological Culture."
C) Place the specimen in a sterile container with saline and label it with the patient's name, date of birth, and "Histopathology."
D) Wrap the specimen in a sterile gauze soaked in saline and label it with the patient's name and date of birth.

Question 126: After a successful laparoscopic cholecystectomy on Mr. Johnson, the surgical technologist is tasked with removing the drapes and other equipment. During this process, what is

the most crucial step to ensure safety when dealing with the cautery device?
A) Turn off the cautery device and unplug it before removing the drapes.
B) Remove the drapes first, then turn off the cautery device.
C) Leave the cautery device on standby mode while removing the drapes.
D) Ask the surgeon to remove the drapes while the cautery device is still on.

Question 127: After a cholecystectomy, Mr. Johnson reports severe abdominal pain, a fever of 102°F, and yellowing of the skin. As a Certified Surgical Technologist, what is the most appropriate action to take?
A) Reassure the patient that these symptoms are normal post-surgery.
B) Administer over-the-counter pain medication and monitor.
C) Report the symptoms immediately to the surgeon.
D) Suggest the patient to increase fluid intake and rest.

Question 128: What is the primary benefit of utilizing online continuing education platforms for Certified Surgical Technologists?
A) Limited access to course materials
B) Inconsistent course quality
C) Flexibility in learning schedule
D) High costs compared to traditional methods

Question 129: Which of the following practices is most effective in ensuring cost containment in the surgical setting?
A) Reusing single-use items after sterilization
B) Implementing a standardized inventory management system
C) Ordering supplies in bulk without considering usage rates
D) Using the most expensive surgical instruments available

Question 130: What is the primary purpose of using a surgical skin antiseptic prior to an incision?
A) To reduce the risk of postoperative infection
B) To remove all resident bacteria from the skin
C) To sterilize the surgical instruments
D) To provide a sterile field for the surgical team

Question 131: Which of the following is the most appropriate suction tip to use during a tonsillectomy procedure to ensure effective removal of blood and debris?
A) Poole suction tip
B) Yankauer suction tip
C) Frazier suction tip
D) Rosen suction tip

Question 132: After a successful appendectomy on Mr. Johnson, the surgical technologist is

responsible for removing the drapes and other equipment. What is the first step in this process?
A) Remove the surgical instruments from the sterile field.
B) Disconnect the suction and electrosurgical units.
C) Remove the drapes by pulling them towards the patient's head.
D) Ensure all counts are correct and accounted for.

Question 133: What is the primary advantage of using an ultrasonic scalpel over traditional electrocautery for hemostasis in surgery?
A) Lower risk of thermal injury to surrounding tissues
B) Higher coagulation temperatures
C) Easier to use
D) More cost-effective

Question 134: Which of the following is the most appropriate step to take before using a pneumatic power drill in surgery?
A) Lubricate the drill with oil
B) Check the air hose for leaks
C) Sterilize the drill using an autoclave
D) Ensure the drill is fully charged

Question 135: During a laparoscopic procedure, which mechanical device is often utilized to control bleeding from small vessels?
A) Laparoscopic stapler
B) Harmonic scalpel
C) Laparoscopic clip applier
D) Bipolar forceps

Question 136: During a surgical procedure, the surgeon asks you to assist in applying a cast to Mr. Johnson's fractured forearm. What is the first step you should take to ensure proper application?
A) Apply padding directly to the skin.
B) Immerse the casting material in water.
C) Position the limb in the desired alignment.
D) Cut the casting material to the appropriate length.

Question 137: Which of the following is a primary reason for using helium in laser technology during intraoperative procedures?
A) Helium is highly reactive and enhances laser precision.
B) Helium is a noble gas that helps stabilize the laser beam.
C) Helium is heavier than air and prevents laser scattering.
D) Helium is used to cool the laser equipment due to its high thermal conductivity.

Question 138: What is the most effective method for ensuring accurate interdepartmental communication regarding surgical schedules?
A) Verbal communication during morning briefings
B) Written memos distributed to all departments
C) Real-time updates through a centralized computer system

D) Weekly departmental meetings

Question 139: During a total hip replacement surgery on a patient named Mrs. Johnson, you notice a small tear in your sterile gown sleeve. What is the most appropriate action to follow standard and universal precautions?
A) Continue the procedure and cover the tear with a sterile drape.
B) Notify the surgeon and replace the gown immediately.
C) Ask the circulating nurse to tape over the tear.
D) Continue the procedure and replace the gown after the surgery.

Question 140: During a total knee arthroplasty, the surgical technologist is responsible for ensuring the power equipment is functioning correctly. Which of the following steps should be performed first when assembling the power equipment?
A) Check the battery charge level.
B) Attach the appropriate blade or bit.
C) Verify the sterilization indicator.
D) Test the equipment for proper operation.

Question 141: Which of the following is the most effective way for a Certified Surgical Technologist to keep track of their continuing education credits using computer technology?
A) Using a paper-based logbook
B) Relying on email notifications from professional organizations
C) Utilizing a dedicated continuing education tracking software
D) Keeping a mental note of completed courses

Question 142: Which of the following is a key administrative duty of a CST in the operating room?
A) Scheduling surgeries
B) Documenting surgical counts
C) Managing patient records
D) Supervising the surgical team

Question 143: During a surgical procedure, a chemical spill occurs in the operating room. What is the first action a Certified Surgical Technologist (CST) should take to ensure safety?
A) Immediately start cleaning up the spill.
B) Evacuate the operating room.
C) Notify the surgical team and follow the facility's spill protocol.
D) Continue with the procedure and address the spill later.

Question 144: Which of the following actions should be taken immediately after a sharps container becomes three-quarters full?
A) Compress the contents to make more room.
B) Continue using the container until it is completely full.
C) Seal the container and replace it with a new one.

D) Transfer the sharps to a larger container.

Question 145: What is the most effective method for a surgical technologist to prevent the transmission of bloodborne pathogens during surgery?
A) Wearing a surgical mask
B) Double-gloving
C) Using a face shield
D) Handwashing before and after the procedure

Question 146: During a preoperative preparation, Sarah, a Certified Surgical Technologist, needs to perform a surgical scrub before assisting in a cardiac surgery. Which of the following steps is crucial to ensure proper aseptic technique?
A) Scrubbing from the elbow to the fingertips
B) Using a nail cleaner under running water before starting the scrub
C) Drying hands and arms with a reusable towel
D) Scrubbing for a minimum of 1 minute

Question 147: Which of the following is the primary reason for wearing a surgical mask during preoperative preparation?
A) To protect the surgical team from splashes
B) To prevent the spread of airborne pathogens from the surgical team to the patient
C) To keep the surgical team warm
D) To enhance communication within the surgical team

Question 148: Sarah, a surgical technologist, is preparing a pneumatic drill for use in a craniotomy. Which of the following actions is

most critical to ensure the drill operates safely and effectively during the procedure?
A) Ensure the drill is properly lubricated.
B) Confirm the air pressure settings are within the recommended range.
C) Check the drill for visible signs of wear and tear.
D) Attach the drill to the air supply line.

Question 149: Which of the following is the most critical step in verifying the availability of surgical equipment before a procedure?
A) Checking the inventory list
B) Confirming equipment functionality
C) Ensuring sterility of instruments
D) Reviewing the surgeon's preference card

Question 150: During an orthopedic surgery, the surgical technologist notices a significant amount of smoke being generated by the electrocautery device. What is the best practice to minimize the potential hazards of surgical smoke?
A) Use high-efficiency particulate air (HEPA) filters in the operating room
B) Ensure all team members wear standard surgical masks
C) Utilize local exhaust ventilation (LEV) systems
D) Increase the room's air exchange rate

ANSWER WITH DETAILED EXPLANATION SET [2]

Question 1: Correct Answer: A) Asking the patient to state their name and date of birth
Rationale: Verifying patient identity by asking them to state their name and date of birth ensures active patient participation and reduces errors. While checking the wristband (B) and confirming with a family member (C) are important, they should complement, not replace, direct patient verification. Reviewing the chart alone (D) lacks patient interaction and increases the risk of errors.

Question 2: Correct Answer: B) To reduce the risk of surgical site infections
Rationale: The primary purpose of performing preoperative skin antisepsis is to reduce the risk of surgical site infections by eliminating or significantly reducing the number of microorganisms on the skin. Options A, C, and D are incorrect because moisturizing the skin, enhancing anesthesia absorption, and identifying skin allergies are not the primary goals of preoperative skin antisepsis. The main focus is infection prevention.

Question 3: Correct Answer: A) Apply the antiseptic to dry hands and rub until dry.
Rationale: Waterless hand antiseptics must be applied to dry hands and rubbed until dry to ensure maximum efficacy. Rinsing with water before or after application (options B and C) can dilute the antiseptic, reducing its effectiveness. Applying to wet hands (option D) can also dilute the product and decrease its antimicrobial activity.

Question 4: Correct Answer: B) Computer navigation system
Rationale: The computer navigation system is crucial for computer-assisted navigation during a total knee arthroplasty. While the tourniquet system and electrocautery unit are standard equipment, they do not address the specific request. The arthroscopy tower is not relevant to this procedure. Ensuring the computer navigation system is available aligns with the surgeon's specific needs, improving surgical precision and outcomes.

Question 5: Correct Answer: B) Matching the graft's mechanical properties to the host tissue
Rationale: When using synthetic tissue grafts, it is crucial to match the graft's mechanical properties to the host tissue to ensure proper function and integration. Option A) is less relevant as radiopacity is not a primary concern. Option C) is incorrect because synthetic grafts typically do not promote rapid vascularization. Option D) is also incorrect as antibacterial properties are not the main consideration in this context.

Question 6: Correct Answer: D) Babcock forceps
Rationale: Babcock forceps are specifically designed for grasping and manipulating delicate tissues such as the gallbladder without causing damage. Metzenbaum scissors are used for cutting delicate tissues, Kocher clamps are for grasping tough tissues, and Maryland dissectors are used for dissection and coagulation. Therefore, Babcock forceps are the most appropriate instrument for this task.

Question 7: Correct Answer: D) Ensure the bone graft is kept moist with a sterile sponge.
Rationale: The first step in preparing an autograft bone is to ensure it remains moist, typically with a sterile sponge. This is crucial to maintain the viability of the graft. Options A and C are incorrect because soaking or irrigating the graft can compromise its integrity. Option B is incorrect because the graft must be properly prepared and kept moist before being passed to the surgeon.

Question 8: Correct Answer: A) Scheduling surgeries
Rationale: Scheduling surgeries is typically the responsibility of administrative staff or a surgical coordinator, not the surgical technologist. Surgical technologists are more directly involved in clinical tasks such as sterilizing surgical instruments (B), maintaining patient records (C), and ordering surgical supplies (D). These tasks ensure that the operating room is prepared and that all necessary materials are available for procedures, but scheduling is outside their usual scope of duties.

Question 9: Correct Answer: D) Inform the circulating nurse and surgeon immediately.
Rationale: The correct action is to inform the circulating nurse and surgeon immediately. This ensures that the discrepancy is addressed promptly, reducing the risk of a retained surgical item. Option B, while partially correct, does not involve the necessary communication with the team. Options A and C are incorrect as they delay addressing the issue, potentially compromising patient safety.

Question 10: Correct Answer: B) Implementing a just-in-time inventory system
Rationale: Implementing a just-in-time inventory system is most effective for cost containment as it reduces waste and storage costs by ensuring supplies are ordered and received only as needed. Reusing single-use items (A) is unsafe and against regulations. Stockpiling supplies (C) can lead to excess inventory and increased costs. Allowing surgeons to use any preferred brand (D) can lead to inconsistent supply costs and inefficiencies.

Question 11: Correct Answer: C) Disconnect the suction tubing, cap the ends, and dispose of it in a biohazard bag.
Rationale: The correct procedure involves disconnecting the suction tubing, capping the ends to prevent contamination, and disposing of it in a biohazard bag. This ensures that any residual fluids are contained and reduces the risk of infection. Option A is incorrect as leaving the tubing attached can lead to contamination. Option B is incorrect as immediate disposal without capping can cause spills. Option D is incorrect as placing it on the sterile field violates sterility protocols.

Question 12: Correct Answer: B) Coordination of voluntary movements
Rationale: The primary function of the cerebellum is the coordination of voluntary movements, including

balance, posture, and fine motor skills. While the regulation of emotions is primarily associated with the limbic system, the production of cerebrospinal fluid occurs in the choroid plexus, and the processing of visual information is managed by the occipital lobe. Therefore, the cerebellum's role in coordinating voluntary movements makes option B the correct answer.

Question 13: Correct Answer: C) Use a backup autoclave to re-sterilize the instruments.

Rationale: The most appropriate immediate action is to use a backup autoclave to re-sterilize the instruments. Continuing with previously sterilized instruments (A) or manually cleaning them with antiseptic solution (B) does not guarantee sterility. Delaying the surgery (D) is not ideal unless no backup autoclave is available. Using a backup autoclave ensures instruments are sterile and patient safety is maintained.

Question 14: Correct Answer: B) Don gown first, then gloves

Rationale: The correct sequence is to don the gown first, then the gloves. This ensures that the sterile field is maintained. Donning gloves first (Option A) can contaminate the gloves. Donning a mask first (Option C) is part of the pre-gowning procedure but not the gowning and gloving sequence. Donning a cap first (Option D) is also part of the pre-gowning procedure but does not follow the correct sequence for gowning and gloving.

Question 15: Correct Answer: B) Remove the hearing aids and place them in a labeled container for safekeeping.

Rationale: The correct action is to remove the hearing aids and place them in a labeled container for safekeeping. This ensures the hearing aids are not lost or damaged during surgery and prevents any potential interference with surgical equipment. Option A is incorrect as hearing aids should not be kept in place during surgery. Option C is incorrect because the surgical technologist should take immediate action. Option D is plausible but less secure than labeling and storing them properly.

Question 16: Correct Answer: B) Hodgkin lymphoma

Rationale: Reed-Sternberg cells are a hallmark of Hodgkin lymphoma, a type of cancer that originates in the lymphatic system. These large, abnormal cells are not found in non-Hodgkin lymphoma, multiple myeloma, or acute myeloid leukemia. The presence of Reed-Sternberg cells helps in differentiating Hodgkin lymphoma from other types of lymphomas and hematologic malignancies.

Question 17: Correct Answer: C) Utilizing a suction device

Rationale: Utilizing a suction device is the most effective method for removing excess blood from the operative site, ensuring a clear view and reducing the risk of complications. Using a sterile gauze pad (A) can be less effective and time-consuming, applying a tourniquet (B) is not suitable for this purpose, and allowing natural coagulation (D) can obstruct the surgical field and delay the procedure. Suction

devices provide continuous and efficient removal of fluids.

Question 18: Correct Answer: A) Common Bile Duct

Rationale: "CBD" stands for Common Bile Duct, which is a crucial structure in the biliary system that transports bile from the liver and gallbladder to the duodenum. Option B (Cystic Bile Duct) and D (Cystic Biliary Duct) are incorrect because the cystic duct specifically connects the gallbladder to the common bile duct. Option C (Common Biliary Drain) is a plausible but incorrect term that does not exist in anatomical terminology.

Question 19: Correct Answer: C) Hand the surgeon a hemostatic clamp and prepare suction.

Rationale: The correct action is to hand the surgeon a hemostatic clamp and prepare suction. This allows the surgeon to quickly control the bleeding and maintain a clear surgical field. Applying direct pressure (A) is impractical in a laparoscopic setting. Increasing insufflation pressure (B) is not an effective method to control arterial bleeding. Converting to an open procedure (D) is a decision for the surgeon, but immediate control of bleeding is critical.

Question 20: Correct Answer: B) Radial artery

Rationale: The radial artery is typically connected to the cephalic vein during AV fistula creation for hemodialysis. The brachial artery (A) and ulnar artery (C) are not commonly used for this connection. The subclavian artery (D) is not involved in this procedure. The radial artery's superficial location and size make it ideal for creating a durable and functional AV fistula, essential for efficient hemodialysis access.

Question 21: Correct Answer: B) Ulna

Rationale: The ulna, along with the humerus and radius, forms the elbow joint. The humerus articulates with the ulna at the trochlear notch, allowing for hinge-like movements. The scapula and clavicle are part of the shoulder girdle, not the elbow. The femur is a bone in the lower limb and does not contribute to the elbow joint. Understanding the specific bones involved in joint formation is crucial for surgical procedures related to the elbow.

Question 22: Correct Answer: B) Estrogen

Rationale: Estrogen is the primary hormone responsible for regulating the menstrual cycle. It works in conjunction with progesterone to prepare the endometrium for potential pregnancy. Testosterone is mainly involved in male reproductive functions, insulin regulates blood sugar levels, and cortisol is a stress hormone. Estrogen's role in the menstrual cycle is crucial, making it the correct answer.

Question 23: Correct Answer: B) To ensure complete hemostasis

Rationale: The primary purpose of using cautery in postoperative procedures is to ensure complete hemostasis, which means stopping bleeding by coagulating blood vessels. This is crucial to prevent postoperative bleeding. While reducing infection risk (A) and minimizing tissue adhesion (C) are important, they are not the primary roles of cautery. Enhancing wound healing (D) is a secondary benefit but not the main purpose of cautery in this context.

Question 24: Correct Answer: B) Coordinate the movement by counting aloud and guiding the team.
Rationale: The primary role of the Certified Surgical Technologist during patient transfer is to coordinate the movement by counting aloud and guiding the team. This ensures synchronized and safe movement. Directing the anesthesia provider (Option A) and holding the patient's head and neck (Option C) are the responsibilities of other team members. Ensuring all surgical instruments are accounted for (Option D) is important but not the primary focus during the transfer process.

Question 25: Correct Answer: C) Suggest a brief pause to discuss the issue and reach a consensus.
Rationale: Suggesting a brief pause to discuss the issue and reach a consensus (Option C) is the best approach. This action promotes open communication, ensures patient safety, and maintains a professional environment. Ignoring the disagreement (Option A) could lead to errors, siding with one party (Option B) might cause further conflict, and reporting immediately (Option D) is unnecessary and could escalate the situation prematurely.

Question 26: Correct Answer: C) Draping the robotic instruments before they are attached to the robotic arms.
Rationale: Draping the robotic instruments before they are attached to the robotic arms (Option C) ensures that the instruments remain sterile and ready for use. Sterilizing the instruments (Option A) is necessary but does not address draping. Draping after attachment (Option B) or simultaneously (Option D) can lead to contamination, compromising the sterile field.

Question 27: Correct Answer: B) To act as the heart's natural pacemaker
Rationale: The sinoatrial (SA) node is responsible for initiating the electrical impulses that set the rhythm of the heart, making it the natural pacemaker. It does not pump blood, receive deoxygenated blood, or prevent backflow of blood. These functions are carried out by the ventricles, atria, and valves, respectively. Understanding the role of the SA node is essential for comprehending cardiac conduction and rhythm.

Question 28: Correct Answer: C) Remove the patient from the immediate danger area.
Rationale: The first priority in the event of a fire in the operating room is to ensure the safety of the patient by removing them from immediate danger. While calling for help, using a fire extinguisher, and turning off electrical equipment are important steps, they come after ensuring the patient's safety. Removing the patient minimizes their risk of injury from the fire, which is the primary concern.

Question 29: Correct Answer: B) Place them in a puncture-resistant sharps container.
Rationale: Contaminated sharps must be disposed of in a puncture-resistant sharps container to prevent injury and reduce the risk of infection. Regular trash bins and biohazard bags do not provide adequate protection against punctures. Autoclaving sharps before disposal is not standard practice and does not address the immediate need for safe containment.

Question 30: Correct Answer: A) Preoperative teaching record
Rationale: The preoperative teaching record is crucial for ensuring that Mrs. Smith has received and understood all necessary preoperative instructions. This document includes information on fasting, medication adjustments, and other preparatory steps. The operative report and postoperative care plan are relevant after the surgery, while the discharge summary is used at the end of the hospital stay.

Question 31: Correct Answer: C) Inspect the suction tubing for kinks or blockages.
Rationale: The first step in troubleshooting inadequate suction is to inspect the suction tubing for kinks or blockages, as these are common issues that can easily be resolved. Option A is incorrect because replacing the canister may not address the root cause. Option B is incorrect as increasing the pressure without identifying the problem can be unsafe. Option D is a last resort after other troubleshooting steps have been taken.

Question 32: Correct Answer: A) Insertion of the laparoscope
Rationale: After establishing pneumoperitoneum, the next step in a laparoscopic cholecystectomy is the insertion of the laparoscope to visualize the abdominal cavity. Clipping the cystic artery and duct (B) and dissecting the gallbladder (C) occur later in the procedure. Closing the port sites (D) is the final step. Thus, option A is the correct sequence step immediately following pneumoperitoneum establishment.

Question 33: Correct Answer: C) 70°F to 75°F
Rationale: Pediatric patients are more susceptible to hypothermia due to their higher body surface area to weight ratio. The recommended operating room temperature for pediatric patients is 70°F to 75°F to ensure their safety and comfort. Option A (60°F to 65°F) is too low and increases hypothermia risk. Option B (68°F to 73°F) is suitable for adults but slightly lower than ideal for pediatric patients. Option D (75°F to 80°F) is too warm and can cause discomfort for the surgical team.

Question 34: Correct Answer: A) Drape the patient first, then cover the laparoscopic equipment with a separate sterile drape.
Rationale: Draping the patient first ensures the surgical field is sterile before introducing the laparoscopic equipment. Covering the equipment with a separate sterile drape maintains sterility throughout the procedure. Option B is incorrect as it risks contaminating the patient. Option C is impractical and may compromise sterility. Option D leaves the patient undraped, violating sterile technique.

Question 35: Correct Answer: B) To prevent delays during the surgery
Rationale: Verifying the availability of surgical equipment before a procedure is crucial to prevent delays during surgery. While familiarity (A) and compliance with policy (C) are important, they are secondary to the primary goal of ensuring that all

necessary equipment is ready and functional to avoid any interruptions. Maintaining cleanliness (D) is also vital but not directly related to the verification process.

Question 36: Correct Answer: B) Recalibrate the navigation system

Rationale: Recalibrating the navigation system is the immediate course of action when a discrepancy is noticed. This step ensures that the system's guidance aligns accurately with the patient's anatomy, maintaining surgical precision. Continuing the surgery and adjusting manually (A) or ignoring minor discrepancies (D) can lead to errors. Restarting the system (C) might not address the calibration issue and could cause delays. Recalibration directly addresses the alignment problem, ensuring accurate guidance.

Question 37: Correct Answer: B) Maintaining the correct intraocular pressure

Rationale: Maintaining the correct intraocular pressure is crucial for the safety and effectiveness of phacoemulsification as it stabilizes the anterior chamber and prevents complications. Option A is incorrect as lasers are not used in phacoemulsification. Option C, while important for infection control, is not directly related to the phacoemulsification process. Option D is unrelated to phacoemulsification and pertains to a different surgical procedure.

Question 38: Correct Answer: A) Sequential compression device (SCD)

Rationale: Sequential compression devices (SCDs) are crucial in preventing deep vein thrombosis (DVT) by promoting blood circulation in the legs during and after surgery. While a pulse oximeter (B) monitors oxygen levels, a Foley catheter (C) aids in urinary drainage, and a nasal cannula (D) provides supplemental oxygen, none of these directly prevent DVT, making SCDs the most appropriate choice for this scenario.

Question 39: Correct Answer: D) Using a sharpness testing device

Rationale: Using a sharpness testing device is the most reliable method to test the sharpness of surgical scissors. This method provides a consistent and objective measure of sharpness. Cutting through gauze and visual inspection are less reliable and can be subjective. Running a finger along the blade is unsafe and not recommended. The sharpness testing device ensures precision and safety in evaluating the instrument's condition.

Question 40: Correct Answer: B) Using the closed gloving technique.

Rationale: The closed gloving technique ensures that the hands do not touch the outside of the gloves, maintaining sterility. Touching the outside of the glove with bare hands (A) and adjusting the glove fit by touching the sterile gown (C) compromise sterility. Donning gloves before the sterile gown (D) is incorrect as the gown should be donned first to maintain aseptic technique.

Question 41: Correct Answer: B) Electrical equipment malfunction

Rationale: Electrical equipment malfunction is a common cause of fires in the operating room due to the presence of various electrical devices. Non-sterile instruments (A) can cause infections but not fires. Inadequate hand hygiene (C) leads to contamination, not fires. Poor lighting conditions (D) can affect visibility but do not directly cause fires. Proper maintenance and regular checks of electrical equipment are essential to prevent such hazards.

Question 42: Correct Answer: A) Check the battery or power supply.

Rationale: The first step is to check the battery or power supply, as this is the most common and easily fixable issue. Replacing the drill (B) or sterilizing a backup drill (D) are more time-consuming actions that should only be taken if the power supply is not the issue. Informing the surgeon (C) is important but should be done after a quick initial assessment.

Question 43: Correct Answer: B) Ultrasonic scalpel

Rationale: The ultrasonic scalpel is most commonly used for tissue dissection and coagulation during laparoscopic surgery. It uses high-frequency ultrasonic vibrations to cut tissue and coagulate blood vessels simultaneously. Cryotherapy (A) is used for freezing tissues, laser ablation (C) uses focused light for cutting or vaporizing tissue, and radiofrequency ablation (D) uses electrical currents to generate heat for tissue destruction. The ultrasonic scalpel is preferred for its precision and minimal thermal spread.

Question 44: Correct Answer: A) The temperature of the irrigation solution.

Rationale: The temperature of the irrigation solution is crucial as it can affect patient outcomes, including tissue damage and hypothermia. While the volume (Option C) and type (Option D) are important, they do not have the immediate impact on patient safety that temperature does. The color (Option B) is generally not a critical factor unless it indicates contamination or improper mixing. Ensuring the solution is at the correct temperature helps maintain physiological stability during surgery.

Question 45: Correct Answer: C) Drop in blood pressure

Rationale: A drop in blood pressure is a critical indicator of significant blood loss and requires immediate intervention. While decreased urine output (A), increased respiratory rate (B), and elevated heart rate (D) are also signs of blood loss, they are not as immediate or critical as a drop in blood pressure, which directly affects perfusion and organ function. Thus, option C is the most critical indicator.

Question 46: Correct Answer: C) Snug, allowing minimal movement but not causing discomfort

Rationale: The safety strap should be applied snugly to allow minimal movement but not cause discomfort, ensuring both safety and comfort. Tight enough to leave an indentation (Option A) can cause pressure injuries, while loose enough to fit a hand underneath easily (Option B) may not provide adequate restraint. Not applying the strap (Option D) is unsafe as it does not prevent accidental movement.

Question 47: Correct Answer: D) Ensuring the

surgical instruments are sterile

Rationale: The Universal Protocol (Time Out) focuses on confirming the patient's identity, verifying the surgical site and procedure, and reviewing any allergies or medical history. Ensuring the surgical instruments are sterile is a critical step but is not part of the Time Out procedure. This step is handled separately by the sterile processing team and surgical technologists before the Time Out.

Question 48: Correct Answer: A) Immediately after use.

Rationale: Contaminated sharps should be disposed of immediately after use to minimize the risk of needlestick injuries and contamination. Option B delays disposal, increasing risk. Option C is incorrect as waiting for the container to be full can lead to overfilling and risk of injury. Option D is incorrect because waiting until the patient leaves the operating room can cause unnecessary delays and potential hazards.

Question 49: Correct Answer: B) Update Dr. Johnson's preference card to reflect the new suture material.

Rationale: Updating Dr. Johnson's preference card ensures that his new preference is consistently followed in future surgeries. Making a mental note (Option A) or relying on verbal reminders (Option C) can lead to errors. Using the new suture material only when asked (Option D) does not guarantee consistency and may cause confusion among the surgical team.

Question 50: Correct Answer: B) To prevent skin irritation and pressure sores.

Rationale: The primary purpose of applying padding before the splint is to prevent skin irritation and pressure sores, ensuring patient comfort and safety. While additional support (A) is a secondary benefit, it is not the primary purpose. Making the splint easier to remove (C) and ensuring it adheres to the skin (D) are not correct; padding actually prevents direct contact with the skin, reducing the risk of complications.

Question 51: Correct Answer: C) Connect the drain to the suction tubing, compress the bulb, then activate the suction.

Rationale: The correct sequence ensures that the JP drain functions properly by creating a vacuum. First, connect the drain to the suction tubing to establish the pathway. Then, compress the bulb to create negative pressure. Finally, activate the suction to maintain continuous drainage. Options A, B, and D either disrupt the vacuum or fail to establish a proper pathway for drainage, leading to ineffective suction.

Question 52: Correct Answer: C) Passing the appropriate instruments to the surgeon

Rationale: The primary responsibility of the surgical technologist during the dissection of the cystic duct and artery is to pass the appropriate instruments to the surgeon. This ensures that the surgeon can efficiently and safely perform the procedure. Adjusting insufflation pressure (A) is typically managed by the anesthesia team, retracting the liver (B) is usually done by the assistant or surgeon, and monitoring vital signs (D) is the responsibility of the anesthesia provider.

Question 53: Correct Answer: B) Use sterile gloves to handle the suture material.

Rationale: Using sterile gloves to handle the suture material is essential to maintain sterility and prevent infection. Opening the suture packet with bare hands (Option A) or placing the suture on a non-sterile surface (Option C) compromises sterility. Cutting the suture with non-sterile scissors (Option D) introduces contaminants. Therefore, Option B is the correct and necessary step to ensure sterility.

Question 54: Correct Answer: B) Electrocardiogram (ECG) leads

Rationale: ECG leads are essential for continuously measuring the cardiac electrical activity during surgery, allowing for the detection of arrhythmias and other cardiac events. Capnography (A) measures exhaled CO2 and is crucial for respiratory monitoring but not for cardiac activity. The pulse oximeter (C) measures oxygen saturation, and the blood pressure cuff (D) measures blood pressure intermittently, neither of which provide continuous cardiac electrical data. Therefore, ECG leads (B) are the correct choice.

Question 55: Correct Answer: B) Temporalis fascia

Rationale: The temporalis fascia is most commonly used for tympanic membrane grafts due to its proximity and similar structure to the tympanic membrane. The nasal septum, buccal mucosa, and palatal mucosa are not typically used for this purpose as they do not provide the necessary structural compatibility. The temporalis fascia offers durability and an optimal healing environment, making it the preferred choice for tympanoplasty.

Question 56: Correct Answer: D) Pass the instrument with the tips facing the surgeon.

Rationale: The correct action is to pass the instrument with the tips facing the surgeon to facilitate immediate use and maintain sterility. Passing the instrument with tips downwards (A) or upwards (B) can cause injury or contamination. A neutral position (C) does not ensure the surgeon can grasp it correctly.

Question 57: Correct Answer: C) Using a high-level disinfectant on all surfaces

Rationale: Using a high-level disinfectant on all surfaces is crucial to eliminate any potential pathogens and prevent cross-contamination. While disposing of sharps (A) and removing linens and waste (D) are important, they do not address the need to disinfect surfaces. Wiping down surgical lights (B) is also necessary but not as comprehensive as disinfecting all surfaces.

Question 58: Correct Answer: B) Verify the medication and dosage with the circulating nurse before preparing it.

Rationale: Verifying the medication and dosage with the circulating nurse before preparing it ensures accuracy and patient safety. Administering immediately (A) or waiting until the end of surgery (D) can lead to errors or delays in necessary treatment. Asking the surgeon to confirm (C) is not the standard protocol for medication verification, which involves the circulating nurse.

Question 59: Correct Answer: C) To maintain accurate fluid balance for the patient

Rationale: Monitoring the amount of solution used is essential for maintaining accurate fluid balance, which is critical for patient stability during surgery. Ensuring enough supplies (A) and preventing contamination (B) are important but secondary to patient safety. Compliance with inventory protocols (D) is necessary but not the primary reason for monitoring solution use. Accurate fluid balance helps prevent complications such as hypovolemia or fluid overload.

Question 60: Correct Answer: C) Monopolar Electrosurgery

Rationale: Monopolar electrosurgery is commonly used in laparoscopic procedures for precise cutting and coagulation. Unlike the Harmonic Scalpel, which uses ultrasonic vibrations, or Bipolar Forceps, which are more suitable for delicate tissues, monopolar electrosurgery provides effective hemostasis. Cryotherapy Probe is not typically used for hemostasis in such procedures. Monopolar electrosurgery ensures efficient and controlled hemostasis, making it the most suitable choice in this scenario.

Question 61: Correct Answer: A) A fracture where the bone is broken into multiple pieces

Rationale: A comminuted fracture involves the bone being shattered into multiple pieces, often due to high-impact trauma. A partially bent bone (B) describes a greenstick fracture, a straight-across break (C) is a transverse fracture, and a spiral pattern break (D) is a spiral fracture. Understanding these distinctions is crucial for appropriate diagnosis and treatment.

Question 62: Correct Answer: C) The graft's size and shape compatibility.

Rationale: The primary consideration is the graft's size and shape compatibility with the surgical site to ensure proper fit and function. Tensile strength (A) and immunogenicity (B) are important but secondary factors. The graft's color and texture (D) are less critical for effectiveness. Proper size and shape (C) ensure the graft fits well, providing structural support and promoting healing.

Question 63: Correct Answer: C) Remove the trocars from the patient's abdomen.

Rationale: The first step in removing equipment after a laparoscopic procedure is to remove the trocars from the patient's abdomen. This ensures that no instruments are left inside and minimizes the risk of injury or complications. Removing the drapes (Option A) or disconnecting the insufflation tubing (Option B) should follow after ensuring all instruments are safely removed. Turning off the electrosurgical unit (Option D) is important but not the immediate first step in this context.

Question 64: Correct Answer: B) Fibrin sealant

Rationale: Fibrin sealant is ideal for controlling capillary bleeding in highly vascular areas because it mimics the final stages of the coagulation cascade, forming a stable clot. Bone wax (A) is used for bone bleeding, a tourniquet (C) is for limb surgeries to control blood flow, and electrocautery (D) is less effective for diffuse capillary bleeding. Fibrin sealant provides targeted hemostasis, ensuring effective control of capillary bleeding without extensive tissue damage.

Question 65: Correct Answer: D) Place instruments back in the instrument tray immediately

Rationale: The correct method is to place instruments back in the instrument tray immediately to maintain organization and ensure that no instruments are left behind. Option A is incorrect as placing instruments on the patient's chest can cause injury and contamination. Option B is incorrect because handing instruments directly to the circulating nurse can be inefficient and increase the risk of contamination. Option C is incorrect as leaving instruments on the drapes can lead to loss or damage during removal.

Question 66: Correct Answer: C) Increase the ultrasound power

Rationale: Increasing the ultrasound power is necessary to effectively emulsify a dense cataract. Decreasing the ultrasound power (Option B) would not provide sufficient energy to break up the cataract. Adjusting the aspiration flow rate (Option A) and irrigation flow rate (Option D) are important but do not directly address the need for more power to emulsify the dense cataract. Therefore, the correct adjustment is to increase the ultrasound power.

Question 67: Correct Answer: C) To check for any gas leakage in the tubing and connections

Rationale: Performing a leak test on a laparoscopic insufflator is essential to ensure there are no gas leaks in the tubing and connections, which could compromise patient safety. Options A, B, and D, while important, do not address the critical issue of gas leakage, which can lead to serious complications during surgery.

Question 68: Correct Answer: B) Paraphrasing the speaker's points

Rationale: Paraphrasing the speaker's points ensures that the listener accurately understands the information being communicated. While nodding occasionally (A) and maintaining eye contact (C) are supportive behaviors, they do not confirm understanding. Taking notes (D) is useful for record-keeping but does not ensure comprehension in real-time. Paraphrasing allows for immediate clarification and demonstrates active engagement.

Question 69: Correct Answer: B) Decrease the aspiration flow rate

Rationale: Decreasing the aspiration flow rate helps stabilize the anterior chamber by reducing the outflow of fluid, preventing chamber collapse. Increasing the irrigation flow rate (Option A) or ultrasound power (Option C) does not directly address the fluid dynamics causing the surge. Decreasing the irrigation flow rate (Option D) could exacerbate the issue by reducing the inflow of fluid. Therefore, the correct action is to decrease the aspiration flow rate.

Question 70: Correct Answer: C) On the thigh

Rationale: The correct placement of the bovie pad is

on a large, muscular area such as the thigh to ensure good electrical contact and minimize the risk of burns. Placing it over a bony prominence (A) or on the upper arm (B) can lead to inadequate contact and potential burns. The abdomen (D) is less ideal due to the presence of visceral organs and potential for movement during surgery.

Question 71: Correct Answer: B) Check the water level in the autoclave reservoir.

Rationale: The first step in troubleshooting an autoclave that fails to reach the required temperature is to check the water level in the reservoir. Insufficient water can prevent the autoclave from generating enough steam to reach the necessary temperature. Replacing the heating element (A) or restarting the cycle (C) may not address the root cause, while contacting biomedical engineering (D) should be done if simpler checks fail.

Question 72: Correct Answer: C) Denial

Rationale: Denial is the stage where the patient refuses to accept the reality of their terminal diagnosis, often as a defense mechanism to cope with overwhelming emotions. Anger (A) involves frustration and questioning, while Depression (B) is marked by deep sadness. Bargaining (D) involves making deals or promises in hopes of reversing the situation. Denial is distinct in its outright refusal to acknowledge the terminal diagnosis, making it the correct answer.

Question 73: Correct Answer: A) To list the surgical instruments and supplies preferred by the surgeon

Rationale: The primary purpose of a surgeon's preference card is to list the surgical instruments and supplies preferred by the surgeon, ensuring that the operating room is prepared according to the surgeon's specific needs. This helps in streamlining the surgical process and minimizing delays. Options B, C, and D are incorrect because they pertain to patient medical history, postoperative care, and billing, which are not the primary focus of a preference card.

Question 74: Correct Answer: D) Cleaning under fingernails

Rationale: Cleaning under fingernails is essential during a medical hand wash to ensure proper asepsis, as it removes debris and microorganisms that could cause infection. Option A is incorrect because a nail brush should be used for the entire duration, not just 30 seconds. Option B is incorrect as hot water can damage skin integrity. Option C is incorrect because hands should be kept higher than elbows to prevent contamination from water running down.

Question 75: Correct Answer: C) Curvilinear array probe

Rationale: The curvilinear array probe is suitable for intraoperative ultrasound in abdominal surgeries due to its ability to provide a wider field of view and penetrate deeper structures. The phased array probe (A) is more suited for cardiac imaging, the linear array probe (B) is better for superficial structures, and the endocavitary probe (D) is designed for internal cavities and not ideal for abdominal assessment.

Question 76: Correct Answer: B) Hip positioner

Rationale: The hip positioner is specifically designed to stabilize and align the leg during hip replacement surgery. The Wilson frame (A) is used for spinal surgeries, knee crutches (C) are for knee procedures, and the Mayfield headrest (D) is for neurosurgical procedures, making them unsuitable for a total hip replacement. The hip positioner ensures the leg remains in the correct position, reducing the risk of complications.

Question 77: Correct Answer: B) The type of ultrasound probe used.

Rationale: The most critical factor for ensuring optimal ultrasound imaging during a liver resection is the type of ultrasound probe used. Different probes offer varying resolutions and penetration depths, which are crucial for accurately locating lesions. While the experience of the surgical technologist (Option C) and the amount of saline used for acoustic coupling (Option D) are important, they are secondary to the choice of probe. The patient's BMI (Option A) is less critical compared to the probe type.

Question 78: Correct Answer: C) To provide a return path for the electrical current

Rationale: The primary purpose of securely attaching the bovie pad is to provide a return path for the electrical current, ensuring patient safety and effective electrosurgery. Preventing movement (A) and maintaining sterility (B) are not the primary purposes. Monitoring heart rate (D) is unrelated to the function of the bovie pad. Proper attachment prevents electrical burns and ensures the current flows safely back to the electrosurgical unit.

Question 79: Correct Answer: C) Laparoscopic camera system

Rationale: The laparoscopic camera system is crucial for a laparoscopic cholecystectomy as it provides the visual field necessary for the surgeon to perform the procedure. While the electrosurgical unit, suction apparatus, and surgical lights are important, the camera system is indispensable for visualization. Without it, the procedure cannot proceed safely or effectively.

Question 80: Correct Answer: C) Olfactory Nerve (I)

Rationale: The olfactory nerve (I) is responsible for the sense of smell. The optic nerve (II) is responsible for vision, the oculomotor nerve (III) controls most of the eye's movements, and the trigeminal nerve (V) is responsible for facial sensation and motor functions such as biting and chewing. Therefore, the olfactory nerve is the correct answer as it specifically transmits sensory information related to smell to the brain.

Question 81: Correct Answer: B) Capnograph

Rationale: A capnograph is essential for monitoring end-tidal CO2 levels, providing crucial information about a patient's ventilatory status. While a pulse oximeter measures oxygen saturation, an ECG monitors heart activity, and a thermometer measures body temperature, none of these devices can measure end-tidal CO2 levels, making the capnograph the correct choice.

Question 82: Correct Answer: C) Inform the surgeon or nurse to re-explain the procedure to the patient.

Rationale: It is crucial for the patient to fully

understand the risks and benefits of the procedure before giving informed consent. The surgical technologist should inform the surgeon or nurse to re-explain the procedure to ensure the patient is well-informed. Option A is incorrect as it is not within the surgical technologist's scope of practice to explain medical procedures. Option B is unethical and illegal. Option D disregards the patient's right to informed consent.

Question 83: Correct Answer: B) Venous bleeding

Rationale: Dark red or maroon blood suggests venous bleeding, which has a lower oxygen content compared to arterial blood. Arterial bleeding (Option A) is bright red due to higher oxygenation. Capillary bleeding (Option C) is usually slow and not characterized by such a dark color. Hemolysis (Option D) refers to the destruction of red blood cells, not the color of blood observed during bleeding. Recognizing these differences aids in identifying the source of bleeding and managing it effectively.

Question 84: Correct Answer: B) Using lead aprons and thyroid shields on the patient

Rationale: Using lead aprons and thyroid shields is the most effective way to minimize a patient's exposure to x-rays. Positioning the x-ray machine close to the patient (Option A) can increase exposure, increasing exposure time (Option C) raises radiation dose, and allowing the patient to hold the x-ray film (Option D) is unsafe and ineffective. Lead aprons and thyroid shields provide a physical barrier that significantly reduces radiation exposure.

Question 85: Correct Answer: C) Immobilization with a cervical collar

Rationale: Immobilization with a cervical collar is essential to prevent further injury to the cervical spine. Immediate removal of the cervical collar (A) could exacerbate the injury, application of a thoracic brace (B) is not appropriate for cervical injuries, and while administration of intravenous fluids (D) is important, it does not address the immediate need to stabilize the cervical spine.

Question 86: Correct Answer: D) Sterile, non-adherent dressing with an antiseptic layer.

Rationale: A sterile, non-adherent dressing with an antiseptic layer is most appropriate as it minimizes infection risk while promoting healing. Gauze dressing without antiseptic (Option A) lacks infection control. Transparent film dressing (Option B) is not suitable for wounds with high exudate. Hydrocolloid dressing (Option C) is better for pressure ulcers, not surgical wounds. The correct option ensures sterility and infection prevention, crucial for postoperative care.

Question 87: Correct Answer: B) Staphylococcus aureus

Rationale: Staphylococcus aureus is the most common cause of surgical site infections due to its ability to colonize the skin and mucous membranes. Escherichia coli and Pseudomonas aeruginosa are also pathogens but are less frequently associated with SSIs. Candida albicans is a fungal pathogen and is not a common cause of SSIs. Understanding the primary pathogens involved in SSIs is crucial for effective infection control and prevention in surgical practice.

Question 88: Correct Answer: C) Shut off the gas supply

Rationale: The most effective immediate action is to shut off the gas supply to prevent the fire from spreading and to eliminate the source of fuel. Evacuating the patient immediately (A) can be dangerous without controlling the fire first. Using a fire extinguisher (B) is important but secondary to stopping the gas flow. Calling for help and waiting (D) wastes critical time needed to control the fire.

Question 89: Correct Answer: B) Patient's consent form

Rationale: Verifying the patient's consent form is the most critical step because it ensures that the patient has been informed about the procedure, understands the risks, and has agreed to proceed. While insurance details, dietary restrictions, and family contact information are important, they do not directly impact the legality and ethicality of performing the surgery. Ensuring consent is a legal requirement and protects both the patient and the surgical team.

Question 90: Correct Answer: C) Drug-induced hypersensitivity

Rationale: Drug-induced hypersensitivity is a primary concern when a widespread rash and fever appear postoperatively. This reaction can be severe and requires immediate attention. Allergic reactions to latex and contact dermatitis typically do not cause fever. A surgical site infection would present with localized symptoms rather than a widespread rash. Thus, C is the most critical condition to address.

Question 91: Correct Answer: B) Reassure the patient by providing accurate information about the procedure.

Rationale: Reassuring the patient by providing accurate information about the procedure helps alleviate anxiety by addressing their concerns directly. Ignoring the patient's concerns (Option A) is unprofessional and neglects patient care. Telling the patient their anxiety will go away on its own (Option C) dismisses their feelings. Suggesting the patient speak to family members (Option D) may not provide the professional reassurance needed. Providing accurate information is the best approach to support the patient.

Question 92: Correct Answer: A) Axillary lymph nodes

Rationale: In breast cancer, the sentinel lymph nodes are typically the axillary lymph nodes because they are the first nodes to which cancer cells are likely to spread from the primary tumor. Inguinal lymph nodes are related to the lower limbs, cervical lymph nodes to the head and neck, and mesenteric lymph nodes to the intestines. Identifying the correct sentinel nodes is critical for accurate staging and treatment planning.

Question 93: Correct Answer: C) The patient might have an increased risk of poor oxygenation during surgery.

Rationale: A hemoglobin level of 8.5 g/dL is significantly lower than the normal range (12-16 g/dL for women), indicating anemia. This can lead to poor oxygenation during surgery, which is a critical concern. Option A is incorrect because anemia does not directly increase infection risk. Option B is incorrect as low hemoglobin does not inherently increase bleeding risk. Option D is incorrect because anemia does not directly cause electrolyte imbalance.

Question 94: Correct Answer: B) Cleaning the wound with sterile saline solution

Rationale: Cleaning the wound with sterile saline solution is essential to maintain sterility and prevent infection. Option A is incorrect because non-sterile gloves can introduce contaminants. Option C is incorrect as bare hands can compromise sterility. Option D is incorrect because using the same dressing for multiple wounds increases the risk of cross-contamination. Proper wound cleaning with sterile materials is crucial for optimal wound care.

Question 95: Correct Answer: A) Anterior to the hilum of the lung

Rationale: The phrenic nerve runs anterior to the hilum of the lung, making this the correct anatomical landmark. Posterior to the hilum (B) is where the vagus nerve is located, lateral to the trachea (C) is incorrect as the phrenic nerve runs more laterally, and medial to the esophagus (D) is incorrect as it is too posterior. Therefore, the correct answer is anterior to the hilum of the lung.

Question 96: Correct Answer: B) Checking expiration dates and rotating stock

Rationale: Checking expiration dates and rotating stock ensures that older supplies are used first, maintaining sterility and reducing waste. Placing new supplies in the front (A) can lead to expired items being overlooked. Storing supplies in their original packaging (C) is important but does not address stock rotation. Ensuring supplies are within easy reach (D) is convenient but not related to sterility and readiness.

Question 97: Correct Answer: C) Midline incision

Rationale: The midline incision provides extensive access to the entire abdominal cavity, making it ideal for exploratory laparotomies. The Pfannenstiel incision is limited to the lower abdomen, the McBurney incision is specific to the right lower quadrant, and the Kocher incision is subcostal and best for upper right quadrant access. While the other options are plausible, they do not offer the comprehensive access needed for a full abdominal exploration.

Question 98: Correct Answer: B) Ultrasonic vibrations

Rationale: The harmonic scalpel uses ultrasonic vibrations to cut and coagulate tissue simultaneously. Unlike electrical cauterization (A), laser energy (C), or radiofrequency waves (D), ultrasonic vibrations generate less heat, reducing thermal damage to surrounding tissues. This makes the harmonic scalpel particularly effective for precise surgical procedures with minimal collateral damage.

Question 99: Correct Answer: B) To enhance the accuracy of implant placement

Rationale: Computer navigation systems are primarily used in orthopedic surgery to enhance the accuracy of implant placement. Unlike option A, which is incorrect because surgical instruments are still necessary, and option C, which is incorrect as the duration of surgery may not necessarily be shortened, option B directly addresses the precision aspect. Option D is also incorrect as imaging techniques are still required for navigation.

Question 100: Correct Answer: B) Disassemble and soak nondisposable instruments in enzymatic cleaner.

Rationale: Nondisposable instruments should be disassembled and soaked in enzymatic cleaner to ensure thorough cleaning before sterilization. Option A is incorrect because sterile water alone does not effectively clean instruments. Option C is incorrect as instruments need to be cleaned before sterilization. Option D is incorrect because instruments must be cleaned and sterilized before reuse, not handed back for immediate reuse.

Question 101: Correct Answer: A) Calibrating the microscope's magnification settings

Rationale: Calibrating the microscope's magnification settings is a critical step in preoperative preparation to ensure accurate visualization during surgery. Option B is incorrect because the microscope does not connect to the anesthesia machine. Option C is incorrect as only the parts of the microscope that will come into contact with the sterile field need to be sterilized, not the entire body. Option D is incorrect because the microscope itself is not placed in the sterile field; only its sterile drape-covered parts are.

Question 102: Correct Answer: B) Anterior chamber

Rationale: The anterior chamber is the fluid-filled space between the cornea and the iris. The vitreous chamber (A) is located behind the lens and filled with vitreous humor. The posterior chamber (C) is the space between the iris and the lens. Aqueous humor (D) is the fluid within the anterior and posterior chambers, but it is not a space. Therefore, the anterior chamber is the correct identification as it specifically refers to the space between the cornea and the iris.

Question 103: Correct Answer: B) Ensuring all equipment is properly grounded

Rationale: Proper grounding of all equipment is essential for electrical safety in the operating room, as it helps prevent electrical shock and equipment malfunction. Option A is incorrect because using extension cords can pose a tripping hazard and may not provide adequate power. Option C is unsafe as overloading circuits can lead to electrical fires. Option D, while promoting safety, is not as critical as proper grounding for preventing electrical hazards.

Question 104: Correct Answer: B) Maintaining sterility

Rationale: Maintaining sterility is the primary consideration when removing equipment to prevent postoperative infections. Speed of removal (Option A) is secondary to sterility. While patient comfort (Option C) is important, it does not supersede the need for sterility. Minimizing noise (Option D) is not a primary concern in this context.

Question 105: Correct Answer: C) Discard the package and obtain a new sterile set
Rationale: Alex should discard the compromised package and obtain a new sterile set to maintain sterility and patient safety. Using instruments from a torn package (Option A) or resealing it (Option B) risks contamination. Informing the surgeon later (Option D) does not address the immediate risk of infection. Ensuring package integrity is crucial to preventing surgical site infections.

Question 106: Correct Answer: A) Ensuring the patient is draped with non-reflective materials
Rationale: Ensuring the patient is draped with non-reflective materials is crucial to prevent laser beam reflections that can cause unintended tissue damage or injury. Standard surgical masks (B) do not protect against laser hazards. Smoke evacuators (C) are important but secondary to preventing reflections. Wet towels (D) help in fire prevention but are less critical than non-reflective draping for laser safety.

Question 107: Correct Answer: B) Check that the suction tubing is securely connected.
Rationale: Ensuring the suction tubing is securely connected is crucial for the functionality of the suction system. An improperly connected tube can lead to loss of suction, which can compromise the procedure. Option A is incorrect because an empty canister is not enough to ensure functionality. Option C is incorrect as the pressure setting should be appropriate for the specific procedure, not a fixed value. Option D, while important, does not directly verify the functionality of the suction system.

Question 108: Correct Answer: B) Clamping and occluding
Rationale: The Kocher clamp is classified as a clamping and occluding instrument because it is designed to control bleeding by clamping blood vessels or tissues. Cutting and dissecting instruments, like scissors, are used for cutting tissues. Grasping and holding instruments, such as forceps, are used to hold tissues. Retracting and exposing instruments, like retractors, are used to hold back tissues to provide better visibility. The Kocher clamp's primary function is to occlude vessels, making it a clamping and occluding instrument.

Question 109: Correct Answer: C) To provide precise information for the patient's medical record
Rationale: Accurately reporting the amount of medication and solution used is crucial for maintaining precise patient medical records, which are essential for ongoing patient care and legal documentation. While ensuring correct postoperative dosage (A), maintaining inventory (B), and complying with policies (D) are important, they are secondary to the primary goal of accurate patient records.

Question 110: Correct Answer: B) To provide a sterile barrier while allowing access to the surgical site.
Rationale: A fenestrated drape is designed with an opening (fenestration) that allows access to the surgical site while maintaining a sterile barrier around it. Option A is incorrect as it does not address sterility.

Option C is incorrect because a single drape may not provide adequate coverage. Option D is incorrect since the primary function of the fenestrated drape is to ensure sterility, not to minimize the use of drapes.

Question 111: Correct Answer: C) Report the low inventory to the supply manager and request a restock based on usage trends.
Rationale: Reporting low inventory and requesting a restock based on usage trends ensures that supplies are managed efficiently and cost-effectively. Ignoring the issue (A) risks running out, ordering excessively (B) can lead to overstock and waste, and borrowing without informing (D) disrupts inventory management and accountability.

Question 112: Correct Answer: C) Utilizing a smoke evacuation system
Rationale: Utilizing a smoke evacuation system is the most effective method for reducing surgical smoke in the operating room. HEPA filters and high-filtration masks provide some protection but do not eliminate smoke at the source. Increasing room ventilation helps but is not as targeted or effective as a dedicated smoke evacuation system. Smoke evacuation systems capture and filter smoke directly at the surgical site, significantly reducing exposure to hazardous particles.

Question 113: Correct Answer: B) Risk of retinal damage to the surgical team.
Rationale: A significant safety concern when using an argon laser is the risk of retinal damage to the surgical team. Argon lasers emit visible blue and green light, which can be harmful to the eyes if proper protective eyewear is not used. Option A is incorrect as argon lasers do not typically cause deep tissue burns; Option C is incorrect as there is no high incidence of postoperative infections specifically associated with argon lasers; Option D is incorrect as excessive smoke production is not a primary concern with argon lasers.

Question 114: Correct Answer: B) Inform the circulating nurse to get the surgeon's signature before proceeding.
Rationale: The surgical technologist must ensure that all required signatures are present on the informed consent form before surgery. The surgeon's signature is crucial as it confirms that the surgeon has explained the procedure and obtained the patient's consent. Option A is incorrect because the surgery cannot proceed without the surgeon's signature. Option C is incorrect as the patient has already signed. Option D is incorrect because the surgeon's signature is essential for legal and ethical reasons.

Question 115: Correct Answer: B) Femoral artery
Rationale: The femoral artery is the primary artery responsible for supplying blood to the lower extremities. The brachial artery supplies blood to the upper arm, the carotid artery supplies blood to the head and neck, and the radial artery supplies blood to the forearm and hand. Understanding the correct anatomical pathways is crucial for surgical technologists to ensure proper vascular management during procedures.

Question 116: Correct Answer: A) Counting the instruments before removing the drapes.
Rationale: Counting the instruments before removing the drapes is crucial to ensure that no instruments are left inside the patient and to maintain an accurate count. Option B is incorrect because counting after removing the drapes can lead to contamination and errors. Option C is incorrect because counting after the patient is transferred can result in missing instruments. Option D is incorrect because counting during extubation can cause distractions and errors.

Question 117: Correct Answer: D) Remove the drapes starting from the surgical site outward.
Rationale: The correct sequence for removing the drapes is to start from the surgical site outward. This method helps to prevent contamination of the surgical site and maintains a sterile field as long as possible. Starting from the head (Option A), feet (Option B), or sides (Option C) does not prioritize the sterile field and could potentially introduce contaminants to the surgical site.

Question 118: Correct Answer: B) Fallopian tube
Rationale: The fallopian tube is responsible for transporting eggs from the ovaries to the uterus. The ureter carries urine from the kidneys to the bladder, the round ligament supports the uterus, and the broad ligament is a peritoneal fold that supports the reproductive organs. Identifying the fallopian tube is crucial to avoid complications during a hysterectomy.

Question 119: Correct Answer: B) Notify the surgeon immediately.
Rationale: The first action in an emergency situation is to notify the surgeon, who will then direct the appropriate interventions. Administering epinephrine (A) or increasing IV fluids (C) requires a physician's order. Chest compressions (D) are only necessary if the patient is in cardiac arrest, which is not indicated by the symptoms described.

Question 120: Correct Answer: A) Filtration of blood
Rationale: The glomerulus is a network of capillaries located at the beginning of a nephron in the kidney, and its primary function is to filter blood, removing waste products and excess substances. Reabsorption of water (B) occurs mainly in the renal tubules, secretion of hormones (C) is not a function of the glomerulus, and concentration of urine (D) occurs in the collecting ducts. Thus, the glomerulus is primarily responsible for blood filtration.

Question 121: Correct Answer: B) Update the preference card in the computer system immediately.
Rationale: Updating the preference card in the computer system immediately ensures that all team members have access to the most current information, reducing the risk of errors. Verbal communication (A) and notes (C) are not reliable for long-term accuracy. Waiting (D) can lead to outdated information being used in surgeries.

Question 122: Correct Answer: C) To prevent surgical complications and ensure proper fit
Rationale: Verifying the correct type and size of implantable items with the surgeon is crucial to prevent surgical complications and ensure the implant fits properly. This step is vital for patient safety and successful surgical outcomes. Option A is incorrect because insurance coverage is not the primary concern in this context. Option B is partially correct but does not address the primary reason. Option D is unrelated to the primary goal of verification.

Question 123: Correct Answer: C) Calibrating the microscope's ocular lenses
Rationale: Calibrating the microscope's ocular lenses is crucial to ensure proper focus and clarity during the procedure. While adjusting light intensity (A), balancing weight distribution (B), and cleaning the objective lens (D) are important, they do not directly address the precise focus needed for optimal visualization. Proper calibration ensures that both ocular lenses are aligned and focused, providing a clear and accurate view of the surgical field.

Question 124: Correct Answer: C) Notify the surgical team and replace the glove immediately.
Rationale: It is crucial to maintain sterility by notifying the surgical team and replacing the glove immediately. This prevents contamination and ensures patient safety. Option A is incorrect as it risks contamination. Option B is partially correct but lacks communication with the team. Option D is incorrect as any tear compromises sterility and must be addressed immediately.

Question 125: Correct Answer: B) Place the specimen in a sterile container without any preservative and label it with the patient's name, date of birth, and "Microbiological Culture."
Rationale: For microbiological cultures, the specimen must be placed in a sterile container without any preservative to prevent contamination and ensure accurate results. Labeling must include the patient's name, date of birth, and "Microbiological Culture." Incorrect options involve preservatives (A), incorrect labeling (C), or inappropriate handling (D), which could affect the culture results.

Question 126: Correct Answer: A) Turn off the cautery device and unplug it before removing the drapes.
Rationale: The most crucial step is to turn off and unplug the cautery device before removing the drapes to prevent accidental burns or electrical hazards. Option B is incorrect because the device should be turned off first. Option C is unsafe as standby mode can still pose risks. Option D is incorrect as it is unsafe to handle drapes with the device still on. Ensuring the device is off and unplugged is the safest practice.

Question 127: Correct Answer: C) Report the symptoms immediately to the surgeon.
Rationale: Severe abdominal pain, fever, and jaundice are abnormal postoperative findings that could indicate complications such as infection or bile duct injury. Immediate reporting to the surgeon is crucial for prompt intervention. Option A is incorrect as these symptoms are not normal. Option B is insufficient as over-the-counter medication will not address the underlying issue. Option D is inadequate since increased fluid intake and rest will not resolve

potential complications.

Question 128: Correct Answer: C) Flexibility in learning schedule

Rationale: The primary benefit of utilizing online continuing education platforms for Certified Surgical Technologists is the flexibility in learning schedule. Online platforms allow professionals to access courses at their convenience, accommodating their work schedules and personal commitments. Limited access to course materials (A) and inconsistent course quality (B) are not inherent to online platforms, and high costs (D) are often mitigated by the reduced need for travel and accommodation compared to traditional methods.

Question 129: Correct Answer: B) Implementing a standardized inventory management system

Rationale: Implementing a standardized inventory management system ensures that supplies are ordered based on actual usage rates, reducing waste and overstocking. Reusing single-use items (A) is against safety regulations. Ordering supplies in bulk (C) without considering usage rates can lead to excess inventory and waste. Using the most expensive instruments (D) unnecessarily increases costs without necessarily improving outcomes.

Question 130: Correct Answer: A) To reduce the risk of postoperative infection

Rationale: The primary purpose of using a surgical skin antiseptic is to reduce the risk of postoperative infection by significantly lowering the number of microorganisms on the skin. Option B is incorrect because it is impossible to remove all resident bacteria. Option C is incorrect as surgical instruments are sterilized through other means. Option D is incorrect because the sterile field is maintained through draping and other sterile techniques, not skin antiseptics.

Question 131: Correct Answer: B) Yankauer suction tip

Rationale: The Yankauer suction tip is specifically designed for effective removal of blood and debris during tonsillectomy procedures. It has a large opening and a curved design, which makes it ideal for oral and pharyngeal suctioning. The Poole suction tip is more suitable for abdominal procedures, the Frazier suction tip is used for neurosurgical and ENT procedures requiring fine suction, and the Rosen suction tip is used in otologic surgeries. Thus, the Yankauer is the most appropriate choice for tonsillectomy.

Question 132: Correct Answer: D) Ensure all counts are correct and accounted for.

Rationale: The first step in removing drapes and other equipment is to ensure all counts are correct and accounted for. This prevents any retained surgical items. Options A, B, and C are incorrect because they do not address the critical safety step of verifying that no instruments or sponges are left inside the patient, which is paramount before removing any equipment.

Question 133: Correct Answer: A) Lower risk of thermal injury to surrounding tissues

Rationale: The primary advantage of using an ultrasonic scalpel over traditional electrocautery is the lower risk of thermal injury to surrounding tissues. Ultrasonic scalpels operate at lower temperatures, reducing collateral damage. Higher coagulation temperatures (B) are not an advantage as they increase the risk of injury. While ease of use (C) and cost-effectiveness (D) are considerations, the key benefit is the reduced thermal spread, making ultrasonic scalpels safer for delicate tissues.

Question 134: Correct Answer: B) Check the air hose for leaks

Rationale: Before using a pneumatic power drill, it is crucial to check the air hose for leaks to ensure proper functionality and safety. Lubricating the drill with oil (A) can cause contamination, sterilizing with an autoclave (C) can damage the equipment, and ensuring the drill is fully charged (D) is irrelevant for pneumatic drills which do not use batteries.

Question 135: Correct Answer: C) Laparoscopic clip applier

Rationale: A laparoscopic clip applier is specifically designed to control bleeding from small vessels during minimally invasive procedures. It provides a mechanical means to occlude vessels quickly and effectively. While a laparoscopic stapler is used for tissue approximation and cutting, the harmonic scalpel uses ultrasonic vibrations for cutting and coagulation, and bipolar forceps use electrical energy. The clip applier is preferred for its precision and ease of use in controlling small vessel bleeding.

Question 136: Correct Answer: C) Position the limb in the desired alignment.

Rationale: The first step in applying a cast is to position the limb in the desired alignment to ensure proper healing. This step is crucial as it affects the overall outcome of the cast application. Applying padding directly to the skin (A) and immersing the casting material in water (B) are subsequent steps. Cutting the casting material (D) is also done later in the process. Proper limb alignment ensures the cast will support the bone correctly as it heals.

Question 137: Correct Answer: B) Helium is a noble gas that helps stabilize the laser beam.

Rationale: Helium, being a noble gas, is chemically inert and does not react with other substances, which helps in stabilizing the laser beam during intraoperative procedures. This stability is crucial for precision. Option A is incorrect because helium is not reactive. Option C is incorrect because helium is lighter than air. Option D, while helium does have high thermal conductivity, its primary role in laser technology is stabilization, not cooling.

Question 138: Correct Answer: C) Real-time updates through a centralized computer system

Rationale: Real-time updates through a centralized computer system ensure that all departments have access to the most current information simultaneously, reducing the risk of miscommunication. Verbal communication (A) and written memos (B) can lead to delays and errors, while weekly meetings (D) are not frequent enough to manage daily changes effectively. This method enhances coordination and efficiency in surgical schedules.

Question 139: Correct Answer: B) Notify the surgeon and replace the gown immediately.

Rationale: The correct action is to notify the surgeon and replace the gown immediately to maintain sterility and prevent contamination. Option A is incorrect because it does not address the breach in sterility. Option C is a common misconception but does not ensure sterility. Option D delays necessary action, risking contamination.

Question 140: Correct Answer: A) Check the battery charge level.

Rationale: The first step in assembling power equipment is to check the battery charge level to ensure the equipment will function throughout the procedure. This is crucial because a low battery can cause delays or complications. While verifying the sterilization indicator (C) and testing the equipment (D) are important, they come after ensuring the battery is charged. Attaching the blade or bit (B) should also follow the battery check to prevent unnecessary handling of sterile components.

Question 141: Correct Answer: C) Utilizing a dedicated continuing education tracking software

Rationale: Utilizing a dedicated continuing education tracking software is the most effective way for a Certified Surgical Technologist to keep track of their continuing education credits. This software can automatically update and remind the user of upcoming deadlines, ensuring accuracy and efficiency. In contrast, paper-based logbooks (A) can be lost or damaged, email notifications (B) can be missed or deleted, and mental notes (D) are unreliable and prone to forgetting.

Question 142: Correct Answer: B) Documenting surgical counts

Rationale: A key administrative duty of a CST is documenting surgical counts to ensure no instruments or sponges are left inside the patient. Scheduling surgeries (A) and managing patient records (C) are typically handled by other administrative staff. Supervising the surgical team (D) is the responsibility of the surgeon or head nurse. Accurate documentation of surgical counts is crucial for patient safety and legal compliance.

Question 143: Correct Answer: C) Notify the surgical team and follow the facility's spill protocol.

Rationale: The first action should be to notify the surgical team and follow the facility's spill protocol to ensure everyone's safety. Immediate cleaning (A) without proper protocol can cause harm. Evacuating the room (B) may not be necessary if the spill is contained. Continuing the procedure (D) without addressing the spill can lead to hazardous exposure.

Question 144: Correct Answer: C) Seal the container and replace it with a new one.

Rationale: Once a sharps container is three-quarters full, it should be sealed and replaced to prevent overfilling, which can lead to sharps injuries. Compressing the contents or continuing to use the container increases the risk of injury. Transferring sharps to another container is unsafe and not recommended.

Question 145: Correct Answer: B) Double-gloving

Rationale: Double-gloving significantly reduces the risk of exposure to bloodborne pathogens by providing an additional barrier. While wearing a surgical mask (A) and using a face shield (C) protect against splashes, they do not prevent direct contact with blood. Handwashing (D) is crucial but does not offer protection during the procedure itself. Double-gloving is the most effective intraoperative measure.

Question 146: Correct Answer: B) Using a nail cleaner under running water before starting the scrub

Rationale: Using a nail cleaner under running water before starting the scrub is crucial to remove debris and reduce microbial load. Scrubbing from the fingertips to the elbow (not elbow to fingertips) ensures contaminants are washed away. Drying hands and arms with a sterile, disposable towel (not reusable) prevents recontamination. The scrub should last 3-5 minutes, not just 1 minute, to be effective.

Question 147: Correct Answer: B) To prevent the spread of airborne pathogens from the surgical team to the patient

Rationale: The primary reason for wearing a surgical mask is to prevent the spread of airborne pathogens from the surgical team to the patient, thereby reducing the risk of surgical site infections. Option A is partially correct but not the primary reason. Option C is incorrect as warmth is not a concern. Option D is incorrect; masks can actually impede communication rather than enhance it.

Question 148: Correct Answer: B) Confirm the air pressure settings are within the recommended range.

Rationale: Confirming the air pressure settings are within the recommended range is most critical to ensure the pneumatic drill operates safely and effectively. Incorrect air pressure can lead to malfunction or insufficient power. While ensuring proper lubrication (A) and checking for wear and tear (C) are important maintenance steps, they do not directly impact immediate operation. Attaching the drill to the air supply line (D) is necessary but should follow verifying the correct air pressure to avoid potential issues during the procedure.

Question 149: Correct Answer: B) Confirming equipment functionality

Rationale: Confirming equipment functionality is the most critical step because non-functional equipment can lead to intraoperative complications and delays. While checking the inventory list (A), ensuring sterility (C), and reviewing the surgeon's preference card (D) are important, they do not address the immediate operability of the equipment, which is crucial for patient safety and surgical success.

Question 150: Correct Answer: C) Utilize local exhaust ventilation (LEV) systems

Rationale: Utilizing local exhaust ventilation (LEV) systems is the best practice to minimize the hazards of surgical smoke by directly capturing and removing it at the source. HEPA filters (A) are not as effective for smoke removal. Standard surgical masks (B) do not provide adequate protection against smoke particles. Increasing the room's air exchange rate (D) does not effectively address the localized nature of surgical smoke. Therefore, option C is the most appropriate and effective measure.

CST Exam Practice Questions [SET 3]

Question 1: During a colorectal surgery on a patient named Sarah, the surgeon requests a circular stapler for anastomosis. What is the most critical action the surgical technologist must perform before handing the stapler to the surgeon?
A) Ensure the stapler is fully assembled.
B) Check the integrity of the anvil and staple cartridge.
C) Lubricate the stapler for smooth operation.
D) Confirm the patient's allergy status.

Question 2: Which instrument is primarily used for clamping blood vessels during surgery?
A) Scalpel
B) Hemostat
C) Retractor
D) Suction tip

Question 3: During a total knee arthroplasty on a 60-year-old patient named Mary, the surgical team must ensure proper alignment of the prosthetic components. Which anatomical landmark is crucial for aligning the femoral component?
A) Tibial tuberosity
B) Medial malleolus
C) Anterior superior iliac spine
D) Femoral epicondyles

Question 4: During a laparoscopic cholecystectomy on Mr. Smith, the surgeon asks you to prepare a Jackson-Pratt (JP) drain for insertion. Which of the following steps is essential to ensure the drain functions properly?
A) Cut the drain to the desired length before insertion.
B) Ensure the bulb is compressed before connecting to the drain.
C) Connect the drain to the suction unit before insertion.
D) Fill the bulb with saline before connecting to the drain.

Question 5: What is the primary reason for documenting a patient's allergy status in the preoperative checklist?
A) To determine the type of anesthesia to be used
B) To prevent the use of contraindicated medications and materials
C) To ensure the patient receives appropriate nutritional support
D) To schedule follow-up appointments post-surgery

Question 6: During the preoperative preparation for a patient named John, the surgical technologist is responsible for preparing the surgical site. Which of the following steps should be performed first?
A) Apply antiseptic solution to the surgical site.
B) Shave the surgical site if necessary.
C) Position the patient on the operating table.
D) Verify the patient's identity and surgical site.

Question 7: During a mass casualty incident, the hospital's disaster plan is activated. As a Certified Surgical Technologist, what is your primary responsibility in the operating room?
A) Triage incoming patients.
B) Assist in the preparation and sterilization of surgical instruments.
C) Coordinate with the hospital's public relations department.
D) Manage the hospital's supply inventory.

Question 8: Which of the following structures is responsible for the production of cerebrospinal fluid (CSF) in the brain?
A) Pineal gland
B) Choroid plexus
C) Hypothalamus
D) Pituitary gland

Question 9: During the preoperative preparation of a patient named Mr. Smith, the surgical technologist is tasked with preparing the surgical site for an abdominal procedure. Which of the following is the correct sequence of steps for preparing the surgical site?
A) Apply antiseptic solution, then shave the area, and finally drape the patient.
B) Shave the area, apply antiseptic solution, and then drape the patient.
C) Drape the patient, apply antiseptic solution, and then shave the area.
D) Apply antiseptic solution, drape the patient, and then shave the area.

Question 10: During a phacoemulsification procedure, the surgical technologist notices that the anterior chamber is collapsing. What should be the first step to address this issue?
A) Increase the irrigation flow rate.
B) Decrease the ultrasound power.
C) Check for leaks in the tubing.
D) Adjust the patient's head position.

Question 11: During a surgical procedure, you notice that the instruments listed on Dr. Johnson's preference card do not match the instruments currently available in the operating room. What is the best course of action?
A) Proceed with the available instruments and inform Dr. Johnson later.
B) Immediately inform the circulating nurse to update the preference card.
C) Substitute the instruments with similar ones without informing anyone.
D) Pause the surgery and search for the correct instruments yourself.

Question 12: What is the primary reason for ensuring that the tubing of a surgical drain is not kinked when connected to a suction apparatus?
A) To prevent air from entering the suction system.
B) To maintain a sterile field.
C) To ensure continuous and effective drainage.
D) To avoid contamination of the surgical site.

Question 13: Which nerve is at risk of being damaged during a thyroidectomy, potentially leading to vocal cord paralysis?
A) Vagus nerve
B) Phrenic nerve
C) Recurrent laryngeal nerve
D) Hypoglossal nerve

Question 14: What is the primary role of a Certified Surgical Technologist (CST) during a hospital-wide disaster drill?
A) Directing patients to the nearest exit
B) Assisting in the triage area
C) Managing the surgical supply inventory
D) Performing administrative duties

Question 15: During the preoperative setup for a patient undergoing a forearm surgery, the surgical technologist must verify the pneumatic tourniquet settings. What is the appropriate action to take to ensure patient safety?
A) Select a tourniquet cuff that is too large to ensure complete occlusion.
B) Inflate the tourniquet to a pressure of 50 mmHg above the patient's diastolic blood pressure.
C) Verify the tourniquet pressure and duration settings with the surgeon before application.
D) Apply the tourniquet cuff loosely to avoid patient discomfort.

Question 16: What is the primary purpose of using a chlorhexidine gluconate (CHG) solution during preoperative skin preparation?
A) To moisturize the skin
B) To reduce the risk of surgical site infections
C) To provide a cooling sensation
D) To remove visible dirt and debris

Question 17: What is the primary purpose of using sequential compression devices (SCDs) in the preoperative setting?
A) To prevent deep vein thrombosis (DVT)
B) To reduce postoperative pain
C) To enhance wound healing
D) To maintain body temperature

Question 18: During a preoperative assessment, Maria, a 45-year-old patient, expresses concerns about the surgical team not understanding her cultural practices and dietary restrictions. How should the surgical technologist address Maria's concerns to ensure cultural competence and patient comfort?
A) Ignore the concerns and proceed with the standard preoperative protocol.
B) Reassure Maria that her concerns will be addressed and communicate them to the surgical team.
C) Suggest Maria follow the hospital's standard dietary guidelines.
D) Inform Maria that cultural practices are not considered in surgical settings.

Question 19: During an abdominal hysterectomy on a 52-year-old patient named Mrs. Johnson, the surgeon decides to use a stapling device to close the fascia. Which stapling device is most appropriate for this task?
A) Skin stapler
B) Linear stapler
C) Circular stapler
D) Fascial stapler

Question 20: Mary, a 60-year-old immunocompromised patient, is undergoing a total knee replacement. Which preoperative intervention is essential to address her immunocompromised status?
A) Scheduling the surgery early in the morning.
B) Administering prophylactic antiviral medication.
C) Isolating the patient in a sterile environment preoperatively.
D) Ensuring all surgical instruments are double-sterilized.

Question 21: During an organ procurement procedure for a patient named John, the surgical technologist is responsible for ensuring that the organs are preserved correctly. Which solution is most commonly used for organ preservation during transport?
A) Normal Saline
B) Ringer's Lactate
C) University of Wisconsin (UW) Solution
D) Dextrose 5% in Water

Question 22: Which of the following is the most critical step in managing a patient with a known latex allergy during preoperative preparation?
A) Administering antihistamines preoperatively
B) Scheduling the patient as the first case of the day
C) Using latex-free gloves and equipment
D) Informing the surgical team about the allergy

Question 23: Which of the following steps is crucial when preparing a wound site for dressing application during surgery?
A) Applying antiseptic ointment directly to the wound
B) Ensuring the wound area is completely dry before dressing
C) Using non-sterile gloves to handle the dressing materials
D) Covering the wound with a non-adhesive dressing

Question 24: What is the primary consideration when selecting instruments for a surgical

procedure?
A) The surgeon's preference
B) The type of surgery being performed
C) The availability of instruments
D) The patient's medical history

Question 25: Which type of joint is characterized by the presence of a fluid-filled cavity that allows for free movement?
A) Fibrous joint
B) Cartilaginous joint
C) Synovial joint
D) Suture joint

Question 26: What is the primary benefit of using active listening techniques during team meetings in a surgical setting?
A) It allows team members to multitask during the meeting
B) It ensures that only the leader's opinions are heard
C) It fosters a collaborative environment and improves team communication
D) It speeds up the decision-making process by reducing discussions

Question 27: Which of the following is the primary purpose of a Ground Fault Circuit Interrupter (GFCI) in a surgical setting?
A) To regulate the voltage supply to electrical equipment
B) To prevent electrical fires by monitoring circuit temperature
C) To protect personnel from electrical shock by interrupting the circuit
D) To ensure the continuous operation of essential medical devices

Question 28: What is the primary ethical responsibility of a surgical technologist when handling patient information?
A) Sharing patient information with colleagues for educational purposes.
B) Discussing patient information only with the surgical team involved in the case.
C) Posting patient information on social media without identifiers.
D) Storing patient information in personal devices for future reference.

Question 29: During an orthopedic surgery on a patient named Mrs. Thompson, the surgical technologist observes that the patient's blood pressure is steadily dropping. What should be the first step taken by the surgical technologist?
A) Increase the IV fluid rate.
B) Inform the surgeon and anesthesia provider immediately.
C) Administer a vasopressor.
D) Check for signs of bleeding at the surgical site.

Question 30: In the event of a natural disaster, the hospital's disaster plan requires all staff to report

to their designated areas. As a Certified Surgical Technologist, where should you report?
A) The hospital's command center
B) The emergency department
C) The operating room
D) The patient registration area

Question 31: During a mass casualty incident, the hospital has activated its disaster plan. As a Certified Surgical Technologist, what is your primary responsibility in this scenario?
A) Triage patients in the emergency department
B) Assist in setting up a temporary morgue
C) Prepare the operating room for incoming trauma cases
D) Provide psychological support to patients' families

Question 32: What is the primary purpose of a Durable Power of Attorney for Health Care in the context of advanced directives?
A) To appoint someone to make financial decisions
B) To designate a healthcare proxy to make medical decisions
C) To outline specific medical treatments a patient wants
D) To provide consent for a surgical procedure

Question 33: Susan is scheduled for an abdominal surgery. What is the correct sequence of actions the surgical technologist should take to prepare the surgical site?
A) Apply antiseptic solution, then shave the site, and finally drape the area.
B) Shave the site, apply antiseptic solution, and then drape the area.
C) Drape the area, shave the site, and then apply antiseptic solution.
D) Apply antiseptic solution, drape the area, and then shave the site.

Question 34: What is the first step a Certified Surgical Technologist should take when preparing to transfer a patient from the operating table to a stretcher?
A) Remove all surgical drapes and equipment from the patient.
B) Ensure the stretcher is locked and at the same height as the operating table.
C) Disconnect all IV lines and catheters before moving the patient.
D) Ask the patient to assist by moving themselves to the stretcher.

Question 35: During a laparoscopic cholecystectomy, the surgeon asks the surgical technologist to prepare a 4-0 absorbable suture for closing the cystic duct. Which of the following is the most appropriate action for the surgical technologist?
A) Prepare a 2-0 non-absorbable suture.
B) Prepare a 4-0 absorbable suture.
C) Prepare a 3-0 absorbable suture.

D) Prepare a 5-0 non-absorbable suture.

Question 36: What is the primary function of the renal cortex in the kidney?
A) Filtration of blood
B) Concentration of urine
C) Storage of urine
D) Regulation of blood pressure

Question 37: During the postoperative cleanup after Mrs. Johnson's surgery, which of the following actions should be taken to properly dispose of contaminated waste?
A) Double-bag the waste in two regular trash bags.
B) Place the waste in a biohazard container without sealing it.
C) Seal the waste in a biohazard bag and then place it in a designated biohazard waste container.
D) Incinerate the waste immediately in the operating room.

Question 38: When applying a cast, what is the primary purpose of using a stockinette?
A) To provide additional support to the injured area
B) To prevent the cast material from sticking to the skin
C) To increase the rigidity of the cast
D) To allow for better ventilation within the cast

Question 39: Which of the following is a key component of effective communication between a preceptor and a new perioperative personnel?
A) Using medical jargon to ensure precision
B) Providing constructive feedback in a timely manner
C) Limiting interactions to formal evaluations
D) Focusing solely on the trainee's mistakes

Question 40: Which of the following is the correct initial step in performing a surgical scrub?
A) Apply sterile gloves.
B) Rinse hands and forearms with water.
C) Clean subungual areas under running water.
D) Dry hands and arms with a sterile towel.

Question 41: Which of the following is a critical step in preventing surgical site infections (SSIs) according to standard and universal precautions?
A) Administering prophylactic antibiotics postoperatively
B) Ensuring proper sterilization of surgical instruments
C) Wearing non-sterile gloves
D) Using alcohol-based hand rubs only after the procedure

Question 42: Which of the following steps is crucial in ensuring the effectiveness of preoperative skin antisepsis?
A) Shaving the surgical site immediately before surgery
B) Applying antiseptic solution in a circular motion from the incision site outward
C) Using sterile water to rinse the antiseptic solution off the skin
D) Allowing the antiseptic solution to dry completely before draping

Question 43: Sarah, a 58-year-old patient, is undergoing aortic valve replacement surgery. During the procedure, the surgical team needs to ensure proper myocardial protection. Which solution is most commonly used for this purpose?
A) Lactated Ringer's solution
B) Normal saline
C) Cardioplegia solution
D) Dextrose 5% in water

Question 44: While preparing for a surgical procedure, a CST notices a chemical spill on the floor. What is the most appropriate personal protective equipment (PPE) to don before addressing the spill?
A) Sterile gloves and surgical mask.
B) Non-sterile gloves, gown, and face shield.
C) Surgical cap and shoe covers.
D) Sterile gloves and gown.

Question 45: Which of the following is the most appropriate action when removing suction equipment from a patient postoperatively?
A) Disconnect the suction tubing while the device is still running.
B) Turn off the suction device before disconnecting the tubing.
C) Remove the suction catheter first, then turn off the device.
D) Leave the suction device on until the patient is fully awake.

Question 46: In the preparation of synthetic tissue grafts, which sterilization method is most appropriate to ensure the material remains biocompatible?
A) Autoclaving
B) Ethylene oxide gas
C) Dry heat
D) Ultraviolet radiation

Question 47: During a postoperative debriefing, the surgical team is discussing the outcomes of Mrs. Lee's orthopedic surgery. How should you, as a Certified Surgical Technologist, use interpersonal skills to contribute effectively to the discussion?
A) Share your thoughts immediately, regardless of the current speaker.
B) Actively listen to others and wait for a pause before contributing.
C) Focus solely on your own tasks and avoid engaging in the discussion.
D) Offer your opinions only if directly asked by the surgeon.

Question 48: Dr. Smith has a specific preference

for the type of suture material used in her surgeries. As a surgical technologist, how should you ensure that her preference is consistently met for every procedure?
A) Memorize Dr. Smith's preferences and recall them during each surgery.
B) Regularly update Dr. Smith's preference card in the computer system.
C) Ask Dr. Smith before each surgery about her suture preference.
D) Use the most commonly used suture material in the hospital.

Question 49: 0 Which of the following best describes the pathogenesis of Clostridium difficile in causing pseudomembranous colitis?
A) Production of endotoxins that cause systemic inflammation
B) Invasion of intestinal mucosa leading to tissue necrosis
C) Production of exotoxins that disrupt the intestinal epithelium
D) Formation of biofilms on the intestinal lining

Question 50: During an orthopedic surgery on a patient named Mrs. Johnson, the anesthesiologist reports a drop in blood pressure and an increase in heart rate. What should the surgical technologist do to assist in managing the patient's blood loss?
A) Increase the lighting in the operating room for better visibility.
B) Hand the surgeon a hemostatic agent to control the bleeding.
C) Adjust the patient's position to improve circulation.
D) Prepare the electrocautery device for use.

Question 51: During a postoperative procedure, the surgical technologist is responsible for reporting the medication and solution amounts used. If a patient named Mr. Smith received 500 ml of saline solution and 2 mg of morphine, what is the correct way to document this in the patient's records?
A) Document only the saline solution amount.
B) Document only the morphine amount.
C) Document both the saline solution and morphine amounts.
D) Document the saline solution amount and note that morphine was administered without specifying the amount.

Question 52: What is the first step in the inspection process of surgical instruments before sterilization?
A) Lubricating the instruments
B) Checking for proper function
C) Cleaning the instruments
D) Assembling the instruments

Question 53: Which of the following is a critical step a CST must take to ensure proper tissue procurement?
A) Ensuring the donor's family has given consent
B) Performing the tissue biopsy
C) Labeling and documenting the harvested tissues accurately
D) Deciding the recipient for the harvested tissue

Question 54: What is the first step a surgical technologist should take upon noticing significant bleeding at the surgical site during the postoperative period?
A) Apply a tourniquet above the surgical site.
B) Notify the surgeon immediately.
C) Increase the patient's IV fluid rate.
D) Administer a dose of anticoagulant.

Question 55: During an orthopedic surgery on Mrs. Smith, the surgeon asks for an instrument to cut small bone fragments. Which instrument should the surgical technologist provide?
A) Rongeur
B) Osteotome
C) Bone curette
D) Bone rasp

Question 56: What is a critical consideration when preparing a geriatric patient for surgery in terms of preoperative assessment?
A) Assessing the patient's nutritional status
B) Evaluating the patient's exercise routine
C) Reviewing the patient's travel history
D) Checking the patient's vaccination records

Question 57: During the preoperative assessment of Mr. Johnson, a 65-year-old patient scheduled for a total knee replacement, which document is essential to verify his current medications and potential allergies?
A) Surgical consent form
B) Anesthesia consent form
C) Preoperative checklist
D) Medication reconciliation form

Question 58: Which of the following is the most critical step in preoperative preparation for a patient with a known latex allergy?
A) Administering prophylactic antibiotics
B) Scheduling the surgery as the first case of the day
C) Using latex-free gloves and equipment
D) Ensuring the patient has fasted for at least 8 hours

Question 59: During a postoperative case debrief, which of the following is a key component to discuss?
A) The surgeon's personal schedule
B) Equipment malfunctions and their impact on the procedure
C) The patient's insurance details
D) The weather conditions on the day of surgery

Question 60: During a surgical procedure, a chemical spill occurs in the operating room. What

is the first action that the Certified Surgical Technologist should take to ensure safety?
A) Call for housekeeping to clean up the spill.
B) Evacuate the operating room immediately.
C) Contain the spill using appropriate materials.
D) Inform the surgeon about the spill.

Question 61: During the postoperative phase, the surgical technologist must remove the drapes from Ms. Smith after a cholecystectomy. Which of the following actions should be taken to ensure the patient's skin integrity is maintained?
A) Quickly pull the drapes off to minimize time under anesthesia.
B) Gently lift the drapes, avoiding any adhesive areas.
C) Cut the drapes away from the patient to avoid movement.
D) Leave the drapes until the patient is fully awake.

Question 62: During an ophthalmic procedure on Mr. Johnson, the surgeon requests the surgical technologist to identify the structure responsible for maintaining the shape of the eyeball and providing protection. Which structure should the surgical technologist identify?
A) Retina
B) Cornea
C) Sclera
D) Lens

Question 63: During a surgical procedure, the surgical technologist, Alex, notices that the sterilization indicator on a pack of instruments has not changed color. What should Alex do next?
A) Use the instruments since they appear clean.
B) Notify the surgeon and replace the instruments with a sterile set.
C) Re-sterilize the instruments immediately.
D) Ignore the indicator and proceed with the surgery.

Question 64: In a total knee arthroplasty, what is the primary role of the surgical technologist during the cementing of the prosthesis?
A) Positioning the limb
B) Mixing the bone cement
C) Holding retractors
D) Suctioning excess cement

Question 65: What is the primary health risk associated with exposure to surgical smoke for operating room personnel?
A) Respiratory infections
B) Eye irritation
C) Carcinogenic effects
D) Skin rashes

Question 66: When should hair removal be performed to best reduce the risk of surgical site infections (SSIs)?
A) Immediately before entering the operating room
B) The night before surgery
C) At least 24 hours before surgery
D) In the preoperative holding area, just before surgery

Question 67: During a craniotomy procedure on a patient named John, the surgeon needs to access the area responsible for motor control. Which lobe of the brain should the surgeon focus on?
A) Temporal Lobe
B) Occipital Lobe
C) Parietal Lobe
D) Frontal Lobe

Question 68: What is the primary reason for using an allograft in orthopedic surgery?
A) It provides a scaffold for bone regeneration.
B) It eliminates the risk of disease transmission.
C) It completely avoids immune rejection.
D) It guarantees faster healing than autografts.

Question 69: In a case of bladder cancer, a cystectomy is planned for a 60-year-old female patient named Mary. Which anatomical structure must be resected along with the bladder to ensure complete removal of the cancerous tissue?
A) Urethra
B) Ureters
C) Pelvic lymph nodes
D) Adrenal glands

Question 70: Which bone is primarily responsible for the articulation with the femur at the hip joint?
A) Tibia
B) Pelvis
C) Fibula
D) Patella

Question 71: During a laparoscopic cholecystectomy on a 45-year-old patient named John, the surgeon needs to identify the structures within the Calot's triangle. Which of the following structures is NOT found within Calot's triangle?
A) Cystic duct
B) Common hepatic duct
C) Cystic artery
D) Common bile duct

Question 72: Which disease process involves the abnormal proliferation of cells in the colon, potentially leading to obstruction and requiring surgical resection?
A) Crohn's Disease
B) Ulcerative Colitis
C) Colorectal Cancer
D) Irritable Bowel Syndrome (IBS)

Question 73: Sarah, a bariatric patient scheduled for surgery, has a history of obstructive sleep apnea (OSA). Which preoperative intervention is most important to reduce her risk of postoperative respiratory complications?
A) Administering a preoperative sedative to reduce

anxiety
B) Ensuring the patient uses her CPAP machine up to the time of surgery
C) Scheduling the surgery early in the morning
D) Providing detailed postoperative pain management instructions

Question 74: During a laparoscopic cholecystectomy on a patient named Mr. Smith, which patient position is most appropriate to optimize the surgical field and minimize complications?
A) Supine with arms tucked
B) Trendelenburg position
C) Reverse Trendelenburg position with slight left tilt
D) Lithotomy position

Question 75: During a laparoscopic cholecystectomy on a patient named Mr. Smith, the surgeon decides to use a harmonic scalpel. What is the primary advantage of using a harmonic scalpel over traditional electrosurgery in this procedure?
A) It provides better hemostasis with less thermal spread.
B) It is more cost-effective than traditional electrosurgery.
C) It requires less training to operate.
D) It eliminates the need for anesthesia.

Question 76: Which of the following actions is most appropriate for a surgical technologist to take if they witness a colleague violating sterile technique during a procedure?
A) Ignore the violation to avoid confrontation.
B) Report the violation to the surgical supervisor immediately.
C) Wait until the procedure is over to address the issue.
D) Correct the colleague privately after the procedure.

Question 77: During a surgical procedure, the surgeon notices that the patient, Mr. Johnson, has a large, inflamed area on his skin with pus formation. The surgeon suspects an abscess. Which layer of the integumentary system is most likely affected in this scenario?
A) Epidermis
B) Dermis
C) Hypodermis
D) Stratum Corneum

Question 78: When should sequential compression devices (SCDs) be applied to a patient undergoing surgery?
A) Immediately after the patient is anesthetized
B) After the surgical incision is made
C) Before the induction of anesthesia
D) During the postoperative recovery phase

Question 79: How should a surgical technologist handle contaminated waste to comply with

Standard Precautions?
A) Double-bag the waste in regular trash bags.
B) Use a single biohazard bag.
C) Incinerate the waste immediately.
D) Place the waste in a biohazard container.

Question 80: Which of the following is a critical aspect of restocking supplies in the operating room?
A) Placing sterile supplies on the floor
B) Ensuring all supplies are within their expiration dates
C) Storing supplies in random order
D) Mixing sterile and non-sterile items

Question 81: What is the primary advantage of using an ultrasonic scalpel over traditional electrocautery in surgical procedures?
A) Lower cost
B) Reduced thermal spread
C) Faster cutting speed
D) Easier to use

Question 82: During a surgical procedure, the lead surgeon, Dr. Smith, becomes visibly frustrated and raises his voice at the scrub tech, Emily, for not anticipating his next instrument request. As a Certified Surgical Technologist, what is the most appropriate response Emily should take to maintain a positive team dynamic?
A) Argue with Dr. Smith to defend her actions.
B) Ignore Dr. Smith and continue with her tasks.
C) Apologize to Dr. Smith and ask for clarification on his preferences.
D) Leave the operating room to avoid further conflict.

Question 83: Emily, a 45-year-old female, presents with severe abdominal pain radiating to her back, nausea, and vomiting. Lab results show elevated serum amylase and lipase levels. What is the most likely diagnosis?
A) Appendicitis
B) Pancreatitis
C) Cholelithiasis
D) Peptic Ulcer Disease

Question 84: When using a thermal cautery device, what is the primary safety concern that a Certified Surgical Technologist should monitor?
A) Infection control
B) Electrical grounding
C) Thermal injury to surrounding tissues
D) Sterility of the device

Question 85: During a total knee arthroplasty on a patient named Sarah, the surgeon needs to control bleeding from the bone surface. Which mechanical method is most appropriate for this situation?
A) Bone wax
B) Electrocautery
C) Gelatin sponge

D) Tourniquet

Question 86: Which of the following is the most appropriate action when a postoperative patient shows signs of respiratory distress?
A) Increase the patient's oxygen flow rate
B) Call for immediate medical assistance
C) Reposition the patient to a more comfortable position
D) Administer pain medication

Question 87: In the midst of a delicate vascular surgery on Mrs. Smith, the surgical technologist notices a slight misalignment in the operating microscope. What is the best immediate action to take?
A) Reposition the patient to align with the microscope
B) Adjust the microscope's fine focus knob
C) Inform the surgeon and assist in realigning the microscope
D) Increase the magnification to compensate for the misalignment

Question 88: What is the correct sequence for donning a sterile gown and gloves in the operating room?
A) Don gloves first, then the gown
B) Don the gown first, then the gloves
C) Don the mask first, then the gown, and finally the gloves
D) Don the cap first, then the gloves, and finally the gown

Question 89: During the postoperative clean-up of an operating room, the surgical technologist notices that several sterile supply packages are torn. What is the most appropriate action to take?
A) Tape the torn packages and place them back in the sterile supply area.
B) Discard the torn packages and document the incident.
C) Use the supplies from the torn packages if they appear uncontaminated.
D) Report the torn packages to the surgeon and seek further instructions.

Question 90: During a surgical procedure on Mr. Johnson, the surgeon decides to use an argon laser for retinal photocoagulation. What is a key characteristic of argon lasers that makes them suitable for this procedure?
A) Argon lasers emit infrared light.
B) Argon lasers are absorbed by melanin.
C) Argon lasers produce a continuous wave beam.
D) Argon lasers are absorbed by the retinal pigment epithelium.

Question 91: During a cholecystectomy, the surgeon asks for the specimen to be sent for a frozen section analysis. What is the correct procedure for verifying, preparing, and labeling the specimen?

A) Place the specimen in formalin and label it with the patient's name and date of surgery.
B) Place the specimen on a dry container and label it with the patient's name, date of surgery, and "frozen section."
C) Place the specimen in saline and label it with the patient's name and type of specimen.
D) Place the specimen in a sterile container and label it with the patient's name, date of surgery, and type of specimen.

Question 92: During a complex surgery, the surgical technologist, Maria, notices a slight burning smell coming from the electrosurgical unit (ESU). What is the most appropriate action for Maria to take to ensure patient safety?
A) Continue using the ESU but monitor it closely.
B) Turn off the ESU immediately and inform the surgeon.
C) Replace the ESU with a backup unit.
D) Move the ESU to a different location in the operating room.

Question 93: During a laparoscopic cholecystectomy, the surgical team notices a significant amount of smoke accumulating in the operative field. What is the most appropriate immediate action to ensure a safe environment for both the patient and the surgical team?
A) Increase the insufflation pressure to clear the smoke.
B) Use a smoke evacuation system to remove the smoke.
C) Open the operating room doors to ventilate the area.
D) Pause the procedure until the smoke dissipates naturally.

Question 94: What is the primary function of the Eustachian tube in the ear?
A) Transmitting sound waves to the inner ear
B) Equalizing air pressure between the middle ear and the atmosphere
C) Producing earwax to protect the ear canal
D) Detecting changes in head position for balance

Question 95: Where should the bovie pad be placed to ensure optimal grounding during an electrosurgical procedure?
A) On the patient's chest
B) On a well-vascularized, muscular area
C) On the patient's forehead
D) On a bony prominence

Question 96: During a preoperative procedure, the surgical team is preparing to position Mr. Johnson for a laparoscopic cholecystectomy. Which of the following actions is most critical to ensure proper positioning and patient safety?
A) Placing a pillow under the patient's knees to prevent hyperextension.
B) Securing the patient's arms at their sides with

padded arm boards.

C) Ensuring the patient's head is elevated to prevent aspiration.

D) Placing the patient in the Trendelenburg position to improve access to the surgical site.

Question 97: Which type of lighting is essential for providing optimal visibility of the surgical site during an operation?
A) Ambient lighting
B) Task lighting
C) Overhead fluorescent lighting
D) Surgical lighting

Question 98: During an open appendectomy on a patient named Ms. Johnson, the surgical field becomes obscured by excessive fluid accumulation. What is the most effective method for the surgical technologist to maintain a clear operative field?
A) Use a Yankauer suction tip to remove the fluid.
B) Continuously irrigate the area with saline.
C) Place multiple sponges around the operative site.
D) Use a Poole suction tip to remove the fluid.

Question 99: What is the primary function of the seminiferous tubules in the male reproductive system?
A) Production of testosterone
B) Storage of sperm
C) Production of sperm
D) Transport of sperm

Question 100: Mrs. Thompson, an 82-year-old patient with a history of hypertension and diabetes, is scheduled for a hip replacement surgery. Which preoperative preparation step is most crucial to minimize the risk of postoperative complications?
A) Administering a high-dose sedative to ensure the patient is calm.
B) Ensuring the patient is well-hydrated and has stable blood glucose levels.
C) Scheduling the surgery late in the day to accommodate the patient's routine.
D) Avoiding the use of compression stockings to prevent discomfort.

Question 101: Which of the following steps is crucial when connecting a Jackson-Pratt drain to a suction apparatus to ensure proper function?
A) Clamping the drain before connection
B) Ensuring the drain is fully compressed before attaching to suction
C) Attaching the drain to the suction apparatus before compressing it
D) Leaving the drain open to air before connection

Question 102: During the postoperative phase for Mrs. Johnson, the surgical technologist must ensure that all equipment is properly removed. What is the correct method for handling the suction canister?
A) Empty the suction canister into the sink and rinse it out.
B) Seal the suction canister and dispose of it in a biohazard container.
C) Leave the suction canister in the operating room for housekeeping to handle.
D) Disconnect the suction canister and store it for future use.

Question 103: During the preoperative assessment of Mr. Johnson, a 65-year-old patient scheduled for elective hip replacement surgery, the surgical technologist notices that he has a history of deep vein thrombosis (DVT). What is the most appropriate preoperative intervention to reduce the risk of thromboembolism?
A) Administer a high dose of aspirin
B) Apply sequential compression devices (SCDs)
C) Encourage early ambulation post-surgery
D) Provide a high-protein diet

Question 104: Which of the following steps is crucial in maintaining retractors during surgery?
A) Sterilizing the retractor mid-procedure
B) Ensuring the retractor is properly positioned and adjusted
C) Frequently changing the retractor
D) Using multiple retractors simultaneously

Question 105: Sarah, a surgical technologist, is preparing the operating room for an orthopedic surgery. She notices that the surgical instruments are not arranged in the correct order. What is the best course of action for Sarah to take?
A) Rearrange the instruments according to the surgeon's preference card.
B) Leave the instruments as they are and inform the surgeon.
C) Ask the circulating nurse to rearrange the instruments.
D) Wait until the surgery starts and then arrange the instruments.

Question 106: When removing drapes and other equipment from the patient postoperatively, what is the primary purpose of using suction?
A) To remove blood clots only.
B) To clear the airway of the patient.
C) To remove all fluids and debris from the surgical site.
D) To dry the surgical site completely.

Question 107: During a surgical procedure to repair a torn rotator cuff, the surgeon asks the surgical technologist to identify the muscle primarily involved in this injury. Which muscle is the surgeon referring to?
A) Deltoid
B) Supraspinatus
C) Biceps brachii
D) Trapezius

Question 108: Sarah is undergoing surgery to relieve pressure caused by a brain tumor. The tumor is located in the area responsible for processing visual information. Which lobe of the brain is affected?
A) Temporal Lobe
B) Occipital Lobe
C) Parietal Lobe
D) Frontal Lobe

Question 109: Which of the following is the most appropriate method for applying light handles during the preoperative preparation?
A) Using sterile gloves to attach the light handles directly
B) Applying the light handles before the patient is draped
C) Using a sterile handle cover to attach the light handles
D) Attaching the light handles after the surgical procedure begins

Question 110: Ms. Garcia, a 45-year-old patient with diabetes, is scheduled for abdominal surgery. During the preoperative preparation, what is the most critical factor the surgical technologist should monitor to prevent complications?
A) Blood glucose levels
B) Blood pressure
C) Heart rate
D) Respiratory rate

Question 111: You are part of a surgical team performing a complex procedure on Mr. Thompson. Midway through the surgery, a new team member makes a suggestion that contradicts the established protocol. How should you diplomatically address this situation?
A) Dismiss the suggestion outright and continue with the protocol.
B) Acknowledge the suggestion and explain why the established protocol is being followed.
C) Implement the new suggestion immediately to show flexibility.
D) Ask the new team member to leave the operating room.

Question 112: What is the primary reason for performing a surgical count of instruments and supplies before a procedure?
A) To ensure all instruments are functioning properly
B) To confirm the availability of all required instruments
C) To prevent retained surgical items
D) To organize instruments in the correct order of use

Question 113: What is the most appropriate method for passing a scalpel to the surgeon during a surgical procedure?
A) Handing it directly to the surgeon's dominant hand

B) Placing it on the Mayo stand for the surgeon to pick up
C) Passing it handle-first with a firm grip
D) Passing it blade-first to ensure quick access

Question 114: During a laparoscopic cholecystectomy on a patient named Mr. Johnson, the surgical technologist notices that the patient's end-tidal CO2 levels are gradually increasing. What should be the immediate action taken by the surgical technologist?
A) Increase the oxygen flow rate.
B) Inform the anesthesia provider immediately.
C) Adjust the position of the patient.
D) Check the insufflation pressure.

Question 115: During an open heart surgery on a 60-year-old patient named Mrs. Smith, the surgical technologist observes bright red blood in the operative field. What does this indicate about the patient's current physiological status?
A) The patient is experiencing hypercapnia.
B) The patient has a high oxygen saturation level.
C) The patient is experiencing acidosis.
D) The patient has a low hemoglobin level.

Question 116: 2 Which of the following is a primary characteristic of Gram-positive bacteria?
A) Thin peptidoglycan layer
B) Outer membrane
C) Thick peptidoglycan layer
D) Presence of lipopolysaccharides

Question 117: Which of the following patient monitoring devices is primarily used to continuously measure the oxygen saturation of a patient's blood during surgery?
A) Electrocardiogram (ECG)
B) Pulse oximeter
C) Capnograph
D) Blood pressure cuff

Question 118: After completing a surgical procedure on Mr. Johnson, the surgical technologist must dispose of the contaminated sharps. What is the correct method for disposing of these sharps in compliance with Standard Precautions?
A) Place the sharps in a red biohazard bag.
B) Place the sharps in a puncture-resistant sharps container.
C) Place the sharps in a regular trash bin.
D) Place the sharps in a sealed plastic bag.

Question 119: Which lymphatic organ is primarily responsible for the maturation of T-lymphocytes?
A) Spleen
B) Thymus
C) Lymph nodes
D) Bone marrow

Question 120: Which of the following actions is

essential to maintain aseptic technique when opening sterile supplies in the operating room?
A) Open the sterile package towards your body.
B) Open the sterile package away from your body.
C) Use your bare hands to open the sterile package.
D) Place the sterile package on a non-sterile surface.

Question 121: During the preoperative preparation of Mr. Johnson, a 65-year-old patient scheduled for a laparoscopic cholecystectomy, what is the most appropriate placement for the safety strap to ensure patient safety?
A) Across the patient's chest
B) Across the patient's thighs
C) Across the patient's ankles
D) Across the patient's hips

Question 122: During a laparoscopic cholecystectomy, the surgeon asks you to connect and activate a Jackson-Pratt (JP) drain to a suction apparatus. Which of the following steps should you perform first?
A) Attach the drain to the suction tubing before securing it to the patient.
B) Secure the drain to the patient before connecting it to the suction tubing.
C) Prime the suction tubing with saline before attaching it to the drain.
D) Ensure the suction apparatus is turned off before connecting the drain.

Question 123: After completing a surgical procedure on Mr. Johnson, the surgical technologist is responsible for performing the room clean-up and restocking supplies. Which of the following steps should be performed first to ensure proper room turnover?
A) Disinfect all surfaces and equipment in the operating room.
B) Remove all soiled linens and waste materials.
C) Restock sterile supplies and instruments.
D) Check and refill the anesthesia cart.

Question 124: Which of the following is the most appropriate action when using a suction device during surgery?
A) Suctioning continuously to keep the site dry
B) Suctioning intermittently to avoid tissue damage
C) Using suction to introduce fluids into the surgical site
D) Avoiding suction to prevent contamination

Question 125: A 5-year-old patient named Emily is scheduled for a tonsillectomy. Which preoperative preparation is most crucial to address her anxiety and ensure her cooperation?
A) Administering a sedative immediately upon arrival
B) Allowing her to bring a favorite toy into the operating room
C) Explaining the procedure in detailed medical terms
D) Restricting food and fluids for 8 hours before surgery

Question 126: After completing a procedure involving cautery on Ms. Smith, the surgical technologist is responsible for removing the drapes and other equipment. What is the best practice to follow to ensure safety and efficiency?
A) Remove the drapes immediately after the procedure without waiting for the surgeon's signal.
B) Disconnect the cautery machine and other electrical equipment before removing the drapes.
C) Leave the cautery machine on while removing the drapes to save time.
D) Ask the circulating nurse to remove the drapes while the technologist handles the cautery machine.

Question 127: What is the primary method for estimating blood loss during surgery?
A) Visual estimation by the surgical team
B) Weighing sponges and drapes before and after use
C) Counting the number of used surgical instruments
D) Measuring the volume of irrigation fluid used

Question 128: During the preoperative preparation for a patient named Ms. Johnson, who is undergoing spinal surgery, the surgical technologist must apply patient safety devices to ensure x-ray safety. Which of the following actions should be taken to protect the surgical team from x-ray exposure?
A) Standing directly behind the x-ray machine
B) Wearing lead aprons and standing behind a lead shield
C) Increasing the distance between the x-ray machine and the surgical team
D) Using a handheld x-ray device for convenience

Question 129: Which of the following strategies is most effective for resolving conflicts within a surgical team?
A) Ignoring the conflict and hoping it resolves itself
B) Addressing the conflict directly and facilitating open communication
C) Assigning blame to the person responsible for the conflict
D) Involving only the senior staff in the resolution process

Question 130: Which of the following is the most effective way for a Certified Surgical Technologist to stay updated with the latest advancements in surgical technology?
A) Attending annual conferences and workshops
B) Relying solely on information from colleagues
C) Using outdated textbooks for reference
D) Ignoring new technologies and techniques

Question 131: During a spinal surgery on a patient named Ms. Johnson, which patient position is most appropriate to ensure optimal access to the surgical site while maintaining patient safety?
A) Prone position with chest rolls
B) Supine position with head elevated

C) Lateral decubitus position
D) Fowler's position

Question 132: During a total hip replacement surgery on a 70-year-old patient named Mary, the surgical team observes a significant drop in the patient's blood pressure. As a Certified Surgical Technologist, what should you do first to assist in identifying the cause of the blood loss?
A) Check the surgical drapes for pooling blood.
B) Increase the IV fluid rate to stabilize blood pressure.
C) Ask the circulating nurse to call for additional blood units.
D) Monitor the patient's urine output for signs of hypovolemia.

Question 133: What is the correct procedure for disposing of contaminated sharps after surgery in compliance with Standard Precautions?
A) Place them in a regular trash bin.
B) Dispose of them in a puncture-resistant, leak-proof sharps container.
C) Leave them on the surgical tray for housekeeping to handle.
D) Wrap them in a towel and place them in the biohazard waste bag.

Question 134: John, a Certified Surgical Technologist, needs to track his continuing education credits efficiently. Which of the following methods best utilizes computer technology for this purpose?
A) Keeping a handwritten logbook of completed courses
B) Using an online continuing education tracking system
C) Relying on email confirmations from course providers
D) Asking his supervisor to keep a record of his credits

Question 135: What is the most appropriate method for sterilizing instruments for immediate use in the operating room?
A) Ethylene oxide gas sterilization
B) Steam sterilization using a gravity displacement autoclave
C) Flash sterilization using a pre-vacuum autoclave
D) Chemical sterilization using glutaraldehyde

Question 136: During a knee replacement surgery for a patient named John, the surgical team needs to prepare a synthetic bone graft. What is the most critical step to ensure the graft's proper integration with the patient's bone?
A) Sterilizing the graft with alcohol.
B) Soaking the graft in saline solution.
C) Ensuring the graft is free of any contaminants.
D) Matching the graft's porosity to the patient's bone density.

Question 137: During a laparoscopic cholecystectomy, what is the primary purpose of insufflating the abdomen with carbon dioxide?
A) To sterilize the abdominal cavity
B) To improve visualization by creating space
C) To reduce the risk of infection
D) To cool the surgical instruments

Question 138: What does bright red blood typically indicate during a surgical procedure?
A) Venous bleeding
B) Arterial bleeding
C) Capillary bleeding
D) Coagulated blood

Question 139: What is the primary responsibility of a surgical technologist in maintaining inventory control in the operating room?
A) Ordering new supplies as needed
B) Sterilizing surgical instruments
C) Tracking and documenting the usage of supplies
D) Assisting in surgical procedures

Question 140: During an abdominal surgery, the surgical technologist notices that the electrocautery device is sparking excessively. What should the surgical technologist do to prevent a potentially harmful situation?
A) Ignore the sparking and continue the procedure.
B) Inform the surgeon immediately and stop using the device.
C) Adjust the settings on the electrocautery device.
D) Replace the electrocautery device with a new one without informing the surgeon.

Question 141: During a postoperative procedure, the surgical technologist is responsible for removing the drapes and other equipment from the patient. Which of the following steps should be performed first to ensure patient safety?
A) Disconnect the suction device from the patient.
B) Remove the surgical drapes carefully.
C) Turn off the suction device.
D) Check the suction canister for proper disposal.

Question 142: During an open abdominal surgery on Ms. Smith, the surgeon needs to control bleeding from a small vessel in the mesentery. Which mechanical method should the surgical technologist prepare?
A) Ligature
B) Argon beam coagulator
C) Topical thrombin
D) Gelatin sponge

Question 143: What is the main advantage of using an allograft over an autograft in surgical procedures?
A) Reduced risk of immune rejection
B) Elimination of donor site morbidity
C) Higher osteogenic potential
D) Immediate availability without the need for

matching

Question 144: During a femoral-popliteal bypass surgery on Mr. Johnson, which anatomical structure must be carefully preserved to prevent nerve damage?
A) Femoral artery
B) Saphenous nerve
C) Popliteal vein
D) Tibial nerve

Question 145: During a laparoscopic cholecystectomy, the surgeon uses a thermal device to achieve hemostasis. Which of the following thermal methods is most appropriate for this procedure?
A) Cryotherapy
B) Electrocautery
C) Ultrasonic scalpel
D) Laser coagulation

Question 146: Which of the following is the most appropriate use of computer technology for a Certified Surgical Technologist (CST) in maintaining patient records?
A) Browsing the internet for medical articles
B) Updating electronic health records (EHR)
C) Playing educational surgical games
D) Watching online surgical tutorials

Question 147: During a surgical procedure, the surgical technologist, Alex, notices that one of the instruments used has visible organic material on it. What is the first step Alex should take to properly decontaminate and clean this instrument?
A) Immediately place the instrument in an ultrasonic

cleaner.
B) Rinse the instrument with cold water to remove organic material.
C) Soak the instrument in a disinfectant solution.
D) Manually scrub the instrument with a brush under running water.

Question 148: Sarah is undergoing a skin graft procedure. The surgeon needs to ensure the graft adheres properly to the underlying tissue. Which layer of the skin provides the necessary support and nourishment for the graft to survive?
A) Epidermis
B) Dermis
C) Stratum basale
D) Subcutaneous tissue

Question 149: Dr. Smith is conducting a research study on postoperative infection rates. As a Certified Surgical Technologist, you are tasked with collecting and entering patient data into a specialized software program. Which of the following actions is most critical to ensure the accuracy and integrity of the data?
A) Entering data as quickly as possible to meet deadlines
B) Double-checking all entries for accuracy before submission
C) Using only pre-approved abbreviations and codes
D) Relying on memory for data entry to save time

Question 150: What does the medical abbreviation "PRN" stand for in a surgical context?
A) Postoperative Recovery Needed
B) As Needed
C) Preoperative Routine Necessary
D) Patient Requires Nutrition

ANSWER WITH DETAILED EXPLANATION SET [3]

Question 1: Correct Answer: B) Check the integrity of the anvil and staple cartridge.
Rationale: Checking the integrity of the anvil and staple cartridge is crucial to ensure proper function and avoid intraoperative complications. Ensuring the stapler is fully assembled (A) is important but secondary to integrity checks. Lubricating the stapler (C) is not typically necessary. Confirming allergy status (D) is essential preoperatively but not specific to stapler use.

Question 2: Correct Answer: B) Hemostat
Rationale: The hemostat is specifically designed for clamping blood vessels to control bleeding during surgery. Unlike the scalpel (A), which is used for cutting, the retractor (C), which is used for holding back tissue, and the suction tip (D), which is used for removing fluids, the hemostat's primary function is to clamp vessels. This makes it the correct choice for this function.

Question 3: Correct Answer: D) Femoral epicondyles
Rationale: The femoral epicondyles are crucial for aligning the femoral component during total knee arthroplasty. The tibial tuberosity (A) is used for tibial alignment, not femoral. The medial malleolus (B) is an ankle landmark, irrelevant to knee surgery. The anterior superior iliac spine (C) is a pelvic landmark, not used for knee alignment. Proper alignment ensures the success of the procedure and patient mobility.

Question 4: Correct Answer: B) Ensure the bulb is compressed before connecting to the drain.
Rationale: Compressing the bulb before connecting it to the drain creates a vacuum that allows for effective drainage of fluids postoperatively. Option A is incorrect because the drain should not be cut; it is pre-sized. Option C is incorrect as the JP drain is typically not connected to a suction unit. Option D is incorrect because filling the bulb with saline would prevent it from creating a vacuum.

Question 5: Correct Answer: B) To prevent the use of contraindicated medications and materials
Rationale: Documenting a patient's allergy status in the preoperative checklist is primarily to prevent the use of contraindicated medications and materials, thereby avoiding allergic reactions. While the type of anesthesia (Option A) and nutritional support (Option C) are important considerations, they are not the primary reasons for documenting allergies. Scheduling follow-up appointments (Option D) is also necessary but unrelated to immediate preoperative allergy management.

Question 6: Correct Answer: D) Verify the patient's identity and surgical site.
Rationale: The first step in preoperative preparation is to verify the patient's identity and surgical site to ensure the correct procedure is performed on the correct patient. This step is crucial to prevent surgical errors. Although applying antiseptic solution (A), shaving the site (B), and positioning the patient (C) are important, they should be done after verifying the patient's identity and surgical site.

Question 7: Correct Answer: B) Assist in the preparation and sterilization of surgical instruments.
Rationale: In a mass casualty incident, the primary responsibility of a Certified Surgical Technologist is to assist in the preparation and sterilization of surgical instruments to ensure that the operating room is ready for an influx of patients requiring surgery. Triage (A) is typically handled by emergency department personnel, coordinating with public relations (C) is not within the surgical technologist's scope, and managing supply inventory (D) is generally the role of the supply chain or materials management department.

Question 8: Correct Answer: B) Choroid plexus
Rationale: The choroid plexus is responsible for the production of cerebrospinal fluid (CSF) in the brain. The pineal gland regulates sleep-wake cycles, the hypothalamus controls various autonomic functions, and the pituitary gland secretes hormones. Thus, the choroid plexus is the only structure that produces CSF, making it the correct answer.

Question 9: Correct Answer: B) Shave the area, apply antiseptic solution, and then drape the patient.
Rationale: The correct sequence is to first shave the area to remove any hair that could harbor bacteria, then apply the antiseptic solution to reduce the microbial load, and finally drape the patient to create a sterile field. Option A is incorrect because applying antiseptic before shaving can lead to contamination. Option C is incorrect as draping before antiseptic application is not sterile practice. Option D is incorrect because shaving should be done before antiseptic application to ensure the area is clean.

Question 10: Correct Answer: A) Increase the irrigation flow rate.
Rationale: The first step to address a collapsing anterior chamber during phacoemulsification is to increase the irrigation flow rate to maintain chamber stability. Decreasing ultrasound power (B) and checking for leaks (C) are secondary steps. Adjusting the patient's head position (D) is unlikely to resolve this issue directly.

Question 11: Correct Answer: B) Immediately inform the circulating nurse to update the preference card.
Rationale: Informing the circulating nurse to update the preference card ensures that the discrepancy is addressed promptly and accurately. Proceeding without the correct instruments (A) or substituting them without informing anyone (C) can compromise patient safety. Pausing the surgery to search for instruments yourself (D) is inefficient and disrupts the surgical flow. The circulating nurse can coordinate the necessary adjustments.

Question 12: Correct Answer: C) To ensure continuous and effective drainage.
Rationale: Kinked tubing can obstruct fluid flow, compromising drainage effectiveness. Option A is partially correct but not the primary reason. Option B is unrelated to tubing kinks, and Option D, while

important, is not the main concern in this context.

Question 13: Correct Answer: C) Recurrent laryngeal nerve

Rationale: The recurrent laryngeal nerve is at risk during a thyroidectomy because it runs close to the thyroid gland and innervates the vocal cords. Damage to this nerve can cause vocal cord paralysis. The vagus nerve, phrenic nerve, and hypoglossal nerve are not as closely associated with the thyroid gland and are less likely to be injured during this procedure.

Question 14: Correct Answer: B) Assisting in the triage area

Rationale: During a hospital-wide disaster drill, a CST's primary role is to assist in the triage area, where they can utilize their medical knowledge to help assess and prioritize patient care. While directing patients (A) and managing supplies (C) are important, they are not the primary responsibilities. Performing administrative duties (D) is also secondary to the immediate need for triage assistance.

Question 15: Correct Answer: C) Verify the tourniquet pressure and duration settings with the surgeon before application.

Rationale: Verifying the tourniquet pressure and duration settings with the surgeon ensures the correct parameters are used, minimizing the risk of complications. Option A is incorrect as an oversized cuff can cause uneven pressure distribution. Option B is incorrect because the inflation pressure should be based on limb occlusion pressure, not diastolic pressure. Option D is incorrect as a loosely applied cuff can lead to ineffective occlusion and increased risk of complications.

Question 16: Correct Answer: B) To reduce the risk of surgical site infections

Rationale: The primary purpose of using chlorhexidine gluconate (CHG) solution during preoperative skin preparation is to reduce the risk of surgical site infections. CHG is a broad-spectrum antimicrobial agent effective against a wide range of pathogens. Option A is incorrect as moisturizing is not the goal. Option C is incorrect as providing a cooling sensation is not relevant. Option D, while partially correct, does not address the primary purpose, which is infection prevention.

Question 17: Correct Answer: A) To prevent deep vein thrombosis (DVT)

Rationale: The primary purpose of using sequential compression devices (SCDs) is to prevent deep vein thrombosis (DVT) by promoting venous blood flow in the legs. While reducing postoperative pain (B), enhancing wound healing (C), and maintaining body temperature (D) are important aspects of perioperative care, they are not the primary functions of SCDs. SCDs specifically target the prevention of blood clots by mimicking natural muscle contractions, which helps to move blood through the veins more effectively.

Question 18: Correct Answer: B) Reassure Maria that her concerns will be addressed and communicate them to the surgical team.

Rationale: Reassuring Maria and communicating her concerns to the surgical team ensures that her cultural practices and dietary restrictions are respected, promoting patient comfort and trust. Ignoring her concerns (Option A) or suggesting standard guidelines (Option C) disregards her cultural needs. Stating that cultural practices are not considered (Option D) is incorrect and dismissive. Addressing her concerns demonstrates cultural competence and patient-centered care.

Question 19: Correct Answer: D) Fascial stapler

Rationale: A fascial stapler is specifically designed for closing the fascia, providing secure and consistent closure with minimal tissue trauma. A skin stapler (A) is used for closing skin incisions, not fascia. A linear stapler (B) is used for gastrointestinal anastomosis and not suitable for fascia. A circular stapler (C) is used for end-to-end anastomosis in colorectal surgery, making it inappropriate for fascia closure.

Question 20: Correct Answer: C) Isolating the patient in a sterile environment preoperatively.

Rationale: Isolating the patient in a sterile environment preoperatively is essential to reduce the risk of infection for immunocompromised patients. Scheduling the surgery early (Option A) does not specifically address infection risk. Prophylactic antiviral medication (Option B) is not generally required unless there is a specific viral risk. Double-sterilizing instruments (Option D) is unnecessary if standard sterilization protocols are followed correctly.

Question 21: Correct Answer: C) University of Wisconsin (UW) Solution

Rationale: The University of Wisconsin (UW) Solution is the most commonly used solution for organ preservation during transport due to its ability to maintain organ viability for extended periods. Normal Saline and Ringer's Lactate are not suitable for long-term organ preservation. Dextrose 5% in Water lacks the necessary components to preserve organ function. The UW Solution contains specific electrolytes and nutrients that help in maintaining the organ's cellular integrity and function during transport.

Question 22: Correct Answer: C) Using latex-free gloves and equipment

Rationale: The most critical step is to use latex-free gloves and equipment to prevent any contact with latex, which could trigger a severe allergic reaction. While scheduling the patient first and informing the team are important, they do not directly prevent exposure. Administering antihistamines is a supportive measure but not a primary preventive strategy.

Question 23: Correct Answer: B) Ensuring the wound area is completely dry before dressing

Rationale: Ensuring the wound area is completely dry before dressing is crucial to prevent bacterial growth and promote proper adhesion of the dressing. Applying antiseptic ointment (A) is not always necessary and can interfere with dressing adherence. Using non-sterile gloves (C) can introduce contaminants, and while non-adhesive dressings (D) are useful, they are not the primary concern in preparation.

Question 24: Correct Answer: B) The type of surgery being performed

Rationale: The primary consideration when selecting instruments for a surgical procedure is the type of surgery being performed. This ensures that the instruments are appropriate for the specific tasks required. While the surgeon's preference (A) and availability of instruments (C) are also important, they are secondary to the surgical requirements. The patient's medical history (D) is crucial for overall care but does not directly influence the choice of surgical instruments.

Question 25: Correct Answer: C) Synovial joint

Rationale: Synovial joints are characterized by a fluid-filled cavity that allows for free movement, making them the most mobile type of joint in the body. Fibrous joints are connected by dense connective tissue and allow little to no movement. Cartilaginous joints are connected by cartilage and permit limited movement. Suture joints are a type of fibrous joint found in the skull, allowing no movement. Thus, synovial joints uniquely provide the greatest range of motion.

Question 26: Correct Answer: C) It fosters a collaborative environment and improves team communication

Rationale: Active listening techniques foster a collaborative environment and improve team communication by ensuring that all team members feel heard and valued. This leads to better decision-making and a more cohesive team. Multitasking (Option A) can lead to misunderstandings, focusing only on the leader's opinions (Option B) can stifle input from other team members, and reducing discussions (Option D) can overlook important details and perspectives.

Question 27: Correct Answer: C) To protect personnel from electrical shock by interrupting the circuit

Rationale: A GFCI is designed to protect personnel from electrical shock by detecting ground faults and interrupting the circuit. Unlike option A, which concerns voltage regulation, or option B, which involves fire prevention, the GFCI's main function is safety. Option D is incorrect as GFCIs may interrupt power to prevent harm, which is contrary to ensuring continuous operation.

Question 28: Correct Answer: B) Discussing patient information only with the surgical team involved in the case.

Rationale: The primary ethical responsibility is to maintain patient confidentiality by discussing information only with the surgical team involved in the case. Sharing information for educational purposes (A), posting on social media (C), or storing on personal devices (D) can lead to breaches of confidentiality and violate HIPAA regulations. Ensuring that patient information is only shared with relevant personnel upholds ethical and legal standards.

Question 29: Correct Answer: B) Inform the surgeon and anesthesia provider immediately.

Rationale: Informing the surgeon and anesthesia provider immediately is essential because they can quickly assess the situation and take appropriate actions to stabilize the patient. Increasing IV fluid rate (A) or administering a vasopressor (C) are actions that require the direction of the anesthesia provider. Checking for signs of bleeding (D) is important but secondary to notifying the surgical and anesthesia team.

Question 30: Correct Answer: C) The operating room

Rationale: In the event of a natural disaster, a Certified Surgical Technologist should report to the operating room. This is where their skills are most needed to prepare for emergency surgeries. Reporting to the command center (A) or patient registration area (D) is not appropriate as these are not areas where surgical technologists are typically required. The emergency department (B) is crucial but does not require the specialized skills of a surgical technologist.

Question 31: Correct Answer: C) Prepare the operating room for incoming trauma cases

Rationale: The primary responsibility of a Certified Surgical Technologist during a mass casualty incident is to prepare the operating room for incoming trauma cases. This ensures that surgical teams are ready to operate immediately, which is critical for saving lives. Triage (A) and psychological support (D) are important but fall outside the scope of a surgical technologist's primary duties. Setting up a temporary morgue (B) is also not within the typical responsibilities of a surgical technologist.

Question 32: Correct Answer: B) To designate a healthcare proxy to make medical decisions

Rationale: A Durable Power of Attorney for Health Care designates a healthcare proxy to make medical decisions on behalf of the patient if they are unable to do so. This differs from financial decisions (A), specific medical treatments (C), and consent for surgical procedures (D). Thus, the primary purpose is to ensure medical decisions align with the patient's wishes through a designated proxy.

Question 33: Correct Answer: B) Shave the site, apply antiseptic solution, and then drape the area.

Rationale: The correct sequence for preparing the surgical site is to first shave the site if necessary, then apply the antiseptic solution, and finally drape the area. Shaving the site (B) first removes hair that could harbor bacteria, applying antiseptic solution (A) reduces microbial load, and draping (C) maintains a sterile field. Options A, C, and D are incorrect as they do not follow the proper sequence.

Question 34: Correct Answer: B) Ensure the stretcher is locked and at the same height as the operating table.

Rationale: Ensuring the stretcher is locked and at the same height as the operating table is crucial for patient safety and ease of transfer. This prevents the stretcher from moving and reduces the risk of injury. Removing drapes and equipment (Option A) and disconnecting IV lines and catheters (Option C) are important but secondary steps. Asking the patient to assist (Option D) is inappropriate, especially if they are under anesthesia or heavily sedated.

Question 35: Correct Answer: B) Prepare a 4-0 absorbable suture.

Rationale: The surgeon specifically requested a 4-0 absorbable suture, which is appropriate for delicate structures like the cystic duct. Option A and D are incorrect because they involve non-absorbable sutures, which are not suitable for this purpose. Option C is incorrect because it does not match the requested size, potentially leading to complications in the closure of the cystic duct. Therefore, Option B is the correct choice.

Question 36: Correct Answer: A) Filtration of blood

Rationale: The renal cortex is primarily responsible for the filtration of blood, which is the initial step in urine formation. The renal medulla, not the cortex, is involved in the concentration of urine (B). The bladder, not the kidney, is responsible for the storage of urine (C). While the kidneys do play a role in regulating blood pressure (D), this function is not specific to the renal cortex. Understanding these functions is essential for surgical technologists working with renal procedures.

Question 37: Correct Answer: C) Seal the waste in a biohazard bag and then place it in a designated biohazard waste container.

Rationale: Sealing the waste in a biohazard bag and placing it in a designated biohazard waste container ensures compliance with Standard Precautions and prevents contamination. Option A is incorrect as regular trash bags are not suitable for biohazardous waste. Option B is incorrect because the waste must be sealed to prevent exposure. Option D is impractical and unsafe as incineration should be done in a controlled environment.

Question 38: Correct Answer: B) To prevent the cast material from sticking to the skin

Rationale: The primary purpose of using a stockinette is to prevent the cast material from sticking to the skin, thereby providing a barrier that enhances patient comfort and skin protection. While additional support (A) and increased rigidity (C) are functions of the cast material itself, and better ventilation (D) is not the primary function of a stockinette.

Question 39: Correct Answer: B) Providing constructive feedback in a timely manner

Rationale: Effective communication involves providing constructive feedback in a timely manner, which helps the trainee improve and learn efficiently. Option A is incorrect as excessive medical jargon can confuse new personnel. Option C is incorrect because ongoing communication is essential. Option D is incorrect as focusing solely on mistakes can be demoralizing and counterproductive.

Question 40: Correct Answer: C) Clean subungual areas under running water.

Rationale: The initial step in performing a surgical scrub is to clean the subungual areas under running water to remove debris and reduce microbial load. This step is crucial before any other actions to ensure thorough decontamination. Options A, B, and D are incorrect as they are subsequent steps in the process. Applying sterile gloves (A) and drying hands (D) occur after the scrub, while rinsing hands and forearms (B) is part of the scrubbing sequence but not the initial step.

Question 41: Correct Answer: B) Ensuring proper sterilization of surgical instruments

Rationale: Proper sterilization of surgical instruments (B) is essential to prevent SSIs by eliminating potential pathogens. Administering prophylactic antibiotics postoperatively (A) is less effective than preoperative administration. Wearing non-sterile gloves (C) does not provide adequate protection. Alcohol-based hand rubs should be used before and after the procedure, not just after (D). Proper sterilization is a critical step in infection control.

Question 42: Correct Answer: D) Allowing the antiseptic solution to dry completely before draping

Rationale: Allowing the antiseptic solution to dry completely before draping is crucial to ensure its effectiveness. This step maximizes the antimicrobial action and reduces the risk of skin irritation. Option A is incorrect as shaving can cause micro-abrasions that increase infection risk. Option B is partially correct but not the most crucial step. Option C is incorrect as rinsing off the antiseptic solution would negate its antimicrobial effect.

Question 43: Correct Answer: C) Cardioplegia solution

Rationale: Cardioplegia solution is specifically designed to induce cardiac arrest and protect the myocardium during open-heart surgeries by reducing metabolic demands. Lactated Ringer's solution (A) and normal saline (B) are used for fluid replacement but do not provide myocardial protection. Dextrose 5% in water (D) is used for energy supply but is not suitable for myocardial protection during surgery. Cardioplegia solution effectively reduces myocardial oxygen consumption, allowing the heart to be safely stopped and protected during the procedure.

Question 44: Correct Answer: B) Non-sterile gloves, gown, and face shield.

Rationale: Non-sterile gloves, gown, and face shield provide comprehensive protection against chemical exposure. Sterile gloves and surgical mask (A) are insufficient for chemical spills. Surgical cap and shoe covers (C) do not protect against chemical exposure. Sterile gloves and gown (D) are intended for maintaining a sterile field, not chemical protection.

Question 45: Correct Answer: B) Turn off the suction device before disconnecting the tubing.

Rationale: Turning off the suction device before disconnecting the tubing ensures patient safety and prevents accidental aspiration or injury. Disconnecting the tubing while the device is still running (Option A) or removing the catheter first (Option C) can cause sudden pressure changes, leading to tissue damage. Leaving the device on until the patient is fully awake (Option D) is unnecessary and can cause discomfort.

Question 46: Correct Answer: B) Ethylene oxide gas

Rationale: Ethylene oxide gas is the most appropriate sterilization method for synthetic tissue grafts because it effectively sterilizes without compromising the material's biocompatibility. Autoclaving and dry heat can degrade synthetic materials, while ultraviolet radiation is not as effective for deep sterilization. Ethylene oxide gas ensures thorough sterilization while maintaining the integrity of the synthetic graft.

Question 47: Correct Answer: B) Actively listen to others and wait for a pause before contributing.
Rationale: Actively listening and waiting for a pause before contributing shows respect for your colleagues and ensures that you understand their perspectives before adding your own. Sharing thoughts immediately (A) can be disruptive, and focusing solely on your tasks (C) or only speaking when asked (D) limits your contribution to the team dynamic. Effective communication involves both listening and timely, respectful participation.

Question 48: Correct Answer: B) Regularly update Dr. Smith's preference card in the computer system.
Rationale: Regularly updating Dr. Smith's preference card in the computer system ensures that her specific preferences are consistently met for each procedure. Memorizing preferences (A) or asking before each surgery (C) can lead to errors or inconsistencies, and using the most common suture material (D) disregards her specific needs. The preference card serves as an official, reliable reference.

Question 49: Correct Answer: C) Production of exotoxins that disrupt the intestinal epithelium
Rationale: Clostridium difficile causes pseudomembranous colitis primarily through the production of exotoxins (Toxin A and Toxin B) that disrupt the intestinal epithelium, leading to inflammation and diarrhea. Endotoxins are associated with Gram-negative bacteria, invasion of mucosa is not the primary mechanism, and biofilm formation is not a key feature of C. difficile pathogenesis. This specific mechanism of exotoxin production distinguishes C. difficile from other pathogenic processes.

Question 50: Correct Answer: B) Hand the surgeon a hemostatic agent to control the bleeding.
Rationale: Handing the surgeon a hemostatic agent (B) directly addresses the source of bleeding and helps control it. Increasing lighting (A) does not directly manage blood loss. Adjusting the patient's position (C) is not a primary intervention for controlling bleeding. Preparing the electrocautery device (D) is useful but secondary to providing immediate hemostatic agents.

Question 51: Correct Answer: C) Document both the saline solution and morphine amounts.
Rationale: The correct documentation involves reporting both the saline solution and morphine amounts used. This ensures accurate medical records and proper postoperative care. Option A and B are incorrect because they only partially document the administered substances. Option D is incorrect as it fails to specify the morphine amount, which is crucial for accurate medical records and patient safety.

Question 52: Correct Answer: C) Cleaning the instruments

Rationale: Cleaning the instruments is the first step in the inspection process before sterilization. This removes any debris or biological material that could interfere with sterilization. Checking for proper function, lubricating, and assembling are subsequent steps that ensure the instruments are in optimal condition for use. Cleaning is crucial as it ensures that the sterilization process will be effective.

Question 53: Correct Answer: C) Labeling and documenting the harvested tissues accurately
Rationale: Labeling and documenting the harvested tissues accurately is a critical step for a CST to ensure proper tissue procurement. This prevents any mix-up or loss of vital information. Option A, while important, is typically handled by the organ procurement organization. Option B is incorrect as CSTs assist but do not perform biopsies. Option D is incorrect because the recipient decision is made by the transplant team, not the CST.

Question 54: Correct Answer: B) Notify the surgeon immediately.
Rationale: The first step upon noticing significant bleeding at the surgical site is to notify the surgeon immediately. This allows the surgeon to assess the situation and take appropriate action. Applying a tourniquet (A) may not be appropriate and could cause further complications. Increasing IV fluid rate (C) and administering anticoagulants (D) are not suitable first responses and could exacerbate the bleeding.

Question 55: Correct Answer: A) Rongeur
Rationale: A rongeur is specifically designed for cutting and removing small bone fragments, making it the correct choice for this scenario. An osteotome is used for cutting bone but requires a mallet and is not ideal for small fragments. A bone curette is used for scraping bone, and a bone rasp is used for smoothing bone surfaces. Therefore, the rongeur is the most suitable instrument for cutting small bone fragments during orthopedic surgery.

Question 56: Correct Answer: A) Assessing the patient's nutritional status
Rationale: Assessing the patient's nutritional status is critical because malnutrition can significantly affect surgical outcomes in geriatric patients. Unlike evaluating exercise routines, travel history, or vaccination records, nutritional status directly impacts wound healing, immune function, and overall recovery. Proper nutritional assessment helps identify deficiencies that can be corrected preoperatively to improve surgical outcomes.

Question 57: Correct Answer: D) Medication reconciliation form
Rationale: The medication reconciliation form is essential for verifying Mr. Johnson's current medications and potential allergies. Unlike the surgical and anesthesia consent forms, which are focused on obtaining patient consent, the medication reconciliation form provides detailed information on the patient's medication history. The preoperative checklist is useful but does not provide the specific details needed for medication and allergy verification.

Question 58: Correct Answer: C) Using latex-free gloves and equipment

Rationale: The most critical step in preoperative preparation for a patient with a known latex allergy is using latex-free gloves and equipment to prevent an allergic reaction. While scheduling the surgery as the first case of the day (Option B) can reduce latex exposure, it is not as crucial as eliminating latex from the environment. Administering prophylactic antibiotics (Option A) and ensuring the patient has fasted (Option D) are important but unrelated to managing latex allergies.

Question 59: Correct Answer: B) Equipment malfunctions and their impact on the procedure

Rationale: Discussing equipment malfunctions and their impact on the procedure is crucial during a postoperative case debrief. This helps identify potential issues and prevent future occurrences. Option A is irrelevant to the debrief. Option C, while important for administrative purposes, is not relevant to surgical improvement. Option D is unrelated to the surgical procedure and its outcomes.

Question 60: Correct Answer: C) Contain the spill using appropriate materials.

Rationale: The first action should be to contain the spill using appropriate materials to prevent it from spreading and causing further harm. This step is crucial to ensure the safety of everyone in the operating room. Evacuating the room (Option B) might be necessary but is not the immediate first step. Calling housekeeping (Option A) and informing the surgeon (Option D) are important but secondary actions after containing the spill.

Question 61: Correct Answer: B) Gently lift the drapes, avoiding any adhesive areas.

Rationale: Gently lifting the drapes and avoiding adhesive areas helps maintain skin integrity and prevents skin tears or irritation. Quickly pulling the drapes (A) can cause injury, while cutting the drapes (C) is unnecessary and could lead to contamination. Leaving the drapes until the patient is fully awake (D) is not practical and can cause discomfort.

Question 62: Correct Answer: C) Sclera

Rationale: The sclera is the tough, fibrous outer layer of the eye that maintains the shape of the eyeball and provides protection. The retina (A) is responsible for receiving light and converting it into neural signals. The cornea (B) is the transparent front part of the eye that refracts light. The lens (D) focuses light onto the retina. Thus, the sclera is the correct answer as it uniquely provides structural support and protection.

Question 63: Correct Answer: B) Notify the surgeon and replace the instruments with a sterile set.

Rationale: The correct action is to notify the surgeon and replace the instruments with a sterile set. The sterilization indicator is a crucial element in confirming that the instruments have been properly sterilized. Using instruments without a confirmed sterilization process can introduce infections. Option A and D are incorrect as they compromise patient safety. Option C is not feasible during surgery and does not address the immediate need for sterile instruments.

Question 64: Correct Answer: B) Mixing the bone cement

Rationale: During total knee arthroplasty, the surgical technologist is primarily responsible for mixing the bone cement to ensure proper consistency and timing for application. Positioning the limb (A) and holding retractors (C) are roles typically managed by the surgeon or assistant. Suctioning excess cement (D) is important but secondary to the critical task of preparing the cement, making option B the correct answer.

Question 65: Correct Answer: C) Carcinogenic effects

Rationale: The primary health risk associated with exposure to surgical smoke is its carcinogenic effects. Surgical smoke contains harmful chemicals and cellular debris, some of which are known carcinogens. Respiratory infections and eye irritation are also concerns but are secondary to the long-term risk of cancer. Skin rashes are less common and not a primary risk. Therefore, minimizing exposure to surgical smoke is crucial for the long-term health of operating room personnel.

Question 66: Correct Answer: D) In the preoperative holding area, just before surgery

Rationale: Hair removal should be performed in the preoperative holding area just before surgery to minimize the time between hair removal and the surgical procedure, thereby reducing the risk of microbial contamination and SSIs. Performing hair removal the night before or 24 hours before surgery increases the risk of bacterial colonization. Immediate removal before entering the operating room can delay the procedure and is less controlled.

Question 67: Correct Answer: D) Frontal Lobe

Rationale: The frontal lobe is responsible for motor control, specifically the precentral gyrus, also known as the primary motor cortex. The temporal lobe is involved in auditory processing, the occipital lobe in visual processing, and the parietal lobe in sensory perception. Therefore, the surgeon should focus on the frontal lobe to access the motor control area.

Question 68: Correct Answer: A) It provides a scaffold for bone regeneration.

Rationale: Allografts are primarily used because they provide a scaffold for bone regeneration, aiding in the natural healing process. Unlike option B, allografts do carry a risk of disease transmission, although it is minimized through rigorous screening and processing. Option C is incorrect because there is still a risk of immune rejection, albeit lower than with xenografts. Option D is incorrect as allografts do not necessarily guarantee faster healing compared to autografts, which are often considered the gold standard for grafting.

Question 69: Correct Answer: C) Pelvic lymph nodes

Rationale: During a cystectomy for bladder cancer, the pelvic lymph nodes must be resected to ensure complete removal of potentially metastatic cancerous tissue. The urethra (A) and ureters (B) are typically preserved unless directly involved by the tumor. The adrenal glands (D) are not related to bladder cancer and do not need to be resected in this procedure.

Question 70: Correct Answer: B) Pelvis

Rationale: The pelvis is the primary bone that articulates with the femur at the hip joint, forming the hip socket (acetabulum). The tibia and fibula are bones in the lower leg, and the patella is the kneecap, none of which are involved in the hip joint articulation. The pelvis provides the necessary socket for the femur to fit into, enabling hip movement.

Question 71: Correct Answer: D) Common bile duct

Rationale: Calot's triangle, also known as the cystohepatic triangle, is bounded by the cystic duct, the common hepatic duct, and the cystic artery. The common bile duct is not part of Calot's triangle. Understanding the anatomy of Calot's triangle is crucial for avoiding injury to these structures during a cholecystectomy. The common bile duct lies outside this anatomical landmark, making option D the correct answer.

Question 72: Correct Answer: C) Colorectal Cancer

Rationale: Colorectal cancer involves the abnormal growth of cells in the colon or rectum, which can lead to obstruction and often requires surgical resection. Crohn's disease and ulcerative colitis are inflammatory bowel diseases that cause inflammation but not abnormal cell proliferation. Irritable Bowel Syndrome (IBS) is a functional disorder without structural abnormalities. Thus, colorectal cancer is the correct answer due to its distinct pathological process involving cell proliferation.

Question 73: Correct Answer: B) Ensuring the patient uses her CPAP machine up to the time of surgery

Rationale: Ensuring the patient uses her CPAP machine up to the time of surgery is critical in managing OSA, which is common in bariatric patients. This reduces the risk of postoperative respiratory complications. Preoperative sedation, surgery timing, and pain management are important but do not directly address the immediate respiratory risks associated with OSA. Using CPAP helps maintain airway patency and reduces the risk of hypoxemia.

Question 74: Correct Answer: C) Reverse Trendelenburg position with slight left tilt

Rationale: The reverse Trendelenburg position with a slight left tilt allows gravity to pull the intestines away from the surgical field, providing better visualization and access to the gallbladder. The supine position with arms tucked (A) does not optimize the surgical field. Trendelenburg (B) is incorrect as it increases venous return and can obscure the view. Lithotomy position (D) is used for gynecological and urological procedures, not for laparoscopic cholecystectomy.

Question 75: Correct Answer: A) It provides better hemostasis with less thermal spread.

Rationale: The harmonic scalpel uses ultrasonic vibrations to cut and coagulate tissue, which results in better hemostasis and less thermal spread compared to traditional electrosurgery. This reduces the risk of damage to surrounding tissues. Option B is incorrect because the harmonic scalpel is generally more expensive. Option C is incorrect because it requires specialized training. Option D is incorrect as

anesthesia is still required for the procedure.

Question 76: Correct Answer: B) Report the violation to the surgical supervisor immediately.

Rationale: Reporting the violation to the surgical supervisor immediately ensures patient safety and maintains the integrity of the sterile field. Ignoring the violation (A) or waiting until after the procedure (C, D) can compromise patient care and increase the risk of infection. Immediate reporting allows for corrective action to be taken promptly, thereby upholding ethical and legal standards in surgical patient care.

Question 77: Correct Answer: B) Dermis

Rationale: The dermis is the layer of the integumentary system most commonly affected by abscesses due to its vascular nature and the presence of hair follicles and sweat glands, which can become infected. The epidermis (A) is the outermost layer and less likely to harbor such infections. The hypodermis (C) is deeper and primarily composed of fat, making it less prone to abscess formation. The stratum corneum (D) is the outermost part of the epidermis and not typically involved in abscesses.

Question 78: Correct Answer: C) Before the induction of anesthesia

Rationale: Sequential compression devices (SCDs) should be applied before the induction of anesthesia to ensure that venous blood flow is maintained throughout the entire perioperative period. Applying SCDs immediately after the patient is anesthetized (A) or after the surgical incision is made (B) delays the initiation of prophylaxis against DVT. Using SCDs only during the postoperative recovery phase (D) misses the opportunity to prevent clot formation during surgery. Proper timing is crucial for effective DVT prevention.

Question 79: Correct Answer: D) Place the waste in a biohazard container.

Rationale: Contaminated waste should be placed in a biohazard container to ensure proper containment and disposal, minimizing the risk of infection. Double-bagging in regular trash bags (Option A) does not meet biohazard standards. Using a single biohazard bag (Option B) may not provide sufficient containment, and immediate incineration (Option C) is not a standard practice in most facilities and requires specialized equipment.

Question 80: Correct Answer: B) Ensuring all supplies are within their expiration dates

Rationale: Ensuring all supplies are within their expiration dates is crucial to maintaining patient safety and preventing infections. Placing sterile supplies on the floor (A) and mixing sterile and non-sterile items (D) compromise sterility. Storing supplies in random order (C) can lead to inefficiencies and errors during procedures.

Question 81: Correct Answer: B) Reduced thermal spread

Rationale: The primary advantage of using an ultrasonic scalpel over traditional electrocautery is the reduced thermal spread, which minimizes damage to surrounding tissues. Lower cost is incorrect as ultrasonic scalpels are generally more expensive.

Faster cutting speed is not the primary advantage, as both methods have comparable speeds. Easier to use is subjective and depends on the surgeon's experience and preference.

Question 82: Correct Answer: C) Apologize to Dr. Smith and ask for clarification on his preferences.
Rationale: Apologizing and asking for clarification helps maintain a positive team dynamic by addressing the issue directly and professionally. Arguing (A) could escalate the situation, ignoring (B) could be seen as unprofessional, and leaving (D) would disrupt the procedure. This approach demonstrates Emily's commitment to improving communication and teamwork.

Question 83: Correct Answer: B) Pancreatitis
Rationale: Elevated serum amylase and lipase levels are indicative of pancreatitis, an inflammation of the pancreas. Appendicitis involves the appendix, cholelithiasis refers to gallstones without inflammation, and peptic ulcer disease involves ulcers in the stomach lining. The symptoms and lab results specifically point to pancreatitis.

Question 84: Correct Answer: C) Thermal injury to surrounding tissues
Rationale: The primary safety concern when using a thermal cautery device is thermal injury to surrounding tissues. This can occur if the device is not used correctly or if excessive heat is applied. Infection control (A) and sterility (D) are always important but are not specific to thermal technology. Electrical grounding (B) is crucial for electrical devices but not the primary concern for thermal cautery. Monitoring and controlling the heat application ensures patient safety and effective outcomes.

Question 85: Correct Answer: A) Bone wax
Rationale: Bone wax is the most appropriate mechanical method for controlling bleeding from bone surfaces during orthopedic procedures. Electrocautery (B) is not effective on bone surfaces. Gelatin sponge (C) is a chemical hemostatic agent, and a tourniquet (D) is used to control blood flow to the entire limb, not localized bleeding from bone. Bone wax works by physically blocking the bleeding channels in the bone.

Question 86: Correct Answer: B) Call for immediate medical assistance
Rationale: When a postoperative patient shows signs of respiratory distress, calling for immediate medical assistance is the most appropriate action. Increasing oxygen flow rate (A) or repositioning the patient (C) might provide temporary relief but do not address the underlying issue. Administering pain medication (D) could potentially worsen the situation by depressing respiration further. Immediate medical intervention is crucial to properly diagnose and treat the cause of respiratory distress.

Question 87: Correct Answer: C) Inform the surgeon and assist in realigning the microscope
Rationale: Informing the surgeon and assisting in realigning the microscope is the best immediate action. This ensures that the surgeon is aware of the issue and can maintain control over the procedure. Repositioning the patient (A) or increasing

magnification (D) could cause further complications. Adjusting the fine focus knob (B) does not address the root cause of the misalignment. Proper realignment is essential for maintaining the accuracy and safety of the surgery.

Question 88: Correct Answer: B) Don the gown first, then the gloves
Rationale: The correct sequence involves donning the gown first to maintain sterility, followed by donning the gloves. This ensures that the hands remain sterile after gowning. Option A is incorrect because donning gloves first can lead to contamination. Option C is partially correct but not specific to gowning and gloving sequence. Option D is incorrect because the cap is donned before entering the sterile field, not in the gowning and gloving sequence.

Question 89: Correct Answer: B) Discard the torn packages and document the incident.
Rationale: Torn sterile packages compromise the sterility of the contents, making them unsafe for use. The correct action is to discard these packages and document the incident to maintain accurate inventory and ensure patient safety. Taping the packages (A) or using the supplies (C) is inappropriate as it risks contamination. Reporting to the surgeon (D) is unnecessary for this standard procedure.

Question 90: Correct Answer: D) Argon lasers are absorbed by the retinal pigment epithelium.
Rationale: Argon lasers are absorbed by the retinal pigment epithelium, making them effective for retinal photocoagulation. This absorption helps in precisely targeting retinal tissues without affecting adjacent structures. Option A is incorrect as argon lasers emit visible blue-green light, not infrared. Option B is partially correct but not the primary reason for retinal use. Option C is incorrect because while argon lasers can produce a continuous wave, it is not the defining characteristic for retinal procedures.

Question 91: Correct Answer: B) Place the specimen on a dry container and label it with the patient's name, date of surgery, and "frozen section."
Rationale: For a frozen section analysis, the specimen must be placed in a dry container to prevent any alteration in tissue structure. It is crucial to label it with the patient's name, date of surgery, and "frozen section" to ensure proper handling and processing. Incorrect options include placing the specimen in formalin (A), which is not suitable for frozen sections, and saline (C), which may alter the tissue. Option D lacks the specific "frozen section" label, which is essential for this procedure.

Question 92: Correct Answer: B) Turn off the ESU immediately and inform the surgeon.
Rationale: The correct action is to turn off the ESU immediately and inform the surgeon to prevent any potential harm to the patient. Continuing to use the ESU (Option A) poses a significant risk. Replacing the ESU (Option C) should only be done after ensuring the cause of the smell is identified and resolved. Moving the ESU (Option D) does not address the potential electrical hazard and could delay necessary intervention.

Question 93: Correct Answer: B) Use a smoke evacuation system to remove the smoke.
Rationale: Utilizing a smoke evacuation system is the most effective and immediate action to ensure a safe environment by removing surgical smoke from the operative field. Increasing insufflation pressure (Option A) can cause complications such as gas embolism. Opening the operating room doors (Option C) compromises the sterile field. Pausing the procedure (Option D) does not actively address the smoke issue and delays the surgery.

Question 94: Correct Answer: B) Equalizing air pressure between the middle ear and the atmosphere
Rationale: The Eustachian tube connects the middle ear to the nasopharynx and helps to equalize air pressure on both sides of the tympanic membrane, which is essential for proper hearing. Transmitting sound waves to the inner ear (A) is the role of the ossicles. Producing earwax (C) is the function of ceruminous glands in the ear canal. Detecting changes in head position (D) is the function of the vestibular system, specifically the semicircular canals.

Question 95: Correct Answer: B) On a well-vascularized, muscular area
Rationale: The bovie pad should be placed on a well-vascularized, muscular area to ensure effective grounding and minimize the risk of burns. Placing it on the chest (A) or forehead (C) is incorrect as these areas are not ideal for grounding due to less muscle mass. Placing it on a bony prominence (D) is also incorrect as bones do not provide effective grounding and increase the risk of burns.

Question 96: Correct Answer: B) Securing the patient's arms at their sides with padded arm boards.
Rationale: Securing the patient's arms at their sides with padded arm boards is critical to prevent brachial plexus injury and ensure patient safety during a laparoscopic cholecystectomy. Options A and C are not specific to this procedure, while D is not appropriate for this type of surgery and can increase the risk of respiratory complications.

Question 97: Correct Answer: D) Surgical lighting
Rationale: Surgical lighting is specifically designed to provide bright, focused, and shadow-free illumination directly onto the surgical site, ensuring optimal visibility for the surgical team. Ambient lighting (A) and overhead fluorescent lighting (C) are too diffuse and not focused enough for detailed surgical work. Task lighting (B) is useful for general tasks but lacks the intensity and focus required for surgical procedures.

Question 98: Correct Answer: D) Use a Poole suction tip to remove the fluid.
Rationale: The Poole suction tip is designed to efficiently remove large volumes of fluid, making it ideal for maintaining a clear operative field during open surgeries. A Yankauer suction tip (A) is less effective for large fluid volumes. Continuous irrigation (B) without adequate suction can exacerbate fluid accumulation. Sponges (C) are less effective than suction for fluid removal and may need frequent replacement.

Question 99: Correct Answer: C) Production of sperm
Rationale: The seminiferous tubules are the site of spermatogenesis, where sperm cells are produced. Option A is incorrect as testosterone is primarily produced by the Leydig cells. Option B is incorrect because sperm is stored in the epididymis. Option D is incorrect as the vas deferens is responsible for the transport of sperm. Therefore, the primary function of the seminiferous tubules is the production of sperm.

Question 100: Correct Answer: B) Ensuring the patient is well-hydrated and has stable blood glucose levels.
Rationale: Ensuring Mrs. Thompson is well-hydrated and has stable blood glucose levels is crucial to minimize postoperative complications, particularly given her history of hypertension and diabetes. High-dose sedatives (A) can increase the risk of respiratory depression, scheduling surgery late in the day (C) can lead to prolonged fasting, and avoiding compression stockings (D) can increase the risk of deep vein thrombosis. Proper hydration and glucose control are essential for optimal surgical outcomes in geriatric patients.

Question 101: Correct Answer: B) Ensuring the drain is fully compressed before attaching to suction
Rationale: Ensuring the drain is fully compressed before attaching to suction is crucial for creating the necessary negative pressure to facilitate fluid drainage. Clamping the drain (A) or attaching it before compressing (C) would not establish the required suction. Leaving the drain open to air (D) would prevent the formation of a vacuum, rendering the drain ineffective.

Question 102: Correct Answer: B) Seal the suction canister and dispose of it in a biohazard container.
Rationale: The correct method is to seal the suction canister and dispose of it in a biohazard container to prevent exposure to potentially infectious materials. Option A is incorrect as emptying the canister into the sink can cause contamination. Option C is incorrect as leaving it for housekeeping does not ensure proper disposal. Option D is incorrect as reusing the canister without proper sterilization is unsafe and against protocols.

Question 103: Correct Answer: B) Apply sequential compression devices (SCDs)
Rationale: Applying sequential compression devices (SCDs) is the most appropriate intervention to reduce the risk of thromboembolism in a patient with a history of DVT. SCDs help promote venous return and prevent blood stasis. Administering a high dose of aspirin (A) is not recommended without physician orders. Encouraging early ambulation (C) is important postoperatively but not a preoperative intervention. Providing a high-protein diet (D) does not directly address thromboembolism risk.

Question 104: Correct Answer: B) Ensuring the retractor is properly positioned and adjusted
Rationale: Proper positioning and adjustment of the retractor are crucial to maintaining its effectiveness during surgery. This prevents tissue damage and maintains a clear surgical field. Sterilizing mid-

procedure (A) is impractical, frequently changing retractors (C) can disrupt the procedure, and using multiple retractors simultaneously (D) can cause unnecessary tissue trauma. Proper positioning and adjustment ensure the retractor functions optimally throughout the surgery.

Question 105: Correct Answer: A) Rearrange the instruments according to the surgeon's preference card.

Rationale: The correct action is to rearrange the instruments according to the surgeon's preference card. This ensures that the instruments are readily available in the correct order, facilitating a smooth and efficient surgery. Leaving the instruments as they are (Option B) or waiting until the surgery starts (Option D) can cause delays and confusion. Asking the circulating nurse (Option C) is not ideal as it is the surgical technologist's responsibility to ensure proper instrument arrangement.

Question 106: Correct Answer: C) To remove all fluids and debris from the surgical site.

Rationale: The primary purpose of using suction postoperatively is to remove all fluids and debris from the surgical site, ensuring a clean and clear area to prevent infection and promote healing. Removing blood clots (A) is part of this process but not the sole purpose. Clearing the airway (B) is not the primary concern during drape removal. Drying the surgical site completely (D) is not necessary and can be harmful.

Question 107: Correct Answer: B) Supraspinatus

Rationale: The supraspinatus muscle is one of the four rotator cuff muscles and is most commonly involved in rotator cuff injuries. The deltoid, biceps brachii, and trapezius muscles, while related to shoulder movement, are not primarily involved in rotator cuff injuries. The deltoid assists in arm abduction, the biceps brachii in elbow flexion and forearm supination, and the trapezius in moving and stabilizing the scapula.

Question 108: Correct Answer: B) Occipital Lobe

Rationale: The occipital lobe is primarily responsible for processing visual information. The temporal lobe is involved in auditory processing, the parietal lobe in sensory perception, and the frontal lobe in motor control and executive functions. Therefore, the tumor affecting Sarah's visual processing is located in the occipital lobe.

Question 109: Correct Answer: C) Using a sterile handle cover to attach the light handles

Rationale: The most appropriate method for applying light handles is using a sterile handle cover. This ensures that the light handles remain sterile and do not compromise the sterile field. Option A could lead to contamination if not done correctly, option B is incorrect as the patient should be draped first, and option D is inappropriate as it disrupts the sterile environment once the procedure has started.

Question 110: Correct Answer: A) Blood glucose levels

Rationale: Monitoring blood glucose levels is crucial for a diabetic patient undergoing surgery to prevent complications such as infections and poor wound healing. Blood pressure (B), heart rate (C), and respiratory rate (D) are also important but do not specifically address the unique risks associated with diabetes. Proper glucose control helps mitigate the risk of perioperative complications, making it the most critical factor in this scenario.

Question 111: Correct Answer: B) Acknowledge the suggestion and explain why the established protocol is being followed.

Rationale: Acknowledging the suggestion and explaining why the established protocol is being followed (Option B) is the most diplomatic approach. It shows respect for the new team member's input while reinforcing the importance of adhering to proven protocols. Dismissing the suggestion (Option A) can be perceived as rude, implementing it immediately (Option C) may compromise patient safety, and asking the new member to leave (Option D) is unnecessarily harsh and unprofessional.

Question 112: Correct Answer: C) To prevent retained surgical items

Rationale: The primary reason for performing a surgical count is to prevent retained surgical items, which can lead to serious complications. While ensuring functionality (Option A) and availability (Option B) are important, they are secondary to the main goal of preventing retained items. Organizing instruments (Option D) is also important but not the primary reason for the surgical count. Thus, preventing retained surgical items is the key objective.

Question 113: Correct Answer: C) Passing it handle-first with a firm grip

Rationale: Passing the scalpel handle-first with a firm grip ensures safety for both the surgical technologist and the surgeon. Handing it directly to the surgeon's dominant hand (A) or placing it on the Mayo stand (B) can lead to accidental injury or delays. Passing it blade-first (D) is dangerous and violates safety protocols.

Question 114: Correct Answer: B) Inform the anesthesia provider immediately.

Rationale: Informing the anesthesia provider immediately is crucial because increasing end-tidal CO2 levels could indicate hypercapnia or other respiratory issues. The anesthesia provider can assess and manage the situation appropriately. Increasing oxygen flow rate (A) or adjusting the patient's position (C) may not directly address the underlying cause. Checking the insufflation pressure (D) is important but secondary to notifying the anesthesia provider.

Question 115: Correct Answer: B) The patient has a high oxygen saturation level.

Rationale: Bright red blood indicates high oxygen saturation, meaning the blood is well-oxygenated. Hypercapnia (A) refers to high carbon dioxide levels and does not directly affect blood color. Acidosis (C) affects blood pH but not color. Low hemoglobin (D) would result in pale or anemic blood, not bright red.

Question 116: Correct Answer: C) Thick peptidoglycan layer

Rationale: Gram-positive bacteria are characterized

by a thick peptidoglycan layer in their cell walls, which retains the crystal violet stain used in Gram staining. In contrast, Gram-negative bacteria have a thin peptidoglycan layer and an outer membrane containing lipopolysaccharides. The presence of an outer membrane and lipopolysaccharides are features of Gram-negative bacteria, not Gram-positive. Therefore, the correct answer is the thick peptidoglycan layer.

Question 117: Correct Answer: B) Pulse oximeter
Rationale: The pulse oximeter is specifically designed to measure the oxygen saturation (SpO2) of a patient's blood continuously and non-invasively. While an ECG monitors heart activity, a capnograph measures CO2 levels, and a blood pressure cuff monitors blood pressure, none of these devices measure oxygen saturation, making the pulse oximeter the correct choice.

Question 118: Correct Answer: B) Place the sharps in a puncture-resistant sharps container.
Rationale: The correct method for disposing of contaminated sharps is to place them in a puncture-resistant sharps container. This ensures that the sharps are contained safely and reduces the risk of injury and contamination. Options A and D are incorrect as they do not provide puncture resistance, and option C is incorrect because it does not comply with Standard Precautions and poses a significant safety hazard.

Question 119: Correct Answer: B) Thymus
Rationale: The thymus is the primary lymphatic organ responsible for the maturation of T-lymphocytes, which are crucial for adaptive immunity. The spleen (option A) filters blood and recycles red blood cells, lymph nodes (option C) filter lymph and house lymphocytes, and bone marrow (option D) is the site of hematopoiesis, including the production of B-lymphocytes. Thus, only the thymus (option B) is correctly identified as the site for T-lymphocyte maturation.

Question 120: Correct Answer: B) Open the sterile package away from your body.
Rationale: Opening the sterile package away from your body ensures that you do not accidentally contaminate the sterile field. Opening it towards your body (Option A) increases the risk of contamination from your clothing or body. Using bare hands (Option C) compromises sterility, and placing the package on a non-sterile surface (Option D) contaminates it.

Question 121: Correct Answer: D) Across the patient's hips
Rationale: The safety strap should be placed across the patient's hips to prevent movement and ensure stability during the procedure. Placing the strap across the chest (Option A) can restrict breathing, across the thighs (Option B) can be ineffective in preventing movement, and across the ankles (Option C) does not provide adequate restraint for the entire body. The hips are the most secure and safe location for the strap.

Question 122: Correct Answer: B) Secure the drain to the patient before connecting it to the suction tubing.
Rationale: Securing the drain to the patient first ensures it is properly positioned and reduces the risk of dislodgement. Option A is incorrect because attaching the drain to the suction tubing first can lead to accidental dislodgement. Option C is incorrect as priming with saline is unnecessary and could introduce contamination. Option D is partially correct but does not address the primary step of securing the drain to the patient.

Question 123: Correct Answer: B) Remove all soiled linens and waste materials.
Rationale: The first step in room turnover is to remove all soiled linens and waste materials to prevent contamination and ensure a clean environment for the next procedure. Disinfecting surfaces (A) and restocking supplies (C) should follow after the initial removal of contaminants. Checking and refilling the anesthesia cart (D) is important but not the first priority in the clean-up process.

Question 124: Correct Answer: B) Suctioning intermittently to avoid tissue damage
Rationale: Suctioning intermittently is essential to avoid tissue damage and ensure effective removal of fluids. Continuous suctioning can cause tissue trauma, making Option A incorrect. Option C is incorrect as suction is used to remove, not introduce, fluids. Option D is incorrect because avoiding suction can lead to fluid accumulation and contamination, compromising the surgical field.

Question 125: Correct Answer: B) Allowing her to bring a favorite toy into the operating room
Rationale: Allowing Emily to bring a favorite toy into the operating room helps reduce her anxiety and provides comfort, which is crucial for pediatric patients. Administering a sedative (A) may be necessary but is not the first step. Explaining the procedure in detailed medical terms (C) is not appropriate for her age. Restricting food and fluids (D) is important but does not address her emotional needs.

Question 126: Correct Answer: B) Disconnect the cautery machine and other electrical equipment before removing the drapes.
Rationale: Disconnecting the cautery machine and other electrical equipment ensures that there is no risk of accidental burns or electrical hazards. Option A is incorrect as it could disrupt the sterile field. Option C is unsafe as it poses a risk of burns. Option D is not ideal because the technologist should manage equipment safety directly.

Question 127: Correct Answer: B) Weighing sponges and drapes before and after use
Rationale: Weighing sponges and drapes before and after use is the primary method for estimating blood loss as it provides a quantifiable measure. Visual estimation (A) is subjective and often inaccurate. Counting instruments (C) does not relate to blood loss. Measuring irrigation fluid (D) helps in fluid balance but not directly in estimating blood loss. This method ensures a more accurate assessment compared to visual estimation, which can be highly

variable.

Question 128: Correct Answer: B) Wearing lead aprons and standing behind a lead shield

Rationale: Wearing lead aprons and standing behind a lead shield is the best practice to protect the surgical team from x-ray exposure. Standing directly behind the x-ray machine (Option A) does not provide adequate protection, increasing distance (Option C) alone is not sufficient without shielding, and using a handheld x-ray device (Option D) can increase exposure risk. Lead aprons and shields effectively block radiation, ensuring the safety of the surgical team.

Question 129: Correct Answer: B) Addressing the conflict directly and facilitating open communication

Rationale: Addressing the conflict directly and facilitating open communication is the most effective strategy for resolving conflicts within a surgical team. This approach encourages transparency and mutual understanding, which are essential for resolving issues. Ignoring the conflict (Option A) can lead to unresolved tensions, assigning blame (Option C) can create a hostile environment, and involving only senior staff (Option D) can exclude valuable perspectives from other team members.

Question 130: Correct Answer: A) Attending annual conferences and workshops

Rationale: Attending annual conferences and workshops is the most effective way for a Certified Surgical Technologist to stay updated with the latest advancements in surgical technology. These events provide access to the latest research, hands-on training, and networking opportunities with experts in the field. Relying solely on colleagues (B) may result in incomplete or outdated information, using outdated textbooks (C) does not provide current advancements, and ignoring new technologies (D) hinders professional growth and patient care quality.

Question 131: Correct Answer: A) Prone position with chest rolls

Rationale: The prone position with chest rolls is ideal for spinal surgery as it provides direct access to the posterior spine while maintaining airway patency and reducing pressure on the abdomen. The supine position with head elevated (B) does not provide access to the posterior spine. The lateral decubitus position (C) is used for thoracic or hip surgeries. Fowler's position (D) is used for head, neck, and shoulder surgeries, not spinal procedures.

Question 132: Correct Answer: A) Check the surgical drapes for pooling blood.

Rationale: Checking the surgical drapes for pooling blood is the first step in identifying the source of blood loss. Increasing the IV fluid rate (Option B) addresses blood pressure but not the source of bleeding. Calling for additional blood units (Option C) is necessary but secondary to identifying the cause. Monitoring urine output (Option D) is important for assessing overall volume status but does not directly identify the bleeding source.

Question 133: Correct Answer: B) Dispose of them in a puncture-resistant, leak-proof sharps container.

Rationale: Contaminated sharps must be disposed of in a puncture-resistant, leak-proof sharps container to prevent injury and contamination. Options A and C are incorrect because they do not ensure safety and compliance with Standard Precautions. Option D is incorrect as wrapping in a towel does not provide adequate protection against punctures and leaks, posing a risk to healthcare workers.

Question 134: Correct Answer: B) Using an online continuing education tracking system

Rationale: Using an online continuing education tracking system (B) allows John to efficiently manage and verify his credits in a centralized, accessible manner. A handwritten logbook (A) and email confirmations (C) can be disorganized and prone to errors. Relying on a supervisor (D) is not practical or reliable. Online systems are designed for accuracy and ease of access.

Question 135: Correct Answer: C) Flash sterilization using a pre-vacuum autoclave

Rationale: Flash sterilization using a pre-vacuum autoclave is the most appropriate method for immediate use as it rapidly achieves high temperatures necessary for sterilization. Ethylene oxide gas sterilization (A) and chemical sterilization using glutaraldehyde (D) require longer processing times, making them unsuitable for immediate use. Steam sterilization using a gravity displacement autoclave (B) is slower compared to a pre-vacuum autoclave, making option C the best choice for urgent situations.

Question 136: Correct Answer: D) Matching the graft's porosity to the patient's bone density.

Rationale: Ensuring the graft's porosity matches the patient's bone density is critical for proper integration and osseointegration. Sterilizing with alcohol (A) and soaking in saline (B) are important but secondary steps. Ensuring the graft is contaminant-free (C) is necessary but does not directly affect integration. Matching porosity (D) ensures the graft supports new bone growth and vascularization, leading to successful integration.

Question 137: Correct Answer: B) To improve visualization by creating space

Rationale: Insufflating the abdomen with carbon dioxide during a laparoscopic cholecystectomy creates space, improving visualization and access to the surgical site. Sterilizing the abdominal cavity (A) and reducing infection risk (C) are not functions of insufflation. Cooling surgical instruments (D) is unrelated to the purpose of insufflation.

Question 138: Correct Answer: B) Arterial bleeding

Rationale: Bright red blood is indicative of arterial bleeding due to its high oxygen content. Venous bleeding (Option A) typically presents as dark red blood because it is deoxygenated. Capillary bleeding (Option C) is usually a slow, oozing type of bleeding, and coagulated blood (Option D) is dark and clotted. Therefore, the bright red color is a clear sign of arterial bleeding.

Question 139: Correct Answer: C) Tracking and documenting the usage of supplies

Rationale: The primary responsibility of a surgical technologist in maintaining inventory control is tracking and documenting the usage of supplies. This ensures that the operating room is adequately stocked and that supplies are available when needed. While ordering new supplies (A) and sterilizing instruments (B) are important, they are not the primary responsibility. Assisting in surgical procedures (D) is a core duty but unrelated to inventory control.

Question 140: Correct Answer: B) Inform the surgeon immediately and stop using the device.

Rationale: The correct action is to inform the surgeon immediately and stop using the device to prevent any potential harm to the patient. Ignoring the sparking (A) or adjusting the settings (C) could lead to further complications. Replacing the device without informing the surgeon (D) could cause confusion and delay in the procedure. Prompt communication ensures patient safety and allows for appropriate measures to be taken.

Question 141: Correct Answer: C) Turn off the suction device.

Rationale: The first step is to turn off the suction device to prevent any accidental suctioning that could harm the patient. Disconnecting the device (Option A) or removing drapes (Option B) before turning off the suction could lead to injury. Checking the suction canister (Option D) is important but should be done after ensuring the suction device is off.

Question 142: Correct Answer: A) Ligature

Rationale: A ligature involves tying off a blood vessel with suture material, a mechanical method of hemostasis suitable for controlling bleeding from a small vessel in the mesentery. The argon beam coagulator (B) is an electrical method, topical thrombin (C) is a chemical method, and a gelatin sponge (D) is an absorbable hemostatic agent. Therefore, a ligature (A) is the most appropriate mechanical method in this context.

Question 143: Correct Answer: B) Elimination of donor site morbidity

Rationale: The main advantage of using an allograft over an autograft is the elimination of donor site morbidity, which means there is no need to harvest tissue from the patient, reducing overall trauma. Reduced risk of immune rejection (Option A) is incorrect as allografts have a higher risk of rejection compared to autografts. Higher osteogenic potential (Option C) is also incorrect as autografts generally have higher osteogenic potential. Immediate availability (Option D) is a benefit but not the main advantage.

Question 144: Correct Answer: B) Saphenous nerve

Rationale: The saphenous nerve must be carefully preserved during a femoral-popliteal bypass to prevent nerve damage, which can lead to sensory loss or neuropathic pain. The femoral artery (A) and popliteal vein (C) are important vascular structures but not directly related to nerve damage. The tibial nerve (D) is not typically at risk in this procedure. Preserving the saphenous nerve is crucial for maintaining sensory function in the lower leg.

Question 145: Correct Answer: B) Electrocautery

Rationale: Electrocautery is the most appropriate thermal method for achieving hemostasis during a laparoscopic cholecystectomy. It uses electrical current to generate heat, which coagulates blood vessels effectively. Cryotherapy is not suitable as it involves freezing tissues. An ultrasonic scalpel, while useful, primarily cuts and coagulates simultaneously and is not typically the first choice for hemostasis alone. Laser coagulation is less commonly used due to its complexity and cost.

Question 146: Correct Answer: B) Updating electronic health records (EHR)

Rationale: Updating electronic health records (EHR) is a crucial administrative duty for a CST, ensuring accurate and up-to-date patient information. Browsing the internet, playing games, and watching tutorials, while potentially educational, do not directly contribute to maintaining patient records. The EHR system is specifically designed for this purpose, making option B the correct choice.

Question 147: Correct Answer: D) Manually scrub the instrument with a brush under running water.

Rationale: The first step in decontaminating an instrument with visible organic material is to manually scrub it with a brush under running water to remove debris. This ensures that the instrument is free of gross contaminants before further cleaning. Option A is incorrect because ultrasonic cleaning is a secondary step. Option B is partially correct but insufficient as it does not involve scrubbing. Option C is incorrect because soaking in disinfectant is not the first step.

Question 148: Correct Answer: B) Dermis

Rationale: The dermis provides the necessary support and nourishment for a skin graft to survive due to its rich blood supply and structural components. The epidermis and stratum basale do not provide sufficient nourishment as they are avascular. The subcutaneous tissue, while providing some support, is not as crucial as the dermis for graft survival.

Question 149: Correct Answer: B) Double-checking all entries for accuracy before submission

Rationale: Double-checking all entries for accuracy before submission is crucial to ensure data integrity and reliability in research. While using pre-approved abbreviations and codes (Option C) is important, it does not guarantee accuracy. Entering data quickly (Option A) and relying on memory (Option D) can lead to errors, compromising the study's validity.

Question 150: Correct Answer: B) As Needed

Rationale: "PRN" is a common medical abbreviation derived from the Latin phrase "pro re nata," which means "as needed." This term is often used in prescribing medications or treatments that are not scheduled but administered based on the patient's condition. Options A, C, and D are incorrect as they do not accurately represent the meaning of "PRN" and are not used in this context.

CST Exam Practice Questions [SET 4]

Question 1: During a laparoscopic cholecystectomy on a patient named Mr. Smith, the surgeon asks for a "Maryland dissector." Which instrument should the surgical technologist hand to the surgeon?
A) Kelly clamp
B) Metzenbaum scissors
C) Maryland dissector
D) Kocher clamp

Question 2: Which of the following enzymes is produced by the pancreas and plays a crucial role in the digestion of proteins?
A) Amylase
B) Lipase
C) Trypsin
D) Pepsin

Question 3: During a postoperative debriefing, which listening barrier is most likely to hinder effective communication among the surgical team?
A) Using medical jargon
B) Interrupting the speaker frequently
C) Asking clarifying questions
D) Providing feedback

Question 4: Mrs. Smith, post-appendectomy, exhibits a sudden drop in blood pressure, increased heart rate, and cold, clammy skin. What should be your immediate course of action?
A) Elevate the patient's legs and wait for improvement.
B) Inform the patient that these symptoms are temporary.
C) Report the symptoms immediately to the surgical team.
D) Administer fluids orally to stabilize blood pressure.

Question 5: What is the primary reason for reviewing the surgeon's preference card during preoperative preparation?
A) To verify the patient's medical history
B) To ensure all required instruments are available
C) To confirm the surgical team's schedule
D) To check the operating room's cleanliness

Question 6: Which of the following is a critical consideration when using a short cycle for sterilizing instruments?
A) Ensuring instruments are pre-cleaned thoroughly
B) Using a lower temperature to avoid instrument damage
C) Sterilizing instruments in large batches
D) Extending the drying time to ensure sterility

Question 7: 4 What is the primary purpose of using a selective culture medium in microbiology?
A) To enhance the growth of all microorganisms
B) To differentiate between types of microorganisms
C) To inhibit the growth of certain microorganisms while allowing others to grow
D) To provide a nutrient-rich environment for fastidious organisms

Question 8: During a preoperative preparation, the surgical technologist, Alex, is about to assist in a procedure involving a patient with a known airborne infection. Which of the following sequences of donning personal protective equipment (PPE) is correct?
A) Gown, gloves, mask, goggles
B) Mask, gown, gloves, goggles
C) Gown, mask, goggles, gloves
D) Mask, goggles, gown, gloves

Question 9: During a total hip arthroplasty, the surgical team needs to control bleeding from the femoral artery. Which thermal method should be used to ensure effective hemostasis?
A) Bipolar electrosurgery
B) Argon beam coagulation
C) Radiofrequency ablation
D) Cryotherapy

Question 10: What is the primary purpose of using a microscope during a surgical procedure?
A) To magnify the surgical field for better visualization
B) To sterilize the surgical instruments
C) To provide illumination in the operating room
D) To monitor the patient's vital signs

Question 11: What is the most appropriate action to take if a surgical technologist notices a small tear in the sterile drape during a procedure?
A) Ignore the tear and continue the procedure.
B) Cover the tear with a sterile towel and continue.
C) Inform the surgeon and replace the drape.
D) Use a non-sterile adhesive to patch the tear.

Question 12: During a laparoscopic appendectomy on a patient named Ms. Smith, the insufflator suddenly stops working. What is the most appropriate immediate action for the surgical technologist to take?
A) Increase the flow rate on the insufflator.
B) Check the gas supply and tubing connections.
C) Switch to a backup insufflator immediately.
D) Inform the surgeon and wait for further instructions.

Question 13: During a laparoscopic procedure, which mechanical device is often used to prevent bleeding from small blood vessels?
A) Harmonic scalpel
B) Ligating clips
C) Fibrin sealant
D) Bone wax

Question 14: Which instrument is specifically designed for clamping blood vessels during surgery?
A) Kocher Forceps
B) Kelly Hemostats
C) Metzenbaum Scissors
D) DeBakey Forceps

Question 15: What is the primary hazard associated with surgical smoke in the operating room?
A) Infection risk
B) Visual impairment
C) Toxic chemical exposure
D) Fire hazard

Question 16: During an intraoperative procedure, the surgical technologist notices that the harmonic scalpel is not performing optimally. What is the most likely cause of this issue?
A) The blade is dull and needs to be replaced.
B) The generator is not properly grounded.
C) The ultrasonic frequency is set too high.
D) The patient's tissue is too dense for the harmonic scalpel to function effectively.

Question 17: When assembling a surgical microscope, what is the most crucial step to ensure optimal visualization during the procedure?
A) Adjusting the height of the microscope stand
B) Calibrating the focus and magnification settings
C) Ensuring the light source is functioning
D) Verifying the cleanliness of the lenses

Question 18: Which of the following is the most effective approach for a surgical technologist to use diplomacy when addressing a conflict between team members in the operating room?
A) Ignore the conflict and focus on the task at hand.
B) Take sides with one of the team members.
C) Address the conflict calmly and facilitate a resolution.
D) Report the conflict to the hospital administration immediately.

Question 19: During the preoperative preparation for Mr. Smith's laparoscopic cholecystectomy, the surgical technologist discovers that the insufflator is malfunctioning. What is the most appropriate action to take to ensure the surgery proceeds as scheduled?
A) Attempt to repair the insufflator on the spot.
B) Inform the surgeon and delay the surgery until the insufflator is fixed.
C) Replace the insufflator with a backup unit from the reserve equipment.
D) Proceed with the surgery without using the insufflator.

Question 20: What is the first step a Certified Surgical Technologist should take when receiving a specimen from the surgical field?
A) Label the specimen container immediately.
B) Verify the specimen type and patient information with the surgeon.
C) Prepare the specimen for transport to the pathology lab.
D) Place the specimen in formalin for preservation.

Question 21: What is the primary purpose of applying a sequential compression device (SCD) to a patient preoperatively?
A) To prevent deep vein thrombosis (DVT)
B) To maintain body temperature
C) To reduce surgical site infection
D) To manage postoperative pain

Question 22: Where should the bovie pad be placed to ensure optimal patient safety during an electrosurgical procedure?
A) Over a bony prominence
B) On a well-vascularized muscle mass
C) On the patient's chest
D) Near the surgical site

Question 23: Which of the following personal protective equipment (PPE) is most essential for a Certified Surgical Technologist to wear when dealing with a chemical spill?
A) Surgical mask
B) Sterile gloves
C) Chemical-resistant gloves
D) Hair cover

Question 24: Sarah, a surgical technologist, is conducting a literature review for a research project on the effectiveness of different sterilization techniques. Which of the following steps should she take first to ensure a comprehensive and relevant review?
A) Search for articles using a single keyword
B) Use multiple databases and a variety of keywords
C) Only review articles from the past year
D) Focus solely on articles from a single journal

Question 25: During a preoperative check, you notice that the power cord of a piece of surgical equipment is frayed. What should be your immediate action?
A) Use the equipment carefully, ensuring the frayed part does not touch anything.
B) Report the issue to the supervisor and tag the equipment as "out of service."
C) Cover the frayed part with electrical tape and proceed with the surgery.
D) Use the equipment only if absolutely necessary and document the issue later.

Question 26: During a total hip replacement surgery for Mr. Johnson, the surgeon asks for a specific type and size of acetabular cup implant. As a Certified Surgical Technologist, what is the

most appropriate action to take before handing the implant to the surgeon?
A) Hand the implant directly to the surgeon without verification.
B) Verify the type and size of the implant with the surgeon before handing it over.
C) Assume the implant size based on the patient's preoperative measurements.
D) Ask the circulating nurse to verify the implant type and size.

Question 27: What is the primary purpose of using a fluid warmer in the perioperative setting?
A) To prevent hypothermia by warming intravenous fluids
B) To cool intravenous fluids for patients with hyperthermia
C) To sterilize intravenous fluids before administration
D) To maintain the viscosity of intravenous fluids

Question 28: Ms. Smith is scheduled for a total hip replacement. During preoperative positioning, what is the most important consideration to prevent complications?
A) Placing the patient in the prone position to improve surgical access.
B) Ensuring the patient's legs are crossed to maintain stability.
C) Positioning the patient in the lateral decubitus position with appropriate padding.
D) Elevating the patient's head to reduce the risk of aspiration.

Question 29: What is the recommended temperature range for an operating room to ensure patient safety and optimal surgical conditions?
A) 60-65°F (15.6-18.3°C)
B) 68-73°F (20-22.8°C)
C) 75-80°F (23.9-26.7°C)
D) 80-85°F (26.7-29.4°C)

Question 30: What postoperative finding should be reported as it may indicate internal bleeding?
A) Light bruising around the surgical site
B) Decreased urine output
C) Increased pain unrelieved by medication
D) Slight increase in heart rate

Question 31: During a surgical procedure, the surgical technologist, Alex, notices that a laparoscopic instrument is not functioning correctly. What is the first step Alex should take to address this issue?
A) Continue using the instrument and report it after the surgery.
B) Inform the surgeon immediately and replace the instrument.
C) Attempt to fix the instrument on the sterile field.
D) Sterilize the instrument again and then use it.

Question 32: During a surgical team debrief,

which listening strategy is most effective for resolving misunderstandings?
A) Interrupting to correct errors
B) Asking open-ended questions
C) Waiting for a pause to speak
D) Providing immediate feedback

Question 33: Which of the following thermoregulatory devices is most commonly used to maintain a patient's core temperature during surgery?
A) Forced-air warming blanket
B) Ice packs
C) Cooling vests
D) Heated intravenous fluids

Question 34: Which type of cell in the integumentary system is primarily responsible for producing melanin, the pigment that gives skin its color?
A) Keratinocytes
B) Melanocytes
C) Langerhans cells
D) Merkel cells

Question 35: What is the primary purpose of utilizing computer technology in surgical research?
A) To automate surgical procedures
B) To enhance data collection and analysis
C) To replace the need for surgical personnel
D) To eliminate the use of physical records

Question 36: During preoperative preparation for a total knee arthroplasty on Mrs. Smith, you need to ensure the bovie pad is correctly positioned. Which of the following is the most critical consideration when placing the bovie pad?
A) Ensuring the pad is placed over a bony prominence
B) Ensuring the pad is placed on clean, dry skin
C) Ensuring the pad is placed near the surgical site
D) Ensuring the pad is placed on an area with hair

Question 37: How can utilizing computer technology enhance the management of surgeon's preference cards?
A) By allowing real-time updates and easy access to preference cards
B) By automatically diagnosing patient conditions
C) By providing a platform for patient-surgeon communication
D) By generating automated surgical reports

Question 38: Which of the following is the most effective method to minimize radiation exposure to the surgical team during intraoperative x-rays?
A) Standing directly next to the x-ray source
B) Wearing a lead apron and thyroid shield
C) Increasing the duration of x-ray exposure
D) Using a higher dose of radiation for clearer images

Question 39: After a successful laparoscopic cholecystectomy, the surgical team is preparing to transfer Mr. Johnson from the operating table to the stretcher. Which of the following steps should be performed first to ensure a safe transfer?
A) Disconnect all IV lines and catheters.
B) Ensure that the stretcher is locked and at the same height as the operating table.
C) Remove all surgical drapes and instruments from the patient.
D) Position the patient's arms across their chest.

Question 40: What is the primary responsibility of a surgical technologist in maintaining sterile technique during a procedure?
A) Ensuring that all team members adhere to sterile technique.
B) Supervising the surgical procedure.
C) Monitoring the patient's vital signs.
D) Documenting the procedure.

Question 41: During an orthopedic surgery, how should a surgical technologist verify the correct size of an implantable device with the surgeon?
A) By checking the implant size against the patient's medical history
B) By confirming the size with the surgeon using the manufacturer's catalog
C) By asking the circulating nurse to verify the size
D) By relying on the preoperative plan without further verification

Question 42: What is the primary responsibility of a surgical technologist in maintaining the sterile field during a surgical procedure?
A) Supervising the surgical team
B) Ensuring all instruments are accounted for
C) Monitoring the patient's vital signs
D) Passing instruments to the surgeon

Question 43: After completing a surgical procedure on Mr. Smith, what is the correct method for disposing of contaminated drapes to ensure compliance with Standard Precautions?
A) Place them in a regular trash bin.
B) Seal them in a biohazard bag and dispose of them in a designated biohazard waste container.
C) Rinse them with water before disposal.
D) Place them in a laundry hamper for cleaning.

Question 44: In preparation for a lengthy orthopedic surgery on a 60-year-old patient named Mrs. Johnson, the surgical technologist must coordinate the use of thermoregulatory devices. Which of the following is the best practice to prevent perioperative hypothermia?
A) Pre-warming the patient with a warming gown
B) Administering cold IV fluids
C) Using a cooling blanket
D) Keeping the operating room temperature low

Question 45: Which type of cautery is most commonly used for precise tissue dissection in delicate surgeries?
A) Monopolar cautery
B) Bipolar cautery
C) Chemical cautery
D) Thermal cautery

Question 46: During a cataract surgery on Mr. Johnson, the surgeon needs to access the anterior chamber of the eye. Which anatomical structure must be incised first to reach this chamber?
A) Retina
B) Sclera
C) Cornea
D) Vitreous humor

Question 47: Which type of cautery is most commonly used for delicate tissue dissection during postoperative procedures?
A) Monopolar cautery
B) Bipolar cautery
C) Chemical cautery
D) Ultrasonic cautery

Question 48: During an open abdominal surgery on a patient named Mrs. Johnson, the surgeon asks the surgical technologist to provide retraction. Which of the following actions should the surgical technologist take to provide effective retraction?
A) Use excessive force to retract the tissue.
B) Hold the retractor steady and in the correct position.
C) Frequently adjust the retractor without the surgeon's direction.
D) Apply minimal pressure to avoid any tissue damage.

Question 49: During a laparoscopic cholecystectomy on a 45-year-old patient named Mr. Smith, the surgical technologist needs to ensure proper thermoregulation. Which device is most appropriate to maintain the patient's core body temperature?
A) Forced-air warming blanket
B) Ice packs
C) Room temperature IV fluids
D) Electric heating pad

Question 50: Mrs. Smith, a patient recovering from a knee replacement surgery, reports increased pain and swelling around the surgical site. Upon examination, the surgical technologist suspects a hematoma. What is the most likely cause of this postoperative complication?
A) Excessive physical activity post-surgery.
B) Inadequate hemostasis during surgery.
C) Allergic reaction to the sutures.
D) Infection at the surgical site.

Question 51: During a knee replacement surgery, the surgeon decides to use an allograft to repair a defect in the patient's femur. Which of the following steps is crucial to ensure the allograft is prepared correctly?
A) Soak the allograft in saline for 5 minutes.
B) Ensure the allograft is thawed to room temperature.
C) Sterilize the allograft using an autoclave.
D) Rinse the allograft with antibiotic solution.

Question 52: During the postoperative phase, the surgical technologist must report the amount of medication and solution used. If a patient named Mrs. Johnson received 1 liter of Ringer's lactate and 50 mcg of fentanyl, how should this be accurately reported?
A) Report only the Ringer's lactate amount.
B) Report only the fentanyl amount.
C) Report both the Ringer's lactate and fentanyl amounts.
D) Report the Ringer's lactate amount and note that fentanyl was administered without specifying the amount.

Question 53: During an intraoperative procedure, which of the following is the best practice to prevent contamination of the sterile field?
A) Reaching over the sterile field to adjust equipment.
B) Keeping sterile instruments below waist level.
C) Ensuring all sterile team members face the sterile field.
D) Allowing non-sterile personnel to pass between sterile fields.

Question 54: Mrs. Johnson is scheduled for surgery and has a known allergy to penicillin. What is the most appropriate step to take regarding her antibiotic prophylaxis?
A) Administer penicillin but monitor for adverse reactions.
B) Substitute penicillin with a cephalosporin.
C) Use an alternative antibiotic such as clindamycin or vancomycin.
D) Avoid administering any antibiotics to prevent an allergic reaction.

Question 55: Which structure in the eye is primarily responsible for focusing light onto the retina?
A) Cornea
B) Lens
C) Iris
D) Sclera

Question 56: What is the primary function of the aqueous humor in the eye?
A) To provide nutrients to the cornea and lens
B) To maintain the shape of the eyeball
C) To transmit light to the retina
D) To control eye movement

Question 57: During a laparoscopic cholecystectomy on a 45-year-old patient named John, the surgeon notices an unexpected increase in blood loss. As a Certified Surgical Technologist, what is the most appropriate immediate action to assist in managing the situation?
A) Increase the insufflation pressure to control bleeding.
B) Hand the surgeon a suction device to clear the field.
C) Inform the anesthesiologist to prepare for a possible transfusion.
D) Apply direct pressure to the bleeding site with a laparoscopic instrument.

Question 58: During the transfer of a patient named John to the operating room table, which of the following steps should be performed first to ensure patient safety?
A) Secure the patient's arms to the arm boards.
B) Confirm the patient's identity and surgical site.
C) Adjust the operating room table to the appropriate height.
D) Apply the safety strap across the patient's thighs.

Question 59: Mr. Johnson is scheduled for a laparoscopic cholecystectomy. During the preoperative assessment, he expresses anxiety about the surgery and concerns about postoperative pain. What is the most appropriate action for the surgical technologist to take?
A) Reassure Mr. Johnson that the surgery is routine and there is nothing to worry about.
B) Inform Mr. Johnson that his concerns will be addressed by the surgeon during the procedure.
C) Acknowledge Mr. Johnson's concerns and inform the perioperative nurse to address them.
D) Tell Mr. Johnson that postoperative pain is minimal and he will receive pain medication.

Question 60: When should the surgical technologist verify the type and size of the implantable item with the surgeon?
A) During the preoperative briefing
B) After the incision is made
C) When the implant is handed to the surgeon
D) During the postoperative debriefing

Question 61: What is the primary purpose of participating in a postoperative case debrief?
A) To assign blame for any complications that occurred
B) To review and improve surgical procedures and teamwork
C) To discuss non-surgical aspects of patient care
D) To finalize billing and administrative paperwork

Question 62: During an anterior cruciate ligament (ACL) reconstruction for Ms. Smith, the surgeon opts for an autograft. Which of the following is a key advantage of using an autograft over an

allograft?
A) Lower risk of disease transmission
B) Faster surgical procedure
C) No need for postoperative rehabilitation
D) Reduced surgical site infection

Question 63: During a laparoscopic cholecystectomy on a 45-year-old patient named John, the surgeon asks for the next instrument after the gallbladder has been dissected and clipped. What instrument should the surgical technologist anticipate?
A) Laparoscopic scissors
B) Laparoscopic grasper
C) Laparoscopic suction/irrigation device
D) Laparoscopic specimen retrieval bag

Question 64: When draping a C-arm fluoroscopy unit, which of the following steps is essential to ensure sterility during a surgical procedure?
A) Drape the entire C-arm, including the wheels.
B) Only drape the portion of the C-arm that will come into contact with the sterile field.
C) Drape the C-arm and the patient together to ensure complete coverage.
D) Use a sterile cover that extends beyond the sterile field to cover the C-arm.

Question 65: Which of the following is the most appropriate initial action for a surgical technologist to take upon noticing a rash on a postoperative patient's skin?
A) Apply a topical antibiotic ointment to the rash
B) Notify the surgeon immediately
C) Document the rash in the patient's chart and continue monitoring
D) Administer an antihistamine to the patient

Question 66: During an orthopedic surgery, the surgeon requests the application of a short arm cast for a patient named John. Which of the following steps is crucial to ensure the cast is properly applied and prevents complications?
A) Applying the cast material directly to the skin without padding.
B) Ensuring the cast is snug but not too tight to allow for swelling.
C) Using hot water to speed up the setting time of the cast material.
D) Wrapping the cast material in a circular motion without overlapping.

Question 67: During a surgical procedure on a patient named John, the surgeon needs to make an incision through the layers of the skin. Which layer of the skin contains the blood vessels that will be encountered first?
A) Epidermis
B) Dermis
C) Subcutaneous tissue
D) Stratum corneum

Question 68: What is the primary purpose of performing a surgical count before the start of a procedure?
A) To ensure all surgical instruments are sterile
B) To verify the availability of all necessary equipment
C) To prevent retained surgical items
D) To confirm the patient's identity

Question 69: What safety measure is essential when using laser technology in the operating room to protect the surgical team?
A) Using standard surgical masks
B) Wearing laser-specific eyewear
C) Applying sunscreen to exposed skin
D) Using lead aprons

Question 70: During a robotic-assisted laparoscopic prostatectomy using the Da Vinci system, what is the most critical step in draping the robotic arms to ensure sterility?
A) Draping the patient first before positioning the robotic arms.
B) Draping the robotic arms first before positioning them over the patient.
C) Draping the robotic arms and patient simultaneously.
D) Draping the robotic arms after they are positioned over the patient.

Question 71: What is the primary consideration when transporting a patient with a suspected spinal injury to the operating room?
A) Ensuring the patient is comfortable
B) Maintaining spinal alignment
C) Monitoring the patient's vital signs
D) Communicating with the surgical team

Question 72: When transferring a patient named Sarah from the stretcher to the operating room table, what is the most important consideration to prevent injury to the patient and staff?
A) Using a draw sheet or transfer board.
B) Asking the patient to move herself if possible.
C) Lifting the patient manually with the help of two staff members.
D) Ensuring the operating room table is locked in place.

Question 73: During a craniotomy procedure on a patient named John, the surgeon asks the surgical technologist to identify the structure responsible for producing cerebrospinal fluid (CSF). Which structure should the surgical technologist identify?
A) Corpus callosum
B) Choroid plexus
C) Amygdala
D) Thalamus

Question 74: What is the primary purpose of a surgeon's preference card in the operating room?
A) To document the patient's medical history

B) To list the surgeon's preferred instruments and supplies
C) To record the surgical procedure's duration
D) To track the anesthesia used during surgery

Question 75: During a laparoscopic cholecystectomy on a patient named Mr. Johnson, the surgeon encounters a small but persistent bleed from a cystic artery branch. Which mechanical method of hemostasis should the surgical technologist prepare to assist the surgeon in controlling the bleed?
A) Electrocautery
B) Hemostatic clips
C) Fibrin sealant
D) Bone wax

Question 76: During a surgical procedure, the surgeon asks for a suture. What is the correct way to pass the suture material to the surgeon?
A) Handing it directly to the surgeon with bare hands
B) Passing it with the needle pointing towards the surgeon
C) Using a needle holder to pass the suture with the needle pointing away from the surgeon
D) Placing it on the sterile field for the surgeon to pick up

Question 77: 0 Mrs. Smith is undergoing an abdominal surgery. The surgical team is concerned about preventing a surgical site infection caused by Staphylococcus aureus. Which of the following preoperative measures is most effective in reducing the risk of infection?
A) Administering a single dose of antibiotics postoperatively
B) Using an alcohol-based antiseptic for skin preparation
C) Shaving the surgical site the night before surgery
D) Applying a povidone-iodine solution immediately before incision

Question 78: What is the first step in removing drapes from a patient postoperatively?
A) Cut the drapes with sterile scissors
B) Remove the drapes in a single motion
C) Ensure all instruments are removed from the drapes
D) Pull the drapes towards the patient's head

Question 79: What is the primary purpose of monitoring a patient's vital signs in the immediate postoperative period?
A) To assess the patient's pain level
B) To detect early signs of complications
C) To ensure the patient is comfortable
D) To determine the patient's nutritional needs

Question 80: Dr. Smith is performing an abdominal hysterectomy and requests a 2-0 silk suture for ligating a vessel. After passing the suture, what is the next appropriate action?

A) Cut the suture immediately after passing it.
B) Hold the suture ends taut for the surgeon.
C) Prepare another suture in anticipation.
D) Wait for the surgeon to request cutting the suture.

Question 81: If a fire breaks out in the operating room, what is the most appropriate initial action for the surgical technologist?
A) Use a fire extinguisher to put out the fire.
B) Evacuate the patient from the operating room.
C) Turn off the oxygen supply.
D) Call for help.

Question 82: During the Time Out procedure, who is responsible for initiating the process?
A) The circulating nurse
B) The anesthesiologist
C) The surgical technologist
D) The surgeon

Question 83: You are mentoring a new perioperative nurse, Maria, who is preparing for her first role as a circulating nurse. Which of the following is the most crucial aspect you should emphasize to Maria regarding her responsibilities?
A) Ensuring all surgical instruments are sterile before the procedure.
B) Maintaining the sterile field throughout the surgery.
C) Documenting the surgical procedure accurately.
D) Assisting the anesthesiologist with patient monitoring.

Question 84: During a surgical procedure, the surgical technologist notices that the sterile field has been compromised. What is the most appropriate immediate action to take?
A) Continue with the procedure and inform the surgeon later.
B) Immediately inform the surgeon and replace the contaminated items.
C) Wait until the procedure is completed to address the issue.
D) Inform the circulating nurse and continue with the procedure.

Question 85: In the preoperative preparation of a bariatric patient, which of the following is essential to minimize the risk of postoperative complications?
A) Administering a high-calorie diet
B) Encouraging increased fluid intake
C) Implementing a preoperative exercise regimen
D) Conducting a thorough respiratory assessment

Question 86: During the transfer of Ms. Davis from the operating table to the stretcher post-appendectomy, she begins to show signs of hypotension. What is the most appropriate immediate action?
A) Complete the transfer quickly to get her to the recovery room.

B) Elevate the patient's legs while still on the operating table.
C) Administer IV fluids immediately.
D) Call for additional staff to assist with the transfer.

Question 87: After a complex orthopedic surgery on Ms. Smith, the surgical team conducts a debrief. Which of the following is a key component that should be included in the debrief discussion?
A) The exact duration of the surgery.
B) The specific instruments used during the procedure.
C) Any deviations from the planned procedure and their outcomes.
D) The personal performance review of each team member.

Question 88: While preparing for an abdominal surgery, the surgical technologist, Maria, finds that the expiration date on a sterile package of drapes has passed. What is the appropriate action for Maria to take?
A) Use the drapes if they appear undamaged and clean
B) Extend the expiration date by 30 days and use the drapes
C) Discard the drapes and obtain a new sterile package
D) Use the drapes and inform the circulating nurse

Question 89: During a laparoscopic cholecystectomy on a patient named Mrs. Johnson, the surgeon asks for an instrument to grasp and manipulate the gallbladder. Which instrument should the surgical technologist hand to the surgeon?
A) Metzenbaum Scissors
B) Babcock Forceps
C) Kocher Clamp
D) Allis Clamp

Question 90: During a laparoscopic cholecystectomy, the surgeon asks the surgical technologist to identify the structure that transports bile from the liver and gallbladder to the duodenum. What is the correct structure?
A) Hepatic artery
B) Common bile duct
C) Portal vein
D) Cystic duct

Question 91: During an intraoperative procedure, which sign is most indicative of potential malignant hyperthermia?
A) Hypotension
B) Tachycardia
C) Bradycardia
D) Hypothermia

Question 92: Mrs. Smith, a postoperative patient, develops a widespread rash on her torso two days

after surgery. What should be your primary concern in this scenario?
A) The rash could be a sign of a latex allergy.
B) The rash is likely a reaction to the surgical dressing.
C) The rash may indicate a systemic infection.
D) The rash is probably due to postoperative stress.

Question 93: Which of the following is the most accurate method for estimating intraoperative blood loss during a surgical procedure?
A) Visual estimation by the surgical team
B) Weighing sponges and measuring suction canisters
C) Counting the number of used surgical sponges
D) Monitoring the patient's vital signs

Question 94: During an open abdominal surgery on a patient named Sarah, the surgeon needs to control diffuse bleeding from a liver laceration. Which thermal method should the surgical technologist prepare?
A) Argon beam coagulation
B) Cryotherapy
C) Bipolar electrosurgery
D) Harmonic scalpel

Question 95: Ms. Johnson, a 58-year-old patient, is being prepared for abdominal surgery. The surgical technologist must ensure the proper application of sequential compression devices (SCDs). Which of the following steps is essential for the effective use of SCDs?
A) Applying the SCDs immediately after the patient is anesthetized
B) Ensuring the SCDs are applied loosely for patient comfort
C) Checking that the SCDs are properly sized and fitted to the patient's legs
D) Removing the SCDs every hour for skin inspection

Question 96: Mrs. Johnson is scheduled for surgery and has a documented allergy to penicillin. Which of the following steps should the surgical technologist take to address this allergy?
A) Ensure the patient wears an allergy bracelet.
B) Administer a test dose of penicillin to confirm the allergy.
C) Use an alternative antibiotic for prophylaxis.
D) Document the allergy in the patient's chart.

Question 97: During an intraoperative procedure involving the use of a harmonic scalpel, the surgical technologist notices that the device is not cutting efficiently. What is the most likely cause of this issue?
A) The device is not properly grounded.
B) The blade is dull or damaged.
C) The power settings are too high.
D) The patient is not properly positioned.

Question 98: Which of the following is the most

important initial step when transferring a patient from the stretcher to the operating room table?
A) Ensure the patient's surgical site is exposed.
B) Verify the patient's identity and surgical procedure.
C) Position the operating room table at the same height as the stretcher.
D) Apply safety straps to secure the patient.

Question 99: Which congenital condition is characterized by the incomplete closure of the spinal column, potentially leading to nerve damage and physical disabilities?
A) Hydrocephalus
B) Spina Bifida
C) Anencephaly
D) Microcephaly

Question 100: Which of the following measures is most effective in reducing the exposure to surgical smoke?
A) Wearing double gloves
B) Using high-filtration surgical masks
C) Employing a smoke evacuation system
D) Increasing room ventilation

Question 101: Which of the following is a primary advantage of using a waterless surgical scrub over traditional methods?
A) Reduced skin irritation
B) Lower cost
C) Longer scrub time
D) Increased bacterial resistance

Question 102: During a tissue graft preparation for a patient named Ms. Smith, the surgical technologist must ensure the graft is kept moist. What is the best method to achieve this?
A) Place the graft in a dry sterile container.
B) Cover the graft with a sterile drape.
C) Soak the graft in an antibiotic solution.
D) Wrap the graft in a saline-moistened gauze.

Question 103: When preparing a Jackson-Pratt (JP) drain for insertion, what is the primary reason for ensuring the bulb is compressed before connecting it to the tubing?
A) To prevent air from entering the wound site
B) To maintain the sterility of the drain
C) To create negative pressure for fluid drainage
D) To ensure the tubing is properly aligned

Question 104: Sarah, a 25-year-old female, presents to the trauma unit after a fall from a height. She is conscious but complains of severe back pain and numbness in her legs. On examination, there is tenderness over the thoracic spine. What is the most appropriate next step in managing this patient?
A) Perform a focused neurological examination
B) Administer high-dose corticosteroids
C) Obtain an urgent MRI of the spine
D) Log-roll the patient to a prone position

Question 105: Mr. Johnson, a 75-year-old patient with mild cognitive impairment, is preparing for a cataract surgery. What is the most important consideration for his preoperative preparation?
A) Providing detailed written instructions for the patient to follow.
B) Ensuring the patient is accompanied by a caregiver who understands the instructions.
C) Minimizing preoperative fasting to avoid confusion and agitation.
D) Avoiding preoperative medications to prevent cognitive decline.

Question 106: Mrs. Johnson is undergoing a total hip arthroplasty. The surgical team decides to place her in the lateral decubitus position. What is the primary reason for choosing this position?
A) To reduce pressure on the lungs
B) To provide better access to the hip joint
C) To prevent deep vein thrombosis
D) To enhance blood circulation to the lower extremities

Question 107: During an emergency surgery, the surgical team needs to sterilize a set of instruments for immediate use. Which of the following methods is most appropriate for achieving this under a short cycle?
A) Ethylene oxide sterilization
B) Steam sterilization using a flash cycle
C) Dry heat sterilization
D) Chemical sterilization with glutaraldehyde

Question 108: Dr. Smith has recently updated his surgical technique for laparoscopic cholecystectomy, preferring a new type of trocar. As a Certified Surgical Technologist, what is the most appropriate action to take regarding Dr. Smith's preference card?
A) Wait until Dr. Smith requests the new trocar during surgery.
B) Update Dr. Smith's preference card immediately to include the new trocar.
C) Inform the surgical team verbally about the change.
D) Use the old trocar until the change is officially documented.

Question 109: What is the most effective active listening technique to ensure understanding during a preoperative team briefing?
A) Nodding occasionally to show agreement
B) Paraphrasing the speaker's points
C) Maintaining eye contact without interruption
D) Taking detailed notes throughout the briefing

Question 110: During an intraoperative procedure, what is the main purpose of using Doppler ultrasound?
A) To measure the density of tissues.
B) To assess blood flow and detect vascular

abnormalities.
C) To provide a detailed image of bone structures.
D) To monitor the patient's vital signs.

Question 111: During a carotid endarterectomy on Ms. Smith, the surgeon needs to temporarily shunt blood flow to maintain cerebral perfusion. Which of the following devices is most suitable for this purpose?
A) Fogarty catheter
B) Javid shunt
C) Penrose drain
D) Hemoclip

Question 112: Sarah, a surgical technologist, is preparing the sterile field for an orthopedic surgery. Which of the following actions ensures that the sterile instruments remain sterile?
A) Reaching over the sterile field to adjust the light.
B) Keeping hands above the waist and within the sterile field.
C) Allowing the edges of the sterile drape to touch non-sterile surfaces.
D) Placing sterile instruments on the edge of the sterile field.

Question 113: Which structure in the ear is primarily responsible for converting sound waves into neural signals?
A) Tympanic membrane
B) Cochlea
C) Eustachian tube
D) Semicircular canals

Question 114: Why is it important to monitor and maintain the temperature within the recommended range in the operating room?
A) To ensure the sterility of surgical instruments
B) To prevent the spread of airborne pathogens
C) To minimize the risk of patient hypothermia
D) To reduce the likelihood of surgical site infections

Question 115: During a total hip replacement surgery for Mr. Johnson, the surgical technologist needs to verify the correct size of the acetabular cup implant. What is the most appropriate action to ensure the correct implant is used?
A) Select the implant size based on the patient's preoperative X-rays.
B) Confirm the implant size with the circulating nurse.
C) Verify the implant size with the surgeon before opening the sterile package.
D) Choose the implant size based on the manufacturer's recommendation.

Question 116: During a surgical procedure on Mr. Johnson, the surgical team must ensure that the environment is free from Clostridium difficile spores. Which of the following measures is most effective in eliminating these spores from the surgical instruments?
A) Standard autoclaving at 121°C for 15 minutes

B) Soaking instruments in 70% isopropyl alcohol for 30 minutes
C) Using ethylene oxide gas sterilization
D) Wiping instruments with a chlorine-based disinfectant

Question 117: During an orthopedic surgery, the surgical technologist is preparing an allograft for implantation in a patient named John. What is the most critical step to ensure the allograft is safe and effective for use?
A) Ensuring the allograft is thawed at room temperature
B) Confirming the allograft is sterilized and free of contaminants
C) Soaking the allograft in saline for 30 minutes
D) Wrapping the allograft in a sterile towel until needed

Question 118: 3 Which type of culture medium is most commonly used to grow and identify Gram-negative bacteria in a clinical laboratory setting?
A) MacConkey agar
B) Blood agar
C) Chocolate agar
D) Sabouraud agar

Question 119: Which of the following is NOT a function of the lymphatic system?
A) Transporting dietary lipids
B) Draining excess interstitial fluid
C) Producing red blood cells
D) Immune response facilitation

Question 120: During a total knee arthroplasty on a 60-year-old patient named Mary, the surgeon is about to cement the prosthetic components. What should the surgical technologist anticipate next?
A) Bone rasp
B) Pulse lavage system
C) Cement mixer and delivery system
D) Tourniquet

Question 121: Which of the following is the most appropriate method for labeling a specimen container in the operating room?
A) Use a pre-printed label with the patient's information.
B) Write the patient's name and date of birth on the container.
C) Include the patient's name, specimen type, and date of collection.
D) Attach a blank label and fill it out later.

Question 122: During a laparoscopic procedure, what is the most critical step a surgical technologist must take when assisting with a laparoscopic stapler?
A) Verifying the stapler's battery charge
B) Ensuring the stapler is properly sterilized
C) Confirming the correct staple size is loaded
D) Checking the stapler's articulation and firing

mechanism

Question 123: When assembling an endoscopic tower, which component is essential for converting the endoscopic image into a format that can be displayed on a monitor?
A) Light source
B) Insufflator
C) Camera control unit (CCU)
D) Suction-irrigation device

Question 124: During an intraoperative procedure, what should a surgical technologist do if they accidentally touch a non-sterile object with a sterile glove?
A) Continue the procedure and avoid touching anything else.
B) Change the glove immediately.
C) Ask a colleague to continue the procedure while they change gloves.
D) Clean the glove with an antiseptic solution.

Question 125: What is the primary reason for ensuring that all suction equipment is properly removed and accounted for after surgery?
A) To maintain a sterile environment in the operating room.
B) To prevent the equipment from being accidentally left inside the patient.
C) To ensure the equipment is ready for the next procedure.
D) To reduce the risk of postoperative infection.

Question 126: When assisting in a total knee arthroplasty, what is the most critical task for the surgical technologist during the cementing of the prosthesis?
A) Ensuring the cement is mixed properly and handed to the surgeon
B) Holding the leg in the correct position
C) Applying the tourniquet
D) Suctioning the blood from the surgical site

Question 127: During preoperative preparation for a knee arthroscopy on Mr. Johnson, the surgical technologist must ensure the pneumatic tourniquet is applied correctly. Which of the following steps is essential to prevent complications?
A) Inflate the tourniquet to 100 mmHg above the patient's systolic blood pressure.
B) Ensure the tourniquet cuff is applied over a single layer of stockinette.
C) Apply the tourniquet cuff directly on the skin without any padding.
D) Inflate the tourniquet immediately after applying the cuff.

Question 128: Sarah, a surgical technologist, is preparing the C-arm for an orthopedic procedure. What is the correct method to drape the C-arm to prevent contamination during surgery?

A) Use a non-sterile cover and ensure it is tightly secured.
B) Drape the C-arm with a sterile cover, ensuring all parts that will be near the sterile field are covered.
C) Only cover the parts of the C-arm that will directly contact the surgical site.
D) Use a sterile cover but leave the bottom part of the C-arm uncovered for mobility.

Question 129: Which type of laser is most commonly used for cutting and coagulating soft tissue during surgical procedures?
A) Carbon Dioxide (CO2) Laser
B) Argon Laser
C) Neodymium-Doped Yttrium Aluminum Garnet (Nd:YAG) Laser
D) Excimer Laser

Question 130: Which of the following is a primary advantage of using an argon laser in surgical procedures?
A) It provides deep tissue penetration.
B) It allows for precise cutting and coagulation.
C) It is the most cost-effective laser option.
D) It has the longest wavelength among surgical lasers.

Question 131: During the preoperative preparation, the surgical technologist, Alex, is responsible for wiping down the operating room and furniture. Which of the following is the most appropriate sequence to ensure a sterile environment?
A) Wipe the surgical table first, then the overhead lights, followed by the floor.
B) Wipe the overhead lights first, then the surgical table, followed by the floor.
C) Wipe the floor first, then the surgical table, followed by the overhead lights.
D) Wipe the surgical table first, then the floor, followed by the overhead lights.

Question 132: Which of the following synthetic materials is most commonly used for bone graft substitutes in orthopedic surgery?
A) Polymethylmethacrylate (PMMA)
B) Hydroxyapatite
C) Silicone
D) Polyethylene

Question 133: What is the primary purpose of applying a bovie pad during an electrosurgical procedure?
A) To monitor the patient's heart rate
B) To ground the patient and complete the electrical circuit
C) To provide a sterile field
D) To administer medication

**Question 134: During a surgical procedure, the surgeon requests a bone graft to be prepared for a patient named Mr. Johnson. What is the first

step the surgical technologist should take to ensure the bone graft is properly prepared?
A) Sterilize the bone graft using an autoclave.
B) Soak the bone graft in saline solution.
C) Verify the bone graft's expiration date and integrity.
D) Shape the bone graft to fit the surgical site.

Question 135: Mr. Smith is undergoing preoperative evaluation for a knee replacement surgery. His laboratory results show a potassium level of 5.8 mEq/L. What should be the surgical technologist's primary concern regarding this lab result?
A) The patient might have an increased risk of cardiac arrhythmias.
B) The patient might have an increased risk of deep vein thrombosis.
C) The patient might have an increased risk of respiratory depression.
D) The patient might have an increased risk of excessive bleeding.

Question 136: During a surgical procedure, you are precepting a new surgical technologist, Alex, who is unsure about the correct sequence of closing counts. What should you instruct Alex to do first?
A) Count the instruments on the Mayo stand.
B) Count the sharps and sponges on the sterile field.
C) Count the instruments on the back table.
D) Count the sponges and sharps off the sterile field.

Question 137: During a preoperative team meeting, Dr. Smith is explaining the surgical procedure to the team. As a Certified Surgical Technologist, what is the most effective listening strategy to ensure you understand the instructions correctly?
A) Nod occasionally to show agreement.
B) Repeat back key points to confirm understanding.
C) Take notes silently without interrupting.
D) Focus on the non-verbal cues of the speaker.

Question 138: Which of the following is a critical step in the preparation of a tissue graft to ensure its viability?
A) Sterilization using high heat
B) Soaking in saline solution
C) Freezing at ultra-low temperatures
D) Coating with antibiotics

Question 139: Which of the following is the most critical factor to monitor in the immediate postoperative period to prevent respiratory complications?
A) Blood pressure
B) Oxygen saturation
C) Urine output
D) Heart rate

Question 140: During the Time Out procedure for Ms. Smith's appendectomy, the circulating nurse realizes that the consent form is missing. What is the most appropriate action to take?
A) Proceed with the surgery and locate the consent form later
B) Pause the Time Out and search for the consent form
C) Continue the Time Out and verbally confirm consent with the patient
D) Halt the procedure until the consent form is found

Question 141: Sarah, a Certified Surgical Technologist, is preparing for a procedure and opts to use a waterless hand antiseptic. What is the recommended duration for rubbing the antiseptic on her hands to achieve proper disinfection?
A) 5 seconds
B) 10 seconds
C) 20 seconds
D) 30 seconds

Question 142: During a coronary artery bypass graft (CABG) surgery, the surgeon asks you to identify the vessel that is commonly used as a graft. Which vessel is most commonly harvested for this purpose?
A) Radial artery
B) Internal mammary artery
C) Femoral artery
D) Carotid artery

Question 143: During a laparoscopic cholecystectomy on a 45-year-old patient named Mr. Smith, the surgeon asks for a suture to close the small incisions in the abdominal wall. Which type of suture is most appropriate for this procedure?
A) Silk suture
B) Polypropylene suture
C) Chromic gut suture
D) Poliglecaprone (Monocryl) suture

Question 144: In the context of laser technology used in intraoperative procedures, why is helium often preferred over other gases?
A) Helium is the most abundant gas in the atmosphere.
B) Helium has a lower ionization energy, making it ideal for laser use.
C) Helium is non-flammable and provides a safe working environment.
D) Helium has a high molecular weight, which enhances laser beam focus.

Question 145: What is the primary reason for performing a count of surgical items before the closure of the surgical site?
A) To ensure all instruments are sterile
B) To confirm the surgical site is free of infection
C) To prevent retained surgical items
D) To verify the patient's identity

Question 146: During the postoperative phase, the surgical technologist is required to report the amount of medication used. In the case of Mrs. Smith, the technologist notices that the recorded amount of anesthetic does not match the actual amount administered. What is the best course of action?
A) Correct the amount in the chart and sign off on it.
B) Inform the anesthesiologist of the discrepancy.
C) Disregard the discrepancy since it is a minor difference.
D) Report the discrepancy to the surgeon during the next scheduled meeting.

Question 147: What is the first step in the room clean-up process after a surgical procedure?
A) Disinfect the surgical instruments
B) Remove all used linens and waste
C) Restock the supply cabinets
D) Mop the floor

Question 148: During a surgical procedure, the surgical technologist, Alex, needs to quickly communicate with the pathology department to confirm the results of a frozen section analysis. Which method of communication would be most efficient and appropriate in this scenario?

A) Sending an email to the pathology department
B) Using the hospital's intercom system
C) Calling the pathology department directly via phone
D) Writing a note and sending it with a runner

Question 149: Which of the following is the primary advantage of using an autograft in surgical procedures?
A) Reduced risk of infection
B) Increased availability of graft material
C) Enhanced integration with host tissue
D) Lower cost compared to synthetic grafts

Question 150: Which computer technology tool is best suited for a Certified Surgical Technologist to access online continuing education courses?
A) Social media platforms
B) Professional organization websites
C) General search engines
D) Personal blogs

ANSWER WITH DETAILED EXPLANATION SET [4]

Question 1: Correct Answer: C) Maryland dissector
Rationale: The Maryland dissector is specifically designed for laparoscopic procedures to dissect and grasp tissues. The Kelly clamp (A) and Kocher clamp (D) are used for clamping and holding tissues but are not appropriate for laparoscopic dissection. Metzenbaum scissors (B) are used for cutting delicate tissues but not for dissection in laparoscopic surgery. Therefore, the correct instrument for the task is the Maryland dissector (C).

Question 2: Correct Answer: C) Trypsin
Rationale: Trypsin, produced by the pancreas, is essential for protein digestion in the small intestine. Amylase breaks down carbohydrates, lipase digests fats, and pepsin, produced by the stomach, also aids in protein digestion but operates in the stomach. Thus, trypsin is the correct enzyme for protein digestion in the small intestine.

Question 3: Correct Answer: B) Interrupting the speaker frequently
Rationale: Interrupting the speaker frequently disrupts the flow of communication and can lead to misunderstandings. Using medical jargon (A) can be a barrier but is less disruptive if the team is familiar with the terms. Asking clarifying questions (C) and providing feedback (D) are essential components of effective listening and communication, enhancing understanding and collaboration.

Question 4: Correct Answer: C) Report the symptoms immediately to the surgical team.
Rationale: A sudden drop in blood pressure, increased heart rate, and cold, clammy skin are signs of potential hemorrhage or shock, which are critical postoperative complications. Immediate reporting to the surgical team is essential for urgent medical intervention. Option A is incorrect as waiting can be dangerous. Option B is misleading since these symptoms are not temporary. Option D is inappropriate because oral fluids are not effective in stabilizing blood pressure in such critical conditions.

Question 5: Correct Answer: B) To ensure all required instruments are available
Rationale: Reviewing the surgeon's preference card is primarily to ensure all required instruments are available, aligning with the surgeon's specific needs for the procedure. Verifying the patient's medical history (A), confirming the surgical team's schedule (C), and checking the operating room's cleanliness (D) are important but pertain to different aspects of preoperative preparation. The preference card directly impacts the readiness and efficiency of the surgical procedure.

Question 6: Correct Answer: A) Ensuring instruments are pre-cleaned thoroughly
Rationale: Ensuring instruments are pre-cleaned thoroughly is critical when using a short cycle for sterilization. Pre-cleaning removes bioburden and ensures effective sterilization. Options B and D are incorrect as they do not align with the principles of short cycle sterilization, and C is incorrect because short cycles are typically used for small, immediate-use loads rather than large batches.

Question 7: Correct Answer: C) To inhibit the growth of certain microorganisms while allowing others to grow
Rationale: Selective culture media contain agents that inhibit the growth of certain bacteria while promoting the growth of others, making it easier to isolate specific types of microorganisms. Enhancing growth of all microorganisms (A) and providing a nutrient-rich environment (D) are not selective. Differentiation (B) is achieved by differential media, not selective media.

Question 8: Correct Answer: D) Mask, goggles, gown, gloves
Rationale: The correct sequence for donning PPE to prevent airborne infection is mask, goggles, gown, and gloves. This ensures the highest level of protection by securing the respiratory tract first. Option A and C incorrectly prioritize the gown and gloves, which do not protect against airborne pathogens. Option B incorrectly places the gloves before the goggles, which can lead to contamination.

Question 9: Correct Answer: A) Bipolar electrosurgery
Rationale: Bipolar electrosurgery is ideal for controlling bleeding from the femoral artery during a total hip arthroplasty. It provides precise coagulation by passing current between two electrodes, minimizing tissue damage. Argon beam coagulation is less precise and more suitable for surface bleeding. Radiofrequency ablation is primarily used for tissue ablation rather than hemostasis. Cryotherapy is inappropriate as it involves freezing and is not effective for arterial bleeding control.

Question 10: Correct Answer: A) To magnify the surgical field for better visualization
Rationale: The primary purpose of using a microscope during a surgical procedure is to magnify the surgical field for better visualization, allowing the surgeon to see small structures and details clearly. Option B is incorrect because sterilization is not a function of the microscope. Option C is incorrect as illumination is provided by surgical lights, not the microscope. Option D is incorrect because monitoring vital signs is done using specialized monitoring equipment, not a microscope.

Question 11: Correct Answer: C) Inform the surgeon and replace the drape.
Rationale: The correct action is to inform the surgeon and replace the drape to maintain the sterile field. Ignoring the tear (A) or covering it with a sterile towel (B) does not fully address the breach in sterility. Using a non-sterile adhesive (D) would further compromise the sterile field. Replacing the drape ensures the highest level of infection control.

Question 12: Correct Answer: B) Check the gas supply and tubing connections.
Rationale: The most appropriate immediate action is to check the gas supply and tubing connections (B) to

ensure there are no obstructions or disconnections causing the insufflator to stop. Increasing the flow rate (A) without checking connections could be dangerous, switching to a backup (C) might not address the root cause, and waiting for instructions (D) could delay the procedure. Ensuring proper gas supply and connection is the first step in troubleshooting.

Question 13: Correct Answer: B) Ligating clips

Rationale: Ligating clips are frequently used in laparoscopic procedures to prevent bleeding from small blood vessels. They provide a reliable mechanical method for vessel occlusion. The harmonic scalpel, while useful, primarily cuts and coagulates tissue using ultrasonic energy. Fibrin sealant and bone wax are chemical and topical agents, respectively, and are not typically used for small vessel hemostasis in laparoscopic surgery. Ligating clips offer precise and effective control of bleeding in these scenarios.

Question 14: Correct Answer: B) Kelly Hemostats

Rationale: Kelly Hemostats are specifically designed for clamping blood vessels during surgery. Kocher Forceps are used for grasping tough tissue, Metzenbaum Scissors are used for cutting delicate tissue, and DeBakey Forceps are used for handling delicate tissues without causing damage. Kelly Hemostats have a locking mechanism and serrated jaws, making them ideal for controlling bleeding by clamping blood vessels, which is not the primary function of the other instruments listed.

Question 15: Correct Answer: C) Toxic chemical exposure

Rationale: The primary hazard associated with surgical smoke is toxic chemical exposure. Surgical smoke contains harmful chemicals such as benzene, hydrogen cyanide, and formaldehyde, which can pose significant health risks to surgical staff. While infection risk (A), visual impairment (B), and fire hazard (D) are concerns, they are not the primary hazard. Infection risk is mitigated by sterile techniques, visual impairment is a secondary issue, and fire hazards are managed through proper equipment and protocols.

Question 16: Correct Answer: A) The blade is dull and needs to be replaced.

Rationale: A dull blade is the most common cause of suboptimal performance in a harmonic scalpel, as it relies on sharpness to effectively cut and coagulate tissue. Option B is incorrect because the harmonic scalpel does not require grounding. Option C is incorrect as the frequency is preset and not adjustable. Option D is incorrect because the harmonic scalpel is designed to handle various tissue densities.

Question 17: Correct Answer: B) Calibrating the focus and magnification settings

Rationale: Calibrating the focus and magnification settings of a surgical microscope is crucial for optimal visualization during a procedure. While options A, C, and D are important for the overall setup, they do not directly impact the clarity and precision of the visual field, which is essential for the surgeon's accuracy and effectiveness.

Question 18: Correct Answer: C) Address the conflict calmly and facilitate a resolution.

Rationale: Addressing the conflict calmly and facilitating a resolution (Option C) is the most effective approach as it promotes teamwork and maintains a positive working environment. Ignoring the conflict (Option A) can lead to unresolved issues and tension. Taking sides (Option B) can create further division. Reporting immediately to administration (Option D) may escalate the situation unnecessarily. Diplomacy involves resolving issues through effective communication and mediation.

Question 19: Correct Answer: C) Replace the insufflator with a backup unit from the reserve equipment.

Rationale: The correct action is to replace the insufflator with a backup unit from the reserve equipment, ensuring the surgery can proceed without delay. Attempting to repair the insufflator (A) could waste valuable time. Informing the surgeon and delaying the surgery (B) is unnecessary if a backup is available. Proceeding without the insufflator (D) is unsafe for a laparoscopic procedure. Having reserve equipment ready is crucial for maintaining the surgical schedule and patient safety.

Question 20: Correct Answer: B) Verify the specimen type and patient information with the surgeon.

Rationale: The first step is to verify the specimen type and patient information with the surgeon to ensure accuracy and prevent any potential errors. Labeling the container (A) and preparing it for transport (C) are subsequent steps. Placing the specimen in formalin (D) is not always appropriate for all specimen types and should be done according to specific guidelines.

Question 21: Correct Answer: A) To prevent deep vein thrombosis (DVT)

Rationale: The primary purpose of applying a sequential compression device (SCD) preoperatively is to prevent deep vein thrombosis (DVT) by promoting blood circulation in the lower extremities. While maintaining body temperature (B), reducing surgical site infection (C), and managing postoperative pain (D) are important perioperative goals, they are not the primary functions of SCDs. SCDs specifically target the prevention of blood clots, which can be a significant risk during and after surgery.

Question 22: Correct Answer: B) On a well-vascularized muscle mass

Rationale: The bovie pad should be placed on a well-vascularized muscle mass to ensure optimal conductivity and reduce the risk of burns. Placing it over a bony prominence (A) or on the chest (C) can increase resistance and risk of burns. Positioning it near the surgical site (D) is not recommended as it may interfere with the surgical field and does not guarantee optimal conductivity.

Question 23: Correct Answer: C) Chemical-resistant gloves

Rationale: Chemical-resistant gloves are essential when dealing with a chemical spill to protect the skin from harmful substances. A surgical mask (A) and hair cover (D) do not provide adequate protection against chemical exposure. Sterile gloves (B) are not designed to resist chemicals and could degrade, offering insufficient protection. Therefore, chemical-resistant gloves are the most appropriate PPE in this scenario.

Question 24: Correct Answer: B) Use multiple databases and a variety of keywords

Rationale: Using multiple databases and a variety of keywords ensures a comprehensive and relevant literature review, capturing a wide range of studies. Searching with a single keyword (A) limits the scope, reviewing only recent articles (C) may miss foundational studies, and focusing on a single journal (D) restricts the diversity of sources. A broad search strategy provides a more thorough understanding of the topic.

Question 25: Correct Answer: B) Report the issue to the supervisor and tag the equipment as "out of service."

Rationale: The immediate action should be to report the issue to the supervisor and tag the equipment as "out of service." This ensures that the equipment is not used until it is repaired, maintaining electrical safety standards. Using the equipment carefully (A) or covering with tape (C) are unsafe practices. Using the equipment only if necessary (D) still poses a risk and is not acceptable.

Question 26: Correct Answer: B) Verify the type and size of the implant with the surgeon before handing it over.

Rationale: The correct action is to verify the type and size of the implant with the surgeon before handing it over. This ensures that the correct implant is used, reducing the risk of complications. Option A is incorrect because it skips verification. Option C is incorrect as preoperative measurements may not always be accurate. Option D is incorrect because the responsibility lies with the technologist to verify directly with the surgeon.

Question 27: Correct Answer: A) To prevent hypothermia by warming intravenous fluids

Rationale: The primary purpose of using a fluid warmer in the perioperative setting is to prevent hypothermia by warming intravenous fluids before they are administered to the patient. Cooling intravenous fluids (option B) is not a common practice in this context. Sterilizing fluids (option C) is not the function of a fluid warmer, and maintaining viscosity (option D) is not a primary concern. Therefore, option A is the correct and most valid answer.

Question 28: Correct Answer: C) Positioning the patient in the lateral decubitus position with appropriate padding.

Rationale: For a total hip replacement, positioning the patient in the lateral decubitus position with appropriate padding is crucial to prevent pressure injuries and maintain proper alignment. Option A is incorrect as the prone position is not suitable for hip surgery. Option B is incorrect because crossing the legs can cause vascular complications. Option D,

while important for other surgeries, is not specific to hip replacement.

Question 29: Correct Answer: B) 68-73°F (20-22.8°C)

Rationale: The recommended temperature range for an operating room is 68-73°F (20-22.8°C) to maintain patient safety and optimal surgical conditions. This range helps prevent hypothermia in patients while also ensuring a comfortable environment for the surgical team. Options A, C, and D are incorrect as they fall outside the recommended range, either being too cold (risking patient hypothermia) or too warm (potentially causing discomfort and increased microbial growth).

Question 30: Correct Answer: C) Increased pain unrelieved by medication

Rationale: Increased pain unrelieved by medication can be a sign of internal bleeding or other serious complications. Light bruising (A) is often expected, decreased urine output (B) can be due to various factors including dehydration, and a slight increase in heart rate (D) can be a normal response to postoperative stress. Persistent, severe pain is a red flag that warrants immediate reporting.

Question 31: Correct Answer: B) Inform the surgeon immediately and replace the instrument.

Rationale: The correct course of action is to inform the surgeon immediately and replace the instrument. Continuing to use a malfunctioning instrument (Option A) can compromise patient safety. Attempting to fix it on the sterile field (Option C) risks contamination. Re-sterilizing the instrument (Option D) is impractical during surgery. Promptly replacing the instrument ensures the procedure continues safely and efficiently.

Question 32: Correct Answer: B) Asking open-ended questions

Rationale: Asking open-ended questions encourages detailed responses and helps clarify misunderstandings. Interrupting to correct errors (A) can be disruptive and may cause defensiveness. Waiting for a pause to speak (C) is polite but does not actively seek clarification. Providing immediate feedback (D) is important but should follow a thorough understanding, which open-ended questions facilitate. This approach promotes a collaborative and clear communication environment.

Question 33: Correct Answer: A) Forced-air warming blanket

Rationale: Forced-air warming blankets are the most commonly used devices to maintain a patient's core temperature during surgery. They provide consistent and controlled warming, which is crucial for preventing hypothermia. Ice packs and cooling vests are used to reduce body temperature, not maintain it. Heated intravenous fluids can help but are not as effective in maintaining core temperature as forced-air warming blankets. Therefore, option A is the most valid and effective choice.

Question 34: Correct Answer: B) Melanocytes

Rationale: Melanocytes are specialized cells located in the basal layer of the epidermis and are responsible for producing melanin, the pigment that gives skin its color. Keratinocytes are primarily involved in producing keratin, Langerhans cells are part of the immune response, and Merkel cells are involved in sensory perception. Therefore, melanocytes are the correct answer as they specifically produce melanin.

Question 35: Correct Answer: B) To enhance data collection and analysis

Rationale: The primary purpose of utilizing computer technology in surgical research is to enhance data collection and analysis. This allows for more accurate, efficient, and comprehensive research outcomes. While automating surgical procedures (A) and replacing surgical personnel (C) are not the main goals, eliminating physical records (D) is a secondary benefit but not the primary purpose.

Question 36: Correct Answer: B) Ensuring the pad is placed on clean, dry skin

Rationale: The bovie pad must be placed on clean, dry skin to ensure proper adhesion and effective grounding. Placing it over a bony prominence (A) or an area with hair (D) can interfere with adhesion and increase the risk of burns. While proximity to the surgical site (C) is a consideration, it is less critical than ensuring the skin is clean and dry for safety and effectiveness.

Question 37: Correct Answer: A) By allowing real-time updates and easy access to preference cards

Rationale: Utilizing computer technology enhances the management of surgeon's preference cards by allowing real-time updates and easy access. This ensures that any changes in preferences are promptly reflected, reducing errors and improving efficiency. Options B, C, and D are incorrect as they do not directly relate to the management of preference cards; diagnosing conditions, patient-surgeon communication, and generating surgical reports are separate functionalities.

Question 38: Correct Answer: B) Wearing a lead apron and thyroid shield

Rationale: Wearing a lead apron and thyroid shield is the most effective method to minimize radiation exposure. Standing directly next to the x-ray source (A) increases exposure, increasing the duration of exposure (C) is counterproductive, and using a higher dose of radiation (D) unnecessarily increases risk. Lead aprons and thyroid shields provide essential protection by absorbing and blocking x-ray radiation.

Question 39: Correct Answer: B) Ensure that the stretcher is locked and at the same height as the operating table.

Rationale: Ensuring that the stretcher is locked and at the same height as the operating table is crucial for a safe transfer. This minimizes the risk of falls and facilitates a smooth transition. Disconnecting IV lines and catheters (A) should be done later to maintain patient stability. Removing surgical drapes and instruments (C) is important but not the first step. Positioning the patient's arms across their chest (D) is also necessary but comes after securing the stretcher.

Question 40: Correct Answer: A) Ensuring that all team members adhere to sterile technique.

Rationale: The primary responsibility of a surgical technologist is to ensure that all team members adhere to sterile technique to prevent infections. Supervising the surgical procedure (B) and monitoring the patient's vital signs (C) are roles typically assigned to other team members. Documenting the procedure (D) is important but secondary to maintaining sterility, which is critical for patient safety and successful surgical outcomes.

Question 41: Correct Answer: B) By confirming the size with the surgeon using the manufacturer's catalog

Rationale: The correct procedure involves confirming the implant size with the surgeon using the manufacturer's catalog to ensure accuracy and compatibility. Option A is incorrect as the patient's medical history does not provide specific implant sizes. Option C is incorrect because the surgical technologist should directly confirm with the surgeon. Option D is incorrect because relying solely on the preoperative plan without verification can lead to errors.

Question 42: Correct Answer: D) Passing instruments to the surgeon

Rationale: The primary responsibility of a surgical technologist in maintaining the sterile field is passing instruments to the surgeon. This ensures that the surgeon can perform the procedure efficiently and without contamination. While ensuring all instruments are accounted for (B) is important, it is secondary to the immediate task of assisting the surgeon. Supervising the surgical team (A) and monitoring the patient's vital signs (C) are roles typically assigned to other personnel, such as the surgical nurse and anesthesiologist.

Question 43: Correct Answer: B) Seal them in a biohazard bag and dispose of them in a designated biohazard waste container.

Rationale: Contaminated drapes must be sealed in a biohazard bag and disposed of in a designated biohazard waste container to prevent the spread of infection. Option A is incorrect as regular trash bins are not appropriate for biohazardous materials. Option C is incorrect because rinsing does not eliminate contamination. Option D is incorrect as laundry hampers are not suitable for biohazardous waste.

Question 44: Correct Answer: A) Pre-warming the patient with a warming gown

Rationale: Pre-warming the patient with a warming gown is the best practice to prevent perioperative hypothermia. Cold IV fluids (B) would decrease body temperature, a cooling blanket (C) is used to lower temperature, and a low operating room temperature (D) increases the risk of hypothermia. Pre-warming helps maintain normothermia by reducing the initial drop in body temperature during anesthesia and surgery.

Question 45: Correct Answer: B) Bipolar cautery

Rationale: Bipolar cautery is most commonly used for precise tissue dissection in delicate surgeries because it allows for controlled and localized coagulation, reducing the risk of damage to surrounding tissues. Monopolar cautery (A) is less precise and can affect a larger area. Chemical cautery (C) and thermal cautery (D) are not typically used for delicate tissue dissection. Thus, B is the correct answer for its precision and control.

Question 46: Correct Answer: C) Cornea
Rationale: The cornea is the transparent, outermost layer of the eye that covers the anterior chamber. To access this chamber, the surgeon must first incise the cornea. The retina and vitreous humor are located in the posterior segment of the eye, and the sclera is the white part of the eye that provides structural support but does not directly cover the anterior chamber.

Question 47: Correct Answer: B) Bipolar cautery
Rationale: Bipolar cautery is most commonly used for delicate tissue dissection because it provides precise control and minimizes thermal damage to surrounding tissues. Monopolar cautery (A) is less precise and can cause more collateral damage. Chemical cautery (C) is not typically used for delicate dissection due to its less controlled nature. Ultrasonic cautery (D) is effective but less commonly used compared to bipolar cautery for this specific purpose.

Question 48: Correct Answer: B) Hold the retractor steady and in the correct position.
Rationale: Effective retraction involves holding the retractor steady and in the correct position as directed by the surgeon. Excessive force (Option A) can cause tissue damage, while frequently adjusting the retractor (Option C) can disrupt the surgical field. Applying minimal pressure (Option D) may not provide adequate exposure. Thus, maintaining a steady and correct position (Option B) ensures optimal surgical conditions and patient safety.

Question 49: Correct Answer: A) Forced-air warming blanket
Rationale: The forced-air warming blanket is the most effective device for maintaining core body temperature during surgery. Ice packs (B) would lower the patient's temperature, room temperature IV fluids (C) do not actively warm the patient, and an electric heating pad (D) may not provide consistent or adequate warming. Forced-air warming blankets distribute warm air evenly over the patient, ensuring stable thermoregulation.

Question 50: Correct Answer: B) Inadequate hemostasis during surgery.
Rationale: A hematoma is often caused by inadequate hemostasis during surgery, leading to blood accumulation in the tissue. Excessive physical activity (A) may worsen an existing hematoma but is not the primary cause. An allergic reaction to sutures (C) and infection (D) can cause swelling and pain but are less likely to result in a hematoma. Proper hemostasis is crucial to prevent this complication.

Question 51: Correct Answer: B) Ensure the allograft is thawed to room temperature.
Rationale: Ensuring the allograft is thawed to room temperature is crucial for proper integration and function. Thawing allows the graft to regain its flexibility and structural integrity. Soaking in saline (A) and rinsing with antibiotic solution (D) are important

but secondary steps. Sterilizing with an autoclave (C) is incorrect as it can damage the tissue structure.

Question 52: Correct Answer: C) Report both the Ringer's lactate and fentanyl amounts.
Rationale: Accurate reporting requires documenting both the Ringer's lactate and fentanyl amounts used. This ensures comprehensive medical records and optimal postoperative care. Option A and B are incorrect as they only partially document the substances used. Option D is incorrect because it does not specify the fentanyl amount, which is essential for maintaining accurate and complete patient records.

Question 53: Correct Answer: C) Ensuring all sterile team members face the sterile field.
Rationale: Ensuring all sterile team members face the sterile field prevents contamination by maintaining constant visual monitoring. Reaching over the sterile field (A) and keeping sterile instruments below waist level (B) can introduce contaminants. Allowing non-sterile personnel to pass between sterile fields (D) disrupts the sterile environment, increasing the risk of contamination.

Question 54: Correct Answer: C) Use an alternative antibiotic such as clindamycin or vancomycin.
Rationale: The correct step is to use an alternative antibiotic such as clindamycin or vancomycin to avoid triggering the penicillin allergy. Administering penicillin (Option A) is unsafe. Cephalosporins (Option B) can cross-react with penicillin. Avoiding antibiotics (Option D) is inappropriate as it increases infection risk.

Question 55: Correct Answer: B) Lens
Rationale: The lens is primarily responsible for focusing light onto the retina. While the cornea also helps in focusing light, it is the lens that fine-tunes this focus, allowing for clear vision. The iris controls the amount of light entering the eye, and the sclera provides structural support but does not focus light.

Question 56: Correct Answer: A) To provide nutrients to the cornea and lens
Rationale: The aqueous humor is a clear fluid that fills the anterior and posterior chambers of the eye, providing nutrients to the avascular structures such as the cornea and lens. While it does help maintain intraocular pressure, its primary function is nutritional. It does not transmit light (a role of the vitreous humor) or control eye movement (a function of the extraocular muscles). Thus, providing nutrients is its main role.

Question 57: Correct Answer: D) Apply direct pressure to the bleeding site with a laparoscopic instrument.
Rationale: Applying direct pressure to the bleeding site with a laparoscopic instrument is the most immediate and effective action to control bleeding. Increasing insufflation pressure (Option A) may not effectively control bleeding and can cause other complications. Handing the surgeon a suction device (Option B) clears the field but does not control the bleeding. Informing the anesthesiologist (Option C) is important but not the immediate action needed to control the bleeding.

Question 58: Correct Answer: B) Confirm the

patient's identity and surgical site.

Rationale: Confirming the patient's identity and surgical site is the first and most crucial step to ensure that the correct procedure is performed on the correct patient. This step prevents wrong-site surgery and other serious errors. While securing the patient's arms (A), adjusting the table height (C), and applying the safety strap (D) are important, they should be done only after confirming the patient's identity and surgical site.

Question 59: Correct Answer: C) Acknowledge Mr. Johnson's concerns and inform the perioperative nurse to address them.

Rationale: Acknowledging the patient's concerns and informing the perioperative nurse ensures that Mr. Johnson's anxiety and pain management needs are appropriately addressed. This approach respects patient autonomy and promotes comprehensive care. Options A and D are dismissive and do not provide a solution. Option B incorrectly implies that the surgeon will address concerns during the procedure, which is not feasible.

Question 60: Correct Answer: A) During the preoperative briefing

Rationale: The verification of the type and size of the implantable item should occur during the preoperative briefing to prevent any delays or errors during the surgery. This ensures that any issues can be addressed before the procedure begins. Options B, C, and D are too late in the process, as verifying after the incision or during the handoff could lead to complications, and postoperative debriefing is not relevant for preoperative verification.

Question 61: Correct Answer: B) To review and improve surgical procedures and teamwork

Rationale: The primary purpose of a postoperative case debrief is to review the surgical procedures and teamwork to identify areas for improvement. This helps enhance patient safety and surgical outcomes. Option A is incorrect as the goal is not to assign blame but to learn and improve. Option C, while important, is not the main focus of the debrief. Option D is administrative and not the primary purpose of the debrief.

Question 62: Correct Answer: A) Lower risk of disease transmission

Rationale: Autografts, such as using Ms. Smith's own tissue, significantly lower the risk of disease transmission compared to allografts, which involve donor tissue. While autografts do not necessarily result in a faster surgical procedure (B) or eliminate the need for postoperative rehabilitation (C), they do offer a reduced risk of immune rejection and disease transmission. Surgical site infection (D) risks are comparable between autografts and allografts.

Question 63: Correct Answer: D) Laparoscopic specimen retrieval bag

Rationale: After the gallbladder is dissected and clipped, the next step is to remove it from the abdominal cavity. The laparoscopic specimen retrieval bag is used for this purpose. Laparoscopic scissors (A) and grasper (B) are used earlier in the procedure

for dissection and manipulation. The suction/irrigation device (C) is used for clearing the surgical field but not for specimen retrieval.

Question 64: Correct Answer: D) Use a sterile cover that extends beyond the sterile field to cover the C-arm.

Rationale: Using a sterile cover that extends beyond the sterile field ensures that the C-arm remains sterile throughout the procedure. This prevents contamination when the C-arm is moved. Option A is incorrect because draping the wheels is unnecessary. Option B is incorrect as it risks contamination when the C-arm is moved. Option C is incorrect because draping the patient and C-arm together can compromise sterility.

Question 65: Correct Answer: B) Notify the surgeon immediately

Rationale: The most appropriate initial action is to notify the surgeon immediately. This ensures that the rash, which could be a sign of an allergic reaction, infection, or other serious condition, is promptly evaluated by a physician. Applying a topical antibiotic (A) or administering an antihistamine (D) without a physician's order is inappropriate and could be harmful. Simply documenting the rash (C) delays necessary medical intervention.

Question 66: Correct Answer: B) Ensuring the cast is snug but not too tight to allow for swelling.

Rationale: Ensuring the cast is snug but not too tight is crucial to accommodate swelling and prevent complications such as compartment syndrome. Option A is incorrect because padding is necessary to protect the skin. Option C is incorrect as hot water can cause burns and speed up setting too quickly. Option D is incorrect because overlapping is necessary to ensure the cast's structural integrity.

Question 67: Correct Answer: B) Dermis

Rationale: The dermis is the layer of the skin that contains blood vessels. The epidermis and stratum corneum are avascular, meaning they do not contain blood vessels. The subcutaneous tissue, while containing larger blood vessels, is located beneath the dermis. Thus, the first blood vessels encountered during an incision are in the dermis.

Question 68: Correct Answer: C) To prevent retained surgical items

Rationale: The primary purpose of performing a surgical count before the start of a procedure is to prevent retained surgical items. This practice ensures that all instruments, sponges, and other materials are accounted for before and after surgery, reducing the risk of leaving items inside the patient. While ensuring sterility (A), verifying equipment availability (B), and confirming patient identity (D) are important, they are not the primary reasons for the surgical count.

Question 69: Correct Answer: B) Wearing laser-specific eyewear

Rationale: Wearing laser-specific eyewear is crucial to protect the surgical team from potential eye damage caused by laser exposure. Standard surgical masks do not offer protection against laser beams, sunscreen is irrelevant for laser safety, and lead aprons protect against ionizing radiation, not laser light. Therefore, laser-specific eyewear is the essential safety measure to prevent ocular injuries during laser procedures.

Question 70: Correct Answer: B) Draping the robotic arms first before positioning them over the patient.

Rationale: Draping the robotic arms first before positioning them over the patient ensures that the sterile field is maintained throughout the procedure. Draping the patient first (Option A) or simultaneously (Option C) can lead to contamination. Draping the arms after positioning them over the patient (Option D) risks breaking sterility due to the movement of the arms.

Question 71: Correct Answer: B) Maintaining spinal alignment

Rationale: Maintaining spinal alignment is crucial to prevent further injury to the spinal cord. While ensuring comfort, monitoring vital signs, and communication are important, they are secondary to preventing additional spinal damage. Proper alignment minimizes the risk of exacerbating the injury, which is the primary concern during transport.

Question 72: Correct Answer: A) Using a draw sheet or transfer board.

Rationale: Using a draw sheet or transfer board is the most important consideration to prevent injury to both the patient and staff during the transfer. This method provides support and reduces the risk of musculoskeletal injuries. Asking the patient to move herself (B) may not be feasible or safe. Lifting manually (C) increases the risk of injury. Ensuring the table is locked (D) is important but secondary to using proper transfer aids.

Question 73: Correct Answer: B) Choroid plexus

Rationale: The choroid plexus is responsible for producing cerebrospinal fluid (CSF). The corpus callosum connects the two cerebral hemispheres, the amygdala is involved in emotion processing, and the thalamus acts as a relay station for sensory information. Identifying the choroid plexus is crucial in understanding CSF dynamics in neurosurgical procedures, making option B the correct choice.

Question 74: Correct Answer: B) To list the surgeon's preferred instruments and supplies

Rationale: A surgeon's preference card is primarily used to list the specific instruments, supplies, and equipment that a surgeon prefers for particular procedures. This ensures that the surgical team is well-prepared and can efficiently set up the operating room according to the surgeon's needs. Options A, C, and D are incorrect because they pertain to patient-specific information or procedural details, not the surgeon's preferences.

Question 75: Correct Answer: B) Hemostatic clips

Rationale: Hemostatic clips are specifically designed for mechanically occluding blood vessels during surgery, making them ideal for controlling a bleed from a cystic artery branch. Electrocautery (A) is an electrical method, fibrin sealant (C) is a chemical method, and bone wax (D) is used primarily in orthopedic procedures to control bleeding from bone

surfaces. Thus, hemostatic clips (B) are the most appropriate mechanical method for this scenario.

Question 76: Correct Answer: C) Using a needle holder to pass the suture with the needle pointing away from the surgeon

Rationale: Using a needle holder to pass the suture with the needle pointing away from the surgeon ensures safety and maintains sterility. Handing it directly with bare hands (A) compromises sterility, while pointing the needle towards the surgeon (B) poses a risk of injury. Placing it on the sterile field (D) is less efficient and can disrupt the workflow.

Question 77: Correct Answer: B) Using an alcohol-based antiseptic for skin preparation

Rationale: Using an alcohol-based antiseptic for skin preparation is most effective in reducing the risk of infection by Staphylococcus aureus. It rapidly reduces skin flora and has a broad-spectrum antimicrobial effect. Administering antibiotics postoperatively does not prevent initial contamination, shaving the night before can cause microabrasions, and povidone-iodine is less effective compared to alcohol-based antiseptics in immediate microbial reduction.

Question 78: Correct Answer: C) Ensure all instruments are removed from the drapes

Rationale: The first step in removing drapes is to ensure all instruments are removed to prevent injury and maintain sterility. Cutting the drapes (Option A) could damage the patient's skin. Removing the drapes in a single motion (Option B) is unsafe as it may dislodge instruments. Pulling the drapes towards the patient's head (Option D) is incorrect as it can cause contamination.

Question 79: Correct Answer: B) To detect early signs of complications

Rationale: Monitoring vital signs in the immediate postoperative period is crucial for detecting early signs of complications such as hemorrhage, infection, or respiratory distress. While assessing pain level (A), ensuring comfort (C), and determining nutritional needs (D) are important, they are not the primary purpose of immediate postoperative vital sign monitoring. Early detection of complications can significantly improve patient outcomes and is therefore the primary focus.

Question 80: Correct Answer: D) Wait for the surgeon to request cutting the suture.

Rationale: The correct action is to wait for the surgeon to request cutting the suture. Cutting the suture immediately (A) or holding the suture ends taut (B) may interfere with the surgeon's technique. Preparing another suture (C) is not necessary until the surgeon indicates. Waiting for the surgeon's instruction ensures the procedure is carried out as directed and maintains the sterile field.

Question 81: Correct Answer: C) Turn off the oxygen supply.

Rationale: The first step in managing an OR fire is to turn off the oxygen supply to prevent the fire from intensifying. Using a fire extinguisher (A) or evacuating the patient (B) are secondary actions. Calling for help (D) is important but not the immediate priority. The oxygen supply must be addressed first to control the fire effectively.

Question 82: Correct Answer: A) The circulating nurse

Rationale: The circulating nurse is responsible for initiating the Time Out procedure. This ensures an impartial party oversees the verification process. While the anesthesiologist, surgical technologist, and surgeon play crucial roles in the surgical team, the circulating nurse's role is specifically designed to manage and coordinate the Time Out to ensure all safety checks are completed. This helps maintain a standardized approach and reduces the likelihood of errors.

Question 83: Correct Answer: C) Documenting the surgical procedure accurately.

Rationale: Accurate documentation (C) is crucial for legal, medical, and continuity of care purposes. Ensuring sterile instruments (A) and maintaining the sterile field (B) are primarily the scrub technologist's responsibilities. Assisting the anesthesiologist (D) is important but secondary to the primary role of documentation for the circulating nurse. This ensures comprehensive patient records and adherence to legal and medical standards.

Question 84: Correct Answer: B) Immediately inform the surgeon and replace the contaminated items.

Rationale: The correct action is to immediately inform the surgeon and replace the contaminated items to maintain patient safety and prevent infection. Continuing with the procedure (A) or waiting until it is completed (C) risks patient safety. Informing the circulating nurse without taking immediate corrective action (D) is insufficient. The priority is to address the contamination immediately to maintain a sterile environment.

Question 85: Correct Answer: D) Conducting a thorough respiratory assessment

Rationale: Conducting a thorough respiratory assessment is essential because bariatric patients are at higher risk for respiratory complications due to obesity-related factors. Ensuring optimal respiratory function preoperatively can significantly reduce postoperative complications. A high-calorie diet (A) is counterproductive, increased fluid intake (B) is standard but not specific to bariatrics, and a preoperative exercise regimen (C) is beneficial but not as critical as respiratory assessment.

Question 86: Correct Answer: B) Elevate the patient's legs while still on the operating table.

Rationale: Elevating the patient's legs while still on the operating table helps to improve blood flow to the heart and stabilize blood pressure. Completing the transfer quickly (A) could exacerbate her condition. Administering IV fluids (C) is important but secondary to immediate physical measures. Calling for additional staff (D) is helpful but not the immediate priority. Elevation provides immediate physiological benefit in hypotensive situations.

Question 87: Correct Answer: C) Any deviations from the planned procedure and their outcomes.

Rationale: A key component of the debrief is discussing any deviations from the planned procedure and their outcomes, as this helps the team understand what happened and how to improve future practices. The exact duration of the surgery (Option A) and specific instruments used (Option B) are less critical. Personal performance reviews (Option D) are not typically part of a debrief and can be addressed separately.

Question 88: Correct Answer: C) Discard the drapes and obtain a new sterile package

Rationale: Maria should discard the expired drapes and obtain a new sterile package to ensure sterility and patient safety. Using expired drapes (Option A) or extending the expiration date (Option B) compromises sterility. Informing the circulating nurse (Option D) without taking immediate action does not mitigate the risk of contamination. Adhering to expiration dates is essential for maintaining sterile conditions.

Question 89: Correct Answer: B) Babcock Forceps

Rationale: Babcock Forceps are designed for atraumatically grasping soft tissues like the gallbladder. Metzenbaum Scissors are used for cutting delicate tissues, Kocher Clamps are for grasping tough tissues or bones, and Allis Clamps are for holding tissues that will be removed. Babcock Forceps are ideal for this procedure as they minimize tissue damage, unlike the other instruments.

Question 90: Correct Answer: B) Common bile duct

Rationale: The common bile duct is responsible for transporting bile from the liver and gallbladder to the duodenum. The hepatic artery supplies blood to the liver, the portal vein carries nutrient-rich blood from the gastrointestinal tract to the liver, and the cystic duct connects the gallbladder to the common bile duct. Misidentifying these structures can lead to surgical complications.

Question 91: Correct Answer: B) Tachycardia

Rationale: Tachycardia is a key early sign of malignant hyperthermia, a life-threatening condition triggered by certain anesthetics. Hypotension, bradycardia, and hypothermia are not primary indicators of this condition. Recognizing tachycardia promptly allows for immediate intervention to prevent severe complications. Misinterpreting other signs could delay diagnosis and treatment, emphasizing the importance of understanding this specific indicator.

Question 92: Correct Answer: C) The rash may indicate a systemic infection.

Rationale: A widespread rash on the torso could be a sign of a systemic infection, which requires immediate attention. While a latex allergy (A) or reaction to the surgical dressing (B) are possible, they are less likely to cause a widespread rash. Postoperative stress (D) is not a common cause of such rashes. Identifying and treating a systemic infection promptly is crucial to prevent further complications.

Question 93: Correct Answer: B) Weighing sponges and measuring suction canisters

Rationale: Weighing sponges and measuring suction canisters provide a quantifiable and objective method for estimating blood loss. Visual estimation (A) is subjective and often inaccurate. Counting used sponges (C) does not provide a measure of the volume of blood loss. Monitoring vital signs (D) can indicate blood loss but does not quantify it. Therefore, option B is the most accurate method.

Question 94: Correct Answer: A) Argon beam coagulation

Rationale: Argon beam coagulation is ideal for controlling diffuse bleeding from a liver laceration as it provides a non-contact method to coagulate large surface areas. Cryotherapy (B) is not suitable for immediate hemostasis. Bipolar electrosurgery (C) is effective for precise coagulation but not for large diffuse bleeding. Harmonic scalpel (D) is used for cutting and coagulation but is less effective for diffuse bleeding control compared to argon beam coagulation.

Question 95: Correct Answer: C) Checking that the SCDs are properly sized and fitted to the patient's legs

Rationale: Proper sizing and fitting of SCDs are essential to ensure effective compression and prevention of DVT. Incorrectly sized devices may not provide adequate compression or could cause discomfort. Option A is incorrect because SCDs should be applied before anesthesia to ensure continuous use. Option B is incorrect as loose SCDs will not provide effective compression. Option D is incorrect because SCDs should not be removed every hour, as this disrupts their effectiveness in preventing DVT.

Question 96: Correct Answer: C) Use an alternative antibiotic for prophylaxis.

Rationale: The correct action is to use an alternative antibiotic for prophylaxis to avoid triggering an allergic reaction. Ensuring the patient wears an allergy bracelet (Option A) and documenting the allergy (Option D) are important but do not address the immediate need to avoid penicillin. Administering a test dose (Option B) is risky and unnecessary if the allergy is already documented. The primary concern is to prevent exposure to the allergen.

Question 97: Correct Answer: B) The blade is dull or damaged.

Rationale: A dull or damaged blade on a harmonic scalpel can significantly reduce its cutting efficiency. Ensuring the blade is sharp and intact is crucial for optimal performance. Option A is incorrect because the harmonic scalpel does not require grounding like traditional electrosurgery. Option C is incorrect as higher power settings would not cause inefficiency in cutting. Option D is irrelevant to the cutting efficiency of the device.

Question 98: Correct Answer: B) Verify the patient's identity and surgical procedure.

Rationale: Verifying the patient's identity and surgical procedure is crucial to ensure patient safety and prevent wrong-site surgery. While positioning the table (C) and applying safety straps (D) are important steps, they come after confirming the patient's identity. Ensuring the surgical site is exposed (A) is not the initial priority.

Question 99: Correct Answer: B) Spina Bifida

Rationale: Spina Bifida is a congenital condition where the spinal column does not close completely, potentially causing nerve damage and physical disabilities. Hydrocephalus involves fluid accumulation in the brain, Anencephaly is the absence of a major portion of the brain, skull, and scalp, and Microcephaly is characterized by a smaller than normal head size. These conditions do not involve the incomplete closure of the spinal column.

Question 100: Correct Answer: C) Employing a smoke evacuation system

Rationale: Employing a smoke evacuation system is the most effective measure in reducing exposure to surgical smoke. These systems capture and filter smoke at the source, significantly reducing the inhalation of harmful chemicals. Wearing double gloves (A) and high-filtration masks (B) provide some protection but do not address airborne particles. Increasing room ventilation (D) helps disperse smoke but does not effectively remove it from the immediate surgical area.

Question 101: Correct Answer: A) Reduced skin irritation

Rationale: Waterless surgical scrubs are formulated to be less irritating to the skin compared to traditional scrubbing methods. This is because they often contain emollients and moisturizers. In contrast, traditional scrubs can cause dryness and irritation due to the repeated use of soap and water. Lower cost (B) and longer scrub time (C) are not accurate, as waterless scrubs are typically more expensive and quicker. Increased bacterial resistance (D) is incorrect, as waterless scrubs are designed to be highly effective against bacteria.

Question 102: Correct Answer: D) Wrap the graft in a saline-moistened gauze.

Rationale: To keep the tissue graft moist, wrapping it in a saline-moistened gauze (D) is the best method. This ensures the graft remains hydrated and viable. Placing the graft in a dry sterile container (A) or covering it with a sterile drape (B) would not maintain moisture. Soaking the graft in an antibiotic solution (C) could be harmful and is not the standard practice for maintaining moisture.

Question 103: Correct Answer: C) To create negative pressure for fluid drainage

Rationale: Compressing the bulb of a Jackson-Pratt drain before connecting it to the tubing creates negative pressure, which is essential for effective fluid drainage from the surgical site. Option A is incorrect as preventing air from entering the wound is not the primary reason. Option B is incorrect because maintaining sterility is a general requirement but not the primary reason for compressing the bulb. Option D is incorrect as tubing alignment does not require bulb compression.

Question 104: Correct Answer: C) Obtain an urgent MRI of the spine

Rationale: An urgent MRI is crucial to assess the extent of spinal injury and plan appropriate management. A focused neurological examination (A) is important but secondary to imaging. High-dose corticosteroids (B) are controversial and not the first step. Log-rolling the patient to a prone position (D) is inappropriate and could exacerbate the injury.

Question 105: Correct Answer: B) Ensuring the patient is accompanied by a caregiver who understands the instructions.

Rationale: Ensuring Mr. Johnson is accompanied by a caregiver who understands the instructions is vital due to his mild cognitive impairment. This ensures compliance and reduces anxiety. Providing detailed written instructions (A) may not be effective due to his cognitive issues. Minimizing preoperative fasting (C) is important but secondary to having a caregiver. Avoiding preoperative medications (D) is not advisable as it could lead to unmanaged pain or anxiety. Having a caregiver ensures all instructions are followed accurately.

Question 106: Correct Answer: B) To provide better access to the hip joint

Rationale: The lateral decubitus position is chosen for total hip arthroplasty to provide optimal access to the hip joint. This position allows the surgeon to expose the hip area adequately. Option A is incorrect as it does not specifically address surgical access. Option C is a general postoperative concern, and D is unrelated to the primary surgical objective.

Question 107: Correct Answer: B) Steam sterilization using a flash cycle

Rationale: Steam sterilization using a flash cycle is the most appropriate method for sterilizing instruments for immediate use in an emergency. It is quick and effective. Ethylene oxide sterilization and dry heat sterilization are too time-consuming for immediate use. Chemical sterilization with glutaraldehyde is not recommended for immediate use due to its longer processing time and potential for residual toxicity.

Question 108: Correct Answer: B) Update Dr. Smith's preference card immediately to include the new trocar.

Rationale: The correct action is to update Dr. Smith's preference card immediately to ensure the surgical team is prepared with the correct instruments. Waiting until the surgery (Option A) or relying on verbal communication (Option C) can lead to confusion and delays. Using the old trocar (Option D) disregards the surgeon's updated technique, potentially compromising patient care.

Question 109: Correct Answer: B) Paraphrasing the speaker's points

Rationale: Paraphrasing the speaker's points ensures that the listener has accurately understood the information and provides an opportunity for clarification. While nodding (A) and maintaining eye contact (C) show engagement, they do not confirm understanding. Taking detailed notes (D) can be helpful but may distract from active listening and immediate clarification.

Question 110: Correct Answer: B) To assess blood flow and detect vascular abnormalities.

Rationale: Doppler ultrasound is primarily used intraoperatively to assess blood flow and detect

vascular abnormalities. This capability is essential for identifying issues such as blood clots or abnormal blood flow patterns. Measuring tissue density (A), imaging bone structures (C), and monitoring vital signs (D) are not the main purposes of Doppler ultrasound. Its primary function is to provide detailed information about vascular conditions, which is critical for surgical decision-making.

Question 111: Correct Answer: B) Javid shunt

Rationale: The Javid shunt is specifically designed for carotid endarterectomy procedures to temporarily divert blood flow and maintain cerebral perfusion. The Fogarty catheter is used for embolectomies, the Penrose drain is used for passive drainage, and the Hemoclip is used for vessel ligation. Therefore, the Javid shunt is the most suitable device for maintaining cerebral perfusion during a carotid endarterectomy.

Question 112: Correct Answer: B) Keeping hands above the waist and within the sterile field.

Rationale: Sarah should keep her hands above the waist and within the sterile field to maintain sterility. Option A is incorrect as reaching over the sterile field can cause contamination. Option C is incorrect because the edges of the sterile drape touching non-sterile surfaces can lead to contamination. Option D is incorrect as placing sterile instruments on the edge of the sterile field risks them falling off and becoming non-sterile.

Question 113: Correct Answer: B) Cochlea

Rationale: The cochlea is the spiral-shaped organ in the inner ear responsible for converting sound waves into neural signals that are then transmitted to the brain. The tympanic membrane (A) vibrates in response to sound waves but does not convert them into neural signals. The Eustachian tube (C) helps equalize pressure in the middle ear, and the semicircular canals (D) are involved in balance, not hearing.

Question 114: Correct Answer: C) To minimize the risk of patient hypothermia

Rationale: Maintaining the operating room temperature within the recommended range is crucial to minimize the risk of patient hypothermia, which can lead to complications such as impaired wound healing and increased infection rates. While options A, B, and D are important considerations in the OR, they are not directly related to temperature management. Sterility of instruments and prevention of airborne pathogens are managed through other means, and surgical site infections are multifactorial, not solely temperature-dependent.

Question 115: Correct Answer: C) Verify the implant size with the surgeon before opening the sterile package.

Rationale: The most appropriate action is to verify the implant size with the surgeon before opening the sterile package. This ensures that the correct implant is used, avoiding potential complications. Option A is incorrect because preoperative X-rays are a guide but not definitive. Option B is incorrect because the circulating nurse may not have the final say. Option D is incorrect because the manufacturer's recommendation does not account for the specific needs of the patient.

Question 116: Correct Answer: C) Using ethylene oxide gas sterilization

Rationale: Ethylene oxide gas sterilization is highly effective in eliminating Clostridium difficile spores, which are resistant to standard autoclaving and alcohol-based disinfectants. Autoclaving at 121°C for 15 minutes may not be sufficient for spores, while 70% isopropyl alcohol and chlorine-based disinfectants are less effective against spore-forming bacteria. Ethylene oxide gas penetrates materials and effectively kills spores, ensuring a sterile environment.

Question 117: Correct Answer: B) Confirming the allograft is sterilized and free of contaminants

Rationale: Ensuring the allograft is sterilized and free of contaminants is critical to prevent infection and ensure the graft's safety and effectiveness. Thawing at room temperature (A) and soaking in saline (C) are not sufficient for sterilization. Wrapping in a sterile towel (D) helps maintain sterility but does not address initial contamination. Proper sterilization is paramount for patient safety and successful graft integration.

Question 118: Correct Answer: A) MacConkey agar

Rationale: MacConkey agar is specifically designed to isolate and differentiate Gram-negative bacteria based on their ability to ferment lactose. Blood agar is used for a wide range of bacteria, including Gram-positive. Chocolate agar is enriched for fastidious organisms, and Sabouraud agar is used for fungi. Therefore, MacConkey agar is the most appropriate for Gram-negative bacteria.

Question 119: Correct Answer: C) Producing red blood cells

Rationale: The lymphatic system is responsible for transporting dietary lipids, draining excess interstitial fluid, and facilitating immune responses. However, the production of red blood cells occurs in the bone marrow, not the lymphatic system. Thus, option C is the correct answer as it is not a function of the lymphatic system, while the other options accurately describe its roles.

Question 120: Correct Answer: C) Cement mixer and delivery system

Rationale: The cement mixer and delivery system (C) are essential for preparing and applying the bone cement to secure the prosthetic components. The bone rasp (A) is used earlier for bone preparation. The pulse lavage system (B) is used to clean the bone surface before cementing. The tourniquet (D) is applied at the beginning of the procedure to control bleeding but is not relevant at this stage.

Question 121: Correct Answer: C) Include the patient's name, specimen type, and date of collection.

Rationale: The most appropriate method for labeling a specimen container is to include the patient's name, specimen type, and date of collection. This ensures all critical information is present. Using a pre-printed label (A) or writing only the patient's name and date of birth (B) lacks necessary details. Attaching a blank label (D) risks incomplete or incorrect information being added later.

Question 122: Correct Answer: D) Checking the stapler's articulation and firing mechanism

Rationale: Checking the stapler's articulation and firing mechanism is essential to ensure it functions correctly during the procedure. While verifying the battery charge (A), ensuring sterilization (B), and confirming the staple size (C) are important, they do not directly impact the immediate functionality of the device during surgery. Proper articulation and firing ensure precise and effective stapling, which is critical for patient safety and surgical success.

Question 123: Correct Answer: C) Camera control unit (CCU)

Rationale: The Camera Control Unit (CCU) is vital for converting the endoscopic image into a digital format that can be displayed on a monitor. The light source (A) provides illumination, the insufflator (B) is used for distending the body cavity, and the suction-irrigation device (D) manages fluids. None of these components are responsible for image conversion, making the CCU the correct answer.

Question 124: Correct Answer: B) Change the glove immediately.

Rationale: The correct action is to change the glove immediately to prevent contamination. Continuing the procedure (A) or asking a colleague to continue (C) does not address the contamination risk. Cleaning the glove with an antiseptic solution (D) is not sufficient to restore sterility. Changing the glove immediately ensures the sterile field is maintained, preventing potential infections.

Question 125: Correct Answer: B) To prevent the equipment from being accidentally left inside the patient.

Rationale: The primary reason for ensuring all suction equipment is properly removed and accounted for is to prevent the equipment from being accidentally left inside the patient, which can lead to severe complications. Maintaining a sterile environment (Option A) and ensuring equipment readiness (Option C) are important but secondary. Reducing postoperative infection risk (Option D) is crucial, but the immediate concern is the physical removal of all equipment from the patient.

Question 126: Correct Answer: A) Ensuring the cement is mixed properly and handed to the surgeon

Rationale: During a total knee arthroplasty, the most critical task for the surgical technologist during the cementing of the prosthesis is to ensure the cement is mixed properly and handed to the surgeon. This step is crucial for the fixation of the prosthesis. Holding the leg (B) is typically done by the assistant, applying the tourniquet (C) is done at the beginning of the procedure, and suctioning blood (D) is important but not the primary task during cementing.

Question 127: Correct Answer: B) Ensure the tourniquet cuff is applied over a single layer of stockinette.

Rationale: Ensuring the tourniquet cuff is applied over a single layer of stockinette prevents direct skin contact, reducing the risk of skin damage. Option A is incorrect because the inflation pressure should be based on limb occlusion pressure, not a fixed value above systolic pressure. Option C is incorrect as direct skin contact can cause injury. Option D is incorrect because the tourniquet should be inflated just before the incision, not immediately after application.

Question 128: Correct Answer: B) Drape the C-arm with a sterile cover, ensuring all parts that will be near the sterile field are covered.

Rationale: The correct method is to drape the C-arm with a sterile cover, ensuring all parts near the sterile field are covered to maintain sterility. Option A is incorrect as a non-sterile cover can lead to contamination. Option C is incorrect because partial coverage can compromise sterility. Option D is incorrect as leaving any part uncovered can risk contamination.

Question 129: Correct Answer: A) Carbon Dioxide (CO2) Laser

Rationale: The Carbon Dioxide (CO2) laser is most commonly used for cutting and coagulating soft tissue due to its high absorption by water in tissues, providing precise cutting and minimal thermal damage. The Argon laser is primarily used for retinal phototherapy, the Nd:YAG laser is often used for deeper tissue penetration, and the Excimer laser is used in ophthalmology for corneal reshaping. Therefore, CO2 laser is the most suitable for soft tissue procedures.

Question 130: Correct Answer: B) It allows for precise cutting and coagulation.

Rationale: The primary advantage of using an argon laser in surgical procedures is its ability to allow for precise cutting and coagulation. Unlike other options, argon lasers emit a specific wavelength that is highly absorbed by hemoglobin and melanin, making it ideal for targeting blood vessels and pigmented tissues. Option A is incorrect as argon lasers do not provide deep tissue penetration; Option C is incorrect as cost-effectiveness is not their primary advantage; Option D is incorrect as argon lasers do not have the longest wavelength among surgical lasers.

Question 131: Correct Answer: B) Wipe the overhead lights first, then the surgical table, followed by the floor.

Rationale: The correct sequence is to wipe the overhead lights first, then the surgical table, followed by the floor. This top-to-bottom approach prevents contaminants from higher surfaces from falling onto already cleaned lower surfaces. Wiping the floor first (Option C) or last (Option D) could recontaminate cleaned areas. Starting with the surgical table (Option A) before the overhead lights could also result in recontamination.

Question 132: Correct Answer: B) Hydroxyapatite

Rationale: Hydroxyapatite is the most commonly used synthetic material for bone graft substitutes due to its biocompatibility and ability to promote bone growth. PMMA is primarily used as bone cement, silicone is used in implants, and polyethylene is used in joint replacements. Hydroxyapatite's osteoconductive properties make it ideal for bone

grafting, unlike the other materials listed.

Question 133: Correct Answer: B) To ground the patient and complete the electrical circuit

Rationale: The primary purpose of the bovie pad is to ground the patient and complete the electrical circuit, ensuring safe and effective use of the electrosurgical unit. Monitoring heart rate (A), providing a sterile field (C), and administering medication (D) are not functions of the bovie pad. These misconceptions can lead to improper use and patient safety risks.

Question 134: Correct Answer: C) Verify the bone graft's expiration date and integrity.

Rationale: The first step in preparing a bone graft is to verify its expiration date and integrity to ensure it is safe and suitable for use. Sterilizing the bone graft using an autoclave (A) is incorrect because bone grafts are typically pre-sterilized. Soaking the bone graft in saline solution (B) and shaping the bone graft (D) are subsequent steps that should only be performed after confirming the graft's viability.

Question 135: Correct Answer: A) The patient might have an increased risk of cardiac arrhythmias.

Rationale: A potassium level of 5.8 mEq/L is above the normal range (3.5-5.0 mEq/L), indicating hyperkalemia, which can cause cardiac arrhythmias. Option B is incorrect because hyperkalemia does not directly increase the risk of deep vein thrombosis. Option C is incorrect as hyperkalemia does not directly cause respiratory depression. Option D is incorrect because hyperkalemia does not increase the risk of excessive bleeding.

Question 136: Correct Answer: B) Count the sharps and sponges on the sterile field.

Rationale: The correct sequence starts with counting sharps and sponges on the sterile field to ensure no items are left inside the patient. Counting instruments on the Mayo stand (A) and back table (C) comes later. Counting sponges and sharps off the sterile field (D) is incorrect as it does not address the immediate concern of retained items in the patient. This ensures patient safety and compliance with surgical protocols.

Question 137: Correct Answer: B) Repeat back key points to confirm understanding.

Rationale: Repeating back key points to confirm understanding ensures that you have accurately received and interpreted the information. This active listening technique helps clarify any misunderstandings immediately. Nodding (A) shows agreement but doesn't verify understanding. Taking notes (C) is helpful but doesn't confirm comprehension in real-time. Focusing on non-verbal cues (D) can provide additional context but is not sufficient for confirming detailed instructions.

Question 138: Correct Answer: C) Freezing at ultra-low temperatures

Rationale: Freezing at ultra-low temperatures is a critical step in the preparation of a tissue graft to ensure its viability. This process preserves the graft's cellular structure and function until it is needed for transplantation. Options A, B, and D are incorrect because high heat sterilization can damage tissue, soaking in saline solution is not sufficient for long-term preservation, and coating with antibiotics does not ensure viability but rather reduces infection risk.

Question 139: Correct Answer: B) Oxygen saturation
Rationale: Monitoring oxygen saturation is crucial in the immediate postoperative period to prevent respiratory complications. While blood pressure, urine output, and heart rate are important, they do not directly indicate respiratory function. Oxygen saturation provides a direct measure of how well the patient is ventilating and oxygenating, which is essential for early detection of hypoxia and other respiratory issues.

Question 140: Correct Answer: D) Halt the procedure until the consent form is found
Rationale: Halting the procedure until the consent form is found is the correct action. The Time Out procedure ensures patient safety by verifying all critical information, including consent. Proceeding without the consent form compromises legal and ethical standards. Pausing the Time Out or verbally confirming consent is insufficient and does not meet the protocol requirements.

Question 141: Correct Answer: D) 30 seconds
Rationale: The recommended duration for rubbing a waterless hand antiseptic is 30 seconds to ensure effective microbial kill. Rubbing for only 5, 10, or 20 seconds (options A, B, and C) is insufficient to achieve proper disinfection, as it does not allow enough contact time for the antiseptic to work effectively.

Question 142: Correct Answer: B) Internal mammary artery
Rationale: The internal mammary artery is most commonly used for coronary artery bypass grafting due to its superior long-term patency rates compared to other vessels. The radial artery (A) is also used but less frequently. The femoral artery (C) and carotid artery (D) are not typically used for this procedure due to their anatomical locations and functions. The internal mammary artery's close proximity to the heart and robust blood flow make it ideal for grafting.

Question 143: Correct Answer: D) Poliglecaprone (Monocryl) suture
Rationale: Poliglecaprone (Monocryl) suture is most appropriate for closing small incisions in the abdominal wall due to its absorbable nature and high tensile strength, which provides adequate wound support during the healing process. Silk sutures (A) are non-absorbable and can cause tissue reaction. Polypropylene sutures (B) are also non-absorbable and more suited for vascular anastomosis. Chromic gut sutures (C) are absorbable but have a shorter absorption period and lower tensile strength compared to Monocryl.

Question 144: Correct Answer: C) Helium is non-flammable and provides a safe working environment.
Rationale: Helium is non-flammable, making it an excellent choice for maintaining a safe environment during laser procedures. This is crucial in a surgical setting where safety is paramount. Option A is incorrect as nitrogen is the most abundant gas. Option B is incorrect because lower ionization energy is not a

primary concern for laser use. Option D is incorrect as helium has a low molecular weight, which does not enhance laser beam focus.

Question 145: Correct Answer: C) To prevent retained surgical items
Rationale: The primary reason for performing a count of surgical items before the closure of the surgical site is to prevent retained surgical items, which can cause serious complications. Options A and B, while important, are not the primary reasons for the count. Option D is unrelated to the purpose of the count. The count ensures that no items are left inside the patient, thereby promoting patient safety.

Question 146: Correct Answer: B) Inform the anesthesiologist of the discrepancy.
Rationale: Informing the anesthesiologist (Option B) ensures that the discrepancy is addressed by the responsible medical professional. Correcting the chart without proper authorization (Option A) is inappropriate and can lead to legal issues. Disregarding the discrepancy (Option C) can result in patient harm. Reporting to the surgeon during the next meeting (Option D) delays necessary corrective action. Immediate communication with the anesthesiologist is crucial for patient safety and accurate documentation.

Question 147: Correct Answer: B) Remove all used linens and waste
Rationale: The first step in the room clean-up process is to remove all used linens and waste to prevent cross-contamination and ensure a clean environment for the next procedure. Disinfecting instruments (A) and mopping the floor (D) are important but come later in the process. Restocking supply cabinets (C) is a final step once the room is clean.

Question 148: Correct Answer: C) Calling the pathology department directly via phone
Rationale: Calling the pathology department directly via phone is the most efficient and appropriate method for urgent communication during a surgical procedure. This allows for immediate feedback and clarification. Email and written notes are too slow for urgent needs, and the intercom system may not provide the privacy or direct contact required for detailed medical communication.

Question 149: Correct Answer: C) Enhanced integration with host tissue
Rationale: Autografts, being derived from the patient's own body, have superior integration with host tissue due to genetic compatibility. This minimizes the risk of rejection and promotes quicker healing. While reduced risk of infection (A) and lower cost (D) are benefits, they are not the primary advantage. Increased availability (B) is incorrect as autografts are limited by the amount of tissue that can be harvested from the patient.

Question 150: Correct Answer: B) Professional organization websites
Rationale: Professional organization websites are the best-suited tool for accessing online continuing education courses because they offer accredited and

relevant courses specifically designed for surgical technologists. Social media platforms (A) and personal blogs (D) may provide unverified information, and general search engines (C) can lead to non-accredited or irrelevant courses. Professional organization websites ensure the courses meet the required standards and are recognized by certifying bodies.

CST Exam Practice Questions [SET 5]

Question 1: What is a common sign that a postoperative hematoma is expanding and may require urgent intervention?
A) Decreased heart rate
B) Increased swelling and pain at the surgical site
C) Improved range of motion
D) Decreased drainage from surgical drains

Question 2: In the context of surgical patient care, which of the following is a legal requirement for obtaining informed consent?
A) The patient must sign the consent form without any explanation.
B) The surgeon must explain the procedure, risks, benefits, and alternatives.
C) The nurse can provide all the necessary information for consent.
D) The patient can give verbal consent without documentation.

Question 3: Emily, a surgical technologist, is preparing the operating room for a procedure that will use a laser. She notices that the laser safety goggles are not available. What should Emily do?
A) Proceed with the procedure and obtain the goggles later.
B) Use regular safety glasses instead of laser-specific goggles.
C) Inform the surgeon and proceed with the procedure.
D) Delay the procedure until the laser safety goggles are available.

Question 4: During a laparoscopic cholecystectomy on a 45-year-old patient named John, the surgeon encounters unexpected bleeding from the cystic artery. Which method of hemostasis is most appropriate to control this bleeding?
A) Manual compression
B) Electrocautery
C) Topical hemostatic agents
D) Ligature

Question 5: During a surgical procedure, the surgeon asks the surgical technologist, Alex, to adjust the lighting. Alex notices that the anesthesiologist, Dr. Smith, is currently busy monitoring the patient's vitals. What should Alex do to ensure effective responsiveness and maintain a smooth workflow?
A) Adjust the lighting himself without informing anyone.
B) Wait until Dr. Smith is free and then ask for permission to adjust the lighting.
C) Inform the circulating nurse about the request and let them handle it.
D) Ignore the request and continue with his current task.

Question 6: Which patient position is most appropriate for a laparoscopic cholecystectomy?
A) Supine
B) Prone
C) Trendelenburg
D) Reverse Trendelenburg

Question 7: What is the primary purpose of using a pneumatic tourniquet in orthopedic surgery?
A) To reduce blood loss by compressing blood vessels
B) To stabilize the bone during drilling
C) To enhance the visibility of the surgical site
D) To prevent infection by isolating the surgical area

Question 8: Which of the following is the primary purpose of using protective padding during surgical procedures?
A) To enhance the patient's comfort
B) To prevent pressure ulcers and nerve damage
C) To absorb excess fluids during surgery
D) To maintain the patient's body temperature

Question 9: During an abdominal surgery, which instrument is most appropriate for retracting the abdominal wall?
A) Gelpi retractor
B) DeBakey forceps
C) Army-Navy retractor
D) Allis clamp

Question 10: Which of the following is a key advantage of using a harmonic scalpel over traditional electrosurgery in intraoperative procedures?
A) Higher risk of electrical burns
B) Increased smoke production
C) Reduced thermal spread
D) Greater blood loss

Question 11: During the postoperative assessment of a patient named Mr. Johnson, the surgical technologist notices a firm, swollen area near the incision site that is painful to touch. What is the most appropriate initial action?
A) Apply a warm compress to the area.
B) Notify the surgeon immediately.
C) Encourage the patient to ambulate.
D) Administer an additional dose of pain medication.

Question 12: Sarah, a surgical technologist, needs to inform the pathology department about a specimen that needs to be analyzed urgently. What is the best method for Sarah to ensure effective interdepartmental communication?
A) Leave a voicemail for the pathology department.
B) Send a message through the hospital's secure messaging system.

C) Write a note and send it via interdepartmental mail.
D) Wait until the pathology department calls back.

Question 13: Which gland is responsible for the secretion of parathyroid hormone (PTH)?
A) Thyroid gland
B) Adrenal gland
C) Parathyroid gland
D) Pituitary gland

Question 14: What is a key strategy for surgical technologists to follow in order to contribute to cost containment?
A) Always using new instruments for every procedure
B) Properly maintaining and handling surgical instruments
C) Frequently changing surgical gloves during a procedure
D) Disposing of all unused supplies after each surgery

Question 15: What is the primary purpose of using an allograft in bone grafting procedures?
A) To reduce the risk of infection
B) To provide structural support and promote bone healing
C) To eliminate the need for additional surgeries
D) To ensure immediate weight-bearing capability

Question 16: After a surgical procedure, the surgical technologist, Jamie, is responsible for cleaning and sterilizing the instruments used. Which of the following is the most effective method for ensuring that all instruments are properly decontaminated before sterilization?
A) Wipe each instrument with an alcohol swab.
B) Use enzymatic cleaner followed by ultrasonic cleaning.
C) Soak instruments in saline solution.
D) Rinse instruments with hot water and air dry.

Question 17: During the preoperative preparation of Mr. Johnson, a 65-year-old patient scheduled for a coronary artery bypass graft (CABG), which patient monitoring device is essential to apply first to ensure continuous assessment of his oxygen saturation levels?
A) Blood pressure cuff
B) Electrocardiogram (ECG) leads
C) Pulse oximeter
D) Temperature probe

Question 18: After a successful appendectomy, the surgical technologist is responsible for removing the drapes and other equipment from the patient, Mr. Johnson. What is the first step the surgical technologist should take in this process?
A) Remove the surgical instruments from the sterile field.
B) Remove the drapes from the patient's body.
C) Ensure all counts are correct and accounted for.
D) Disconnect the patient from all monitoring equipment.

Question 19: When mixing medications for a surgical procedure, which of the following is the primary reason for labeling the mixed solution immediately?
A) To comply with hospital policy
B) To prevent contamination
C) To ensure accurate administration
D) To avoid confusion with other medications

Question 20: During the preoperative assessment of a 7-year-old boy named Jacob scheduled for an appendectomy, what is the most important factor to consider to ensure his safety and comfort?
A) Ensuring he understands the risks of the surgery
B) Confirming he has no allergies to medications
C) Discussing the surgical procedure with his parents only
D) Allowing him to choose his post-operative meal

Question 21: During a laparoscopic appendectomy on a patient named John, the surgeon asks the surgical technologist to provide a linear stapler for the resection of the appendix. Which of the following steps should the surgical technologist take first?
A) Load the stapler with staples.
B) Hand the stapler directly to the surgeon.
C) Verify the staple size and load the stapler.
D) Test fire the stapler to ensure proper function.

Question 22: Which layer of the skin is primarily responsible for providing a barrier against pathogens and environmental damage?
A) Epidermis
B) Dermis
C) Hypodermis
D) Subcutaneous tissue

Question 23: Which of the following is a key characteristic of CO2 beam coagulators that makes them suitable for delicate surgical procedures?
A) High penetration depth
B) Low absorption by water
C) High precision and control
D) High scatter of the laser beam

Question 24: During a laparoscopic procedure to remove ovarian cysts, the surgeon asks the surgical technologist to identify the structure that provides blood supply to the ovaries. Which structure should the surgical technologist identify?
A) Uterine artery
B) Ovarian artery
C) Internal iliac artery
D) Superior mesenteric artery

Question 25: When utilizing computer technology for research in a surgical setting, which software is most commonly used for statistical analysis?

A) Microsoft Word
B) Adobe Photoshop
C) SPSS
D) AutoCAD

Question 26: When adding sterile instruments to a sterile field, which of the following is the correct procedure?
A) Drop the instruments from a height of 12 inches.
B) Drop the instruments gently from a height of 6 inches.
C) Place the instruments directly onto the sterile field with your hands.
D) Slide the instruments onto the sterile field.

Question 27: During preoperative preparation, which component of the Da Vinci system is specifically draped to ensure sterility?
A) The surgeon console
B) The patient cart
C) The vision cart
D) The operating room lights

Question 28: A patient named Mr. Johnson has been diagnosed with terminal cancer and has a life expectancy of less than six months. The surgical team needs to discuss end-of-life care options with him. Which of the following is the most appropriate approach for the surgical technologist to take in this situation?
A) Discuss the patient's prognosis and treatment options in detail with him.
B) Provide emotional support and refer the patient to a palliative care specialist.
C) Avoid discussing the prognosis to prevent causing distress.
D) Encourage the patient to seek a second opinion from another oncologist.

Question 29: During a surgical procedure, the lead surgeon, Dr. Smith, becomes increasingly frustrated with the progress and begins to raise his voice at the surgical team. As a Certified Surgical Technologist, how should you respond to maintain a positive group dynamic and ensure the procedure continues smoothly?
A) Ignore the surgeon's behavior and continue your tasks silently.
B) Respond to the surgeon with a calm and respectful tone, acknowledging his concerns.
C) Leave the operating room to avoid further conflict.
D) Ask another team member to address the surgeon's behavior.

Question 30: During a team meeting, you notice that one of the new surgical technologists, Alex, is not participating in the discussion and seems hesitant to share ideas. How should you diplomatically encourage Alex to contribute?
A) Directly ask Alex why they are not participating.
B) Criticize Alex for not being a team player.
C) Create an open and inclusive environment by

asking for everyone's input, including Alex's.
D) Ignore Alex's behavior and continue with the meeting.

Question 31: What is the primary purpose of applying a sterile dressing to a surgical wound site immediately after surgery?
A) To keep the wound dry and free from moisture
B) To prevent the wound from being exposed to air
C) To protect the wound from infection and absorb exudate
D) To promote the formation of a scab

Question 32: What is the first step in checking the integrity of a sterile package before use in the operating room?
A) Inspect the expiration date
B) Check for any visible tears or holes
C) Verify the sterilization indicator
D) Confirm the package contents

Question 33: After a laparoscopic cholecystectomy, Mr. Johnson is experiencing severe shoulder pain. As a Certified Surgical Technologist, what is the most appropriate initial action to alleviate his discomfort?
A) Administering a muscle relaxant
B) Encouraging ambulation and deep breathing exercises
C) Applying a heating pad to the shoulder
D) Increasing the dosage of his pain medication

Question 34: During a surgical procedure, the surgical technologist notices that several sterile instruments were opened but not used. What is the best course of action to follow proper cost containment processes?
A) Discard all unused instruments immediately.
B) Re-sterilize and reuse the instruments for the next surgery.
C) Return the unused instruments to the sterile supply area.
D) Report the unused instruments to the supervisor and follow the facility's policy for handling unused sterile items.

Question 35: Mrs. Smith is undergoing a mastectomy, and the surgeon instructs you to connect a Hemovac drain to the suction apparatus. What is the correct method to ensure the Hemovac drain is activated properly?
A) Compress the Hemovac reservoir before connecting it to the tubing.
B) Connect the Hemovac drain to the suction tubing and then compress the reservoir.
C) Fill the Hemovac reservoir with saline before connecting it to the tubing.
D) Ensure the Hemovac reservoir is fully expanded before connecting it to the tubing.

Question 36: Which type of incision is typically used for an appendectomy?

A) Midline incision
B) McBurney's incision
C) Pfannenstiel incision
D) Subcostal incision

Question 37: Which of the following postoperative findings should be reported immediately as it indicates a potential complication?
A) Slight redness around the incision site
B) Mild swelling of the extremities
C) Persistent high fever
D) Small amount of serous drainage from the wound

Question 38: During a total knee arthroplasty procedure, the surgical technologist is responsible for assembling and testing the power equipment. Which of the following steps should be performed first to ensure the equipment is functioning correctly?
A) Connect the power equipment to the power source.
B) Verify the equipment settings are correct.
C) Check the integrity of the power cord and connections.
D) Test the equipment on a sterile surface.

Question 39: During the postoperative cleanup after Mrs. Smith's surgery, the surgical technologist encounters a blood-soaked drape. What is the correct procedure for disposing of this contaminated drape in compliance with Standard Precautions?
A) Place the drape in a regular laundry hamper.
B) Incinerate the drape immediately.
C) Place the drape in a designated biohazard waste container.
D) Wash the drape with disinfectant before disposal.

Question 40: During a phacoemulsification procedure on a patient named Mr. Smith, the surgeon notices that the ultrasound handpiece is not effectively emulsifying the lens material. What is the most likely cause of this issue?
A) The irrigation fluid is too warm.
B) The phaco tip is clogged.
C) The aspiration flow rate is too high.
D) The power settings are too low.

Question 41: During a laparoscopic cholecystectomy for a patient named Mr. Johnson, when should the surgical technologist perform the first instrument count with the circulator?
A) Before the patient enters the operating room.
B) After the initial incision is made.
C) Before the surgical procedure begins.
D) After the surgical procedure is completed.

Question 42: During a recent surgery, Dr. Johnson requested a different type of retractor than what was listed on his preference card. As a Certified Surgical Technologist, what should you do to ensure the preference card is accurate for future
surgeries?
A) Make a note of the change and update the preference card after confirming with Dr. Johnson.
B) Ignore the change since it was a one-time request.
C) Update the preference card immediately without confirmation.
D) Wait for the nurse to update the preference card.

Question 43: What is the primary reason for using a laser safety officer (LSO) in the operating room?
A) To operate the laser equipment
B) To ensure compliance with laser safety protocols
C) To assist the surgeon during the procedure
D) To monitor the patient's vital signs

Question 44: After a surgical procedure, the surgical technologist is responsible for reporting the amount of medication and solution used. During the postoperative phase, the technologist notices that the amount of saline solution recorded in the patient's chart for Mr. Johnson does not match the actual amount used. What should the technologist do next?
A) Ignore the discrepancy and proceed with the documentation.
B) Report the discrepancy to the circulating nurse immediately.
C) Adjust the recorded amount to match the actual usage without informing anyone.
D) Wait until the end of the shift to report the discrepancy.

Question 45: Which of the following veins is most commonly used for coronary artery bypass grafting (CABG)?
A) Femoral vein
B) Basilic vein
C) Great saphenous vein
D) Cephalic vein

Question 46: Sarah, a surgical technologist, is preparing for an initial surgical scrub before assisting in a major surgery. What is the recommended duration for the initial surgical scrub to ensure proper asepsis?
A) 1 minute
B) 3 minutes
C) 5 minutes
D) 7 minutes

Question 47: During the preoperative check for Ms. Johnson's total knee arthroplasty, the surgical technologist finds that the power drill is not functioning. What should be the immediate next step?
A) Notify the surgeon and wait for their instructions.
B) Use a manual drill instead of the power drill.
C) Replace the malfunctioning power drill with a reserved backup.
D) Cancel the surgery and reschedule for another day.

Question 48: When transferring a patient to the operating room table, which technique is recommended to prevent musculoskeletal injuries among the surgical team?
A) Use a draw sheet and coordinate movements.
B) Lift the patient manually using proper body mechanics.
C) Slide the patient using a friction-reducing device.
D) Ask the patient to assist by scooting over.

Question 49: During a high-stress surgical procedure, how should a surgical technologist respond to a surgeon's abrupt and demanding behavior to maintain effective interpersonal dynamics?
A) Respond with equal intensity to assert authority.
B) Maintain composure and respond calmly to the surgeon's requests.
C) Ignore the surgeon's behavior and focus solely on the task.
D) Leave the operating room to avoid confrontation.

Question 50: During a laparoscopic cholecystectomy on a 45-year-old patient named Mr. Smith, the surgeon identifies an abnormal anatomical structure that appears to be a duplicated gallbladder. What is the most appropriate initial step for the surgical technologist to assist the surgeon in managing this abnormality?
A) Proceed with the removal of both structures.
B) Convert to an open cholecystectomy for better visualization.
C) Perform an intraoperative cholangiogram to clarify the anatomy.
D) Stop the procedure and refer the patient for further imaging studies.

Question 51: Which of the following is a key component of a computer navigation system used in surgery?
A) Electromagnetic field generator
B) Ultrasound transducer
C) Fiber optic camera
D) Laser scalpel

Question 52: During the postoperative room cleanup after a surgery on Ms. Smith, the surgical technologist notices that the sterile supply cart is low on certain items. What should the technologist do to ensure the room is properly restocked?
A) Notify the central supply department and wait for them to restock
B) Restock the cart with items from another operating room
C) Replenish the cart with supplies from the central sterile supply area
D) Leave a note for the next shift to restock the cart

Question 53: Sarah, a 45-year-old patient, is scheduled for a hysterectomy. The surgeon

instructs the surgical technologist to prepare for the removal of the "uterus and adnexa." What does "adnexa" refer to in this context?
A) Ovaries and fallopian tubes
B) Uterine lining
C) Cervix
D) Vaginal canal

Question 54: Which of the following steps is essential immediately after completing the surgical hand scrub?
A) Dry hands with a sterile towel
B) Apply hand lotion
C) Put on sterile gloves directly
D) Rinse hands with water

Question 55: During a laparoscopic cholecystectomy, the surgical technologist notices that the patient's arm is positioned in a way that could potentially lead to nerve damage. What is the most appropriate action to take to ensure protective padding is applied correctly?
A) Place a rolled towel under the patient's wrist.
B) Use a gel pad under the patient's elbow.
C) Secure the arm with a strap without additional padding.
D) Place a foam pad under the patient's shoulder.

Question 56: When positioning a safety strap on a patient, where should it be placed to ensure maximum effectiveness?
A) Across the patient's chest
B) Across the patient's thighs
C) Across the patient's abdomen
D) Across the patient's ankles

Question 57: What is the primary purpose of using an allograft in orthopedic surgery?
A) To reduce the risk of infection
B) To provide a scaffold for bone growth
C) To eliminate the need for autograft harvesting
D) To accelerate the healing process

Question 58: Why is it important for a Certified Surgical Technologist to understand cultural diversity in the operating room?
A) To ensure that all surgical procedures are performed uniformly.
B) To enhance communication and teamwork among a diverse surgical team.
C) To minimize the need for interpreters in the operating room.
D) To reduce the time spent on preoperative preparations.

Question 59: While preparing Ms. Johnson for a total knee replacement, the surgical technologist notices that the bovie pad is not adhering well to the skin. What is the most appropriate action to take?
A) Apply more adhesive to the bovie pad
B) Shave the area and reapply the bovie pad

C) Place the bovie pad on a different area without shaving
D) Use a different type of electrosurgical unit

Question 60: Which of the following is the most appropriate use of computer technology in the management of surgical inventory?
A) Tracking surgical team schedules
B) Monitoring patient vital signs
C) Managing surgical instrument inventory
D) Documenting patient consent forms

Question 61: 3 During a surgical procedure on Mr. Johnson, the surgical technologist notices that the sterile field has been compromised by a small tear in one of the drapes. Which immediate action should the surgical technologist take to maintain the principles of surgical microbiology?
A) Ignore the tear and continue with the procedure.
B) Cover the tear with another sterile drape.
C) Inform the surgeon and replace the compromised drape.
D) Move the tear to a less critical area of the sterile field.

Question 62: During a laparoscopic procedure to treat endometriosis in a 32-year-old patient named Sarah, the surgeon asks the surgical technologist to identify the structure that transports ova from the ovaries to the uterus. Which structure should the surgical technologist identify?
A) Ureter
B) Fallopian Tube
C) Round Ligament
D) Urethra

Question 63: During a femoral-popliteal bypass surgery on Mr. Johnson, the surgeon asks for a vascular clamp to control bleeding from the femoral artery. Which of the following clamps is most appropriate for this procedure?
A) DeBakey clamp
B) Satinsky clamp
C) Bulldog clamp
D) Fogarty clamp

Question 64: During the postoperative removal of equipment, which instrument is essential for ensuring that all surgical instruments are accounted for and no foreign objects are left in the patient?
A) Sponge forceps
B) Needle holder
C) Instrument counting tray
D) Retractor

Question 65: What is the primary benefit of using active listening skills during team meetings in a surgical setting?
A) It allows the listener to prepare their response while others are speaking
B) It helps in accurately understanding and

interpreting the speaker's message
C) It reduces the time needed for meetings by quickly moving through the agenda
D) It ensures that the loudest team member's opinions are prioritized

Question 66: A 45-year-old patient named John presents with severe abdominal pain, nausea, and vomiting. Upon examination, he has a positive Murphy's sign. Which surgical pathology is most likely responsible for John's symptoms?
A) Appendicitis
B) Cholecystitis
C) Pancreatitis
D) Diverticulitis

Question 67: If a fire occurs in the operating room, what is the most appropriate initial action for the surgical technologist?
A) Evacuate the patient immediately.
B) Use a fire extinguisher to put out the fire.
C) Turn off the oxygen supply.
D) Call for help.

Question 68: What is the primary reason for using a smoke evacuator during laser surgery?
A) To reduce the risk of fire
B) To maintain a sterile field
C) To remove airborne contaminants
D) To enhance visibility for the surgeon

Question 69: During an orthopedic surgery, the surgical technologist notices that the smoke evacuation system is not functioning properly. What should be the technologist's next step to maintain a safe environment?
A) Inform the surgeon and switch to a backup smoke evacuation system.
B) Continue the procedure and use a handheld suction device to remove smoke.
C) Increase the room ventilation by adjusting the HVAC system.
D) Ignore the issue as the smoke will eventually dissipate.

Question 70: Which muscle is involved in the dorsiflexion of the foot at the ankle joint?
A) Gastrocnemius
B) Soleus
C) Tibialis Anterior
D) Peroneus Longus

Question 71: During a total knee arthroplasty for Mr. Johnson, the surgical team decides to use an autograft for ligament reconstruction. Which of the following is the most appropriate source for the autograft in this scenario?
A) Allograft from a cadaver
B) Synthetic ligament
C) Patellar tendon from the patient
D) Xenograft from a pig

Question 72: Emily, a surgical technologist, is preparing instruments for an upcoming surgery. She notices that one of the instruments has a small crack. What should Emily do with this instrument?

A) Use the instrument as it is since the crack is small.
B) Report the defect and remove the instrument from the set.
C) Sterilize the instrument again to ensure it is safe to use.
D) Use the instrument but inform the surgeon about the crack.

Question 73: Which of the following is the primary consideration when positioning a patient in the lithotomy position for a gynecological procedure?

A) Ensuring the patient's arms are tucked at their sides
B) Preventing pressure on the peroneal nerve
C) Keeping the patient's head elevated
D) Ensuring the patient's legs are fully extended

Question 74: During the preoperative preparation for a patient named Mr. Johnson undergoing a total knee arthroplasty, the surgical technologist must ensure proper protective padding is applied to prevent pressure injuries. Which area is most critical to pad to prevent common pressure injuries during this procedure?

A) The patient's lower back.
B) The patient's heels.
C) The patient's upper arms.
D) The patient's neck.

Question 75: A 32-year-old male named John is brought to the emergency room after a motorcycle accident. He is experiencing severe pain in his right leg, which appears deformed and swollen. Upon examination, there is an open wound with bone protruding. What is the most appropriate initial management step for this patient?

A) Apply a tourniquet above the injury
B) Administer intravenous antibiotics
C) Perform immediate surgical debridement
D) Immobilize the leg and cover the wound with a sterile dressing

Question 76: During an orthopedic surgery on a patient named Mrs. Smith, the surgical technologist accidentally brushes against a non-sterile surface. What is the most appropriate action to take to maintain aseptic technique?

A) Continue with the procedure and avoid touching the sterile field.
B) Inform the circulating nurse and replace the contaminated items.
C) Wipe the area with a sterile cloth and continue.
D) Ask another team member to take over while you scrub out and re-gown.

Question 77: During the preoperative check for Ms. Smith's total knee arthroplasty, the surgical technologist discovers that the power drill is not functioning. What should be the technologist's immediate course of action?

A) Inform the circulating nurse
B) Proceed with the surgery using manual instruments
C) Attempt to repair the drill
D) Check for a backup power drill

Question 78: During a laparoscopic cholecystectomy on Mr. Johnson, the surgical technologist notices that the insufflation tubing is kinked, which could lead to inadequate pneumoperitoneum. What should the surgical technologist do to prevent a potentially harmful situation?

A) Straighten the tubing and continue the procedure.
B) Inform the surgeon and assist in replacing the tubing.
C) Increase the insufflation pressure to compensate for the kink.
D) Ignore the kink and monitor the patient's vital signs closely.

Question 79: During a preoperative preparation for a spinal surgery, the surgical technologist is responsible for draping the C-arm. Which of the following steps is crucial to ensure the sterility of the C-arm during the procedure?

A) Drape the C-arm with a sterile cover before the patient is brought into the operating room.
B) Ensure the C-arm is draped with a sterile cover after the surgical site is prepped and draped.
C) Position the C-arm in the operating room and then drape it with a sterile cover.
D) Sterilize the C-arm with a disinfectant spray before draping it with a sterile cover.

Question 80: What is the most effective first step to take when a fire breaks out in the operating room?

A) Use a fire extinguisher immediately
B) Evacuate the patient and staff
C) Shut off the oxygen supply
D) Call for help

Question 81: Who is primarily responsible for obtaining informed consent from a patient before surgery?

A) The surgical technologist
B) The anesthesiologist
C) The surgeon
D) The nurse

Question 82: During the preoperative preparation, Sarah, a Certified Surgical Technologist, is about to perform a medical hand wash. Which of the following steps is essential to ensure proper aseptic technique?

A) Use a nail brush to scrub under the nails for 15 seconds.
B) Wash hands and forearms up to the elbows for at least 2 minutes.

C) Dry hands with a reusable cloth towel.
D) Apply lotion immediately after washing to prevent skin dryness.

Question 83: Sarah, a surgical technologist, is asked by her supervisor to falsify a patient's surgical record to cover up a minor error that did not harm the patient. What is the most appropriate action for Sarah to take?
A) Comply with the supervisor's request to avoid conflict.
B) Refuse to falsify the record and report the request to the hospital's compliance officer.
C) Alter the record but document the changes in a personal log.
D) Discuss the situation with the patient and seek their consent.

Question 84: During a surgical procedure, what is the best preventative action to avoid patient burns from electrosurgical equipment?
A) Placing the grounding pad on a bony prominence.
B) Ensuring the grounding pad is properly placed on a well-vascularized muscle mass.
C) Using the lowest power setting on the electrosurgical unit.
D) Frequently checking the temperature of the electrosurgical unit.

Question 85: What is the primary reason for using a battery-powered surgical saw over a pneumatic one?
A) Battery-powered saws are more powerful
B) Battery-powered saws are quieter
C) Battery-powered saws eliminate the need for air hoses
D) Battery-powered saws are less expensive

Question 86: What is the recommended duration for performing a medical hand wash before a surgical procedure?
A) 10 seconds
B) 20 seconds
C) 2 minutes
D) 5 minutes

Question 87: During a total knee arthroplasty, the surgeon needs to access the quadriceps tendon. Which muscle group does the quadriceps tendon belong to?
A) Hamstrings
B) Adductors
C) Quadriceps femoris
D) Gastrocnemius

Question 88: 2 During a surgical procedure, a sample is taken from a patient named Ms. Smith for anaerobic culture. Which of the following conditions is essential for the accurate growth of anaerobic bacteria?
A) Exposure to room air
B) Incubation in a CO2 incubator

C) Use of an anaerobic chamber
D) Immediate freezing of the sample

Question 89: During tissue procurement from a deceased donor, the surgical technologist must ensure proper labeling and documentation. What is the primary reason for this meticulous process?
A) To ensure the tissue is used within the same hospital
B) To prevent legal issues
C) To maintain traceability and ensure compatibility
D) To expedite the procurement process

Question 90: During the cardiac cycle, which phase is characterized by the ventricles contracting and ejecting blood into the arteries?
A) Atrial systole
B) Ventricular systole
C) Atrial diastole
D) Ventricular diastole

Question 91: What is the primary function of a Bovie electrosurgical pencil in the operating room?
A) Cutting and coagulating tissue
B) Holding sutures
C) Retracting tissue
D) Suctioning fluids

Question 92: During a laparoscopic cholecystectomy on a patient named Mr. Smith, the surgeon accidentally nicks a blood vessel, causing a significant amount of blood to spill onto the surgical field. As the surgical technologist, what is the most appropriate immediate action to follow standard and universal precautions?
A) Continue assisting the surgeon without changing gloves.
B) Immediately change gloves and continue assisting.
C) Use a suction device to clear the blood and then change gloves.
D) Notify the circulating nurse and step away from the field.

Question 93: After a laparoscopic cholecystectomy, Mr. Smith is in the recovery room. The nurse notices that he has a significant amount of drainage from his surgical site. What is the most appropriate initial action for the surgical technologist to take?
A) Apply a new sterile dressing and notify the surgeon.
B) Increase the flow rate of IV fluids.
C) Administer pain medication as prescribed.
D) Encourage the patient to ambulate.

Question 94: Which chemical agent is used to achieve hemostasis by causing vasoconstriction and is often combined with local anesthetics?
A) Epinephrine
B) Protamine Sulfate

C) Fibrin Sealant
D) Vitamin K

Question 95: During the preparation of a Jackson-Pratt drain, what is the correct method to ensure it functions properly?
A) Attach the bulb to the tubing before insertion
B) Ensure the tubing is clamped before insertion
C) Prime the tubing with saline before insertion
D) Compress the bulb after insertion to create suction

Question 96: During a surgical procedure on Mr. Johnson, the surgeon needs to locate the phrenic nerve to avoid damaging it. Which anatomical landmark is the most reliable for identifying the phrenic nerve?
A) Anterior to the scalene muscle
B) Posterior to the sternocleidomastoid muscle
C) Lateral to the trachea
D) Medial to the carotid artery

Question 97: During a laparoscopic cholecystectomy, the surgeon requests that the patient, Mr. Smith, be placed in the reverse Trendelenburg position. What is the primary purpose of this position in this procedure?
A) To reduce venous return to the heart
B) To improve access to the upper abdomen
C) To prevent aspiration
D) To enhance visualization of the pelvic organs

Question 98: Which of the following is the primary consideration when preparing an allograft for implantation during surgery?
A) Ensuring the allograft is sourced from a living donor
B) Confirming the allograft is free from infectious agents
C) Matching the allograft size exactly to the recipient's defect
D) Ensuring the allograft is cryopreserved

Question 99: Which part of the gastrointestinal tract is primarily responsible for nutrient absorption?
A) Stomach
B) Small intestine
C) Large intestine
D) Esophagus

Question 100: Which hormone is primarily responsible for regulating the body's metabolism and energy production?
A) Insulin
B) Thyroxine
C) Cortisol
D) Glucagon

Question 101: Which thermal method is most commonly used for achieving hemostasis during laparoscopic surgery?
A) Cryotherapy

B) Electrocautery
C) Ultrasonic scalpel
D) Laser coagulation

Question 102: What does the term "hemostasis" refer to in surgical terminology?
A) The process of blood formation
B) The cessation of bleeding
C) The inflammation of a blood vessel
D) The destruction of red blood cells

Question 103: Which instrument is primarily used for grasping and holding tissues during surgery?
A) Metzenbaum scissors
B) Allis forceps
C) Babcock forceps
D) Mayo scissors

Question 104: Dr. Smith is preparing for an urgent surgical procedure and requires a set of instruments to be sterilized quickly. Which of the following best describes the key steps to ensure effective sterilization using a short cycle?
A) Load instruments loosely, use a high temperature, and ensure adequate drying time
B) Pack instruments tightly, use a low temperature, and skip drying time
C) Load instruments loosely, use a high temperature, and skip drying time
D) Pack instruments tightly, use a high temperature, and ensure adequate drying time

Question 105: Which of the following actions should be taken when transporting a patient with a chest tube to the operating room?
A) Clamping the chest tube
B) Keeping the drainage system below chest level
C) Removing the chest tube before transport
D) Placing the patient in a prone position

Question 106: During a thyroidectomy procedure on a patient named John, the surgeon accidentally damages the parathyroid glands. Which immediate postoperative complication is the surgical technologist most concerned about?
A) Hypercalcemia
B) Hypocalcemia
C) Hyperthyroidism
D) Hypothyroidism

Question 107: Which of the following best describes the role of cultural competence in patient care within the surgical setting?
A) It ensures that all patients receive identical treatment regardless of their background.
B) It helps in tailoring patient care to meet the specific cultural needs of each patient.
C) It eliminates the need for cultural sensitivity training for the surgical team.
D) It focuses solely on language barriers between patients and healthcare providers.

Question 108: After completing a surgical procedure on Mr. Johnson, the surgical technologist is responsible for cleaning the operating room. Which of the following steps is the most critical to ensure proper room turnover?
A) Wiping down the surgical lights and tables
B) Disposing of all sharps and biohazard materials
C) Restocking the sterile supply cart
D) Mopping the floor with a disinfectant solution

Question 109: During a surgical procedure, the surgical technologist is responsible for draping the patient, Mr. Johnson, who is undergoing an abdominal surgery. What is the correct sequence of draping to ensure a sterile field?
A) Place the fenestrated drape first, followed by the four towels.
B) Place the four towels first, followed by the fenestrated drape.
C) Place the fenestrated drape first, followed by the laparotomy sheet.
D) Place the laparotomy sheet first, followed by the fenestrated drape.

Question 110: Sarah, a surgical technologist, is tasked with managing the surgical schedule and ensuring all team members are aware of their responsibilities. What is the most effective method Sarah should use to communicate the surgical schedule to the team?
A) Verbally inform each team member individually.
B) Post the schedule on the bulletin board in the break room.
C) Send an email with the schedule to all team members.
D) Rely on team members to check the electronic scheduling system.

Question 111: During a laparoscopic cholecystectomy, the surgeon asks for a stapling device to secure the cystic duct. Which stapling device is most appropriate for this procedure?
A) Linear stapler
B) Circular stapler
C) Skin stapler
D) Endoscopic clip applier

Question 112: Sarah, a Certified Surgical Technologist, is required to complete continuing education credits to maintain her certification. She decides to utilize computer technology for this purpose. Which of the following actions best demonstrates the effective use of computer technology for continuing education?
A) Attending in-person workshops and conferences
B) Watching surgical technique videos on YouTube
C) Enrolling in accredited online courses and webinars
D) Reading surgical journals in the hospital library

Question 113: Mrs. Smith, a 60-year-old patient, reports a rash and itching around her surgical incision site three days after a knee replacement surgery. What is the most appropriate immediate action for a Certified Surgical Technologist?
A) Apply a topical antibiotic ointment
B) Notify the surgeon immediately
C) Advise the patient to take an antihistamine
D) Clean the area with antiseptic solution

Question 114: Which of the following is a critical step when assembling a powered surgical drill?
A) Ensuring the drill is fully charged
B) Verifying the correct drill bit is securely attached
C) Applying lubricant to the drill motor
D) Testing the drill on a sample material

Question 115: Which of the following muscles is primarily responsible for the abduction of the shoulder joint?
A) Deltoid
B) Biceps Brachii
C) Trapezius
D) Pectoralis Major

Question 116: During a laparoscopic cholecystectomy on Mrs. Johnson, the surgical technologist is responsible for assembling and testing the insufflator. Which step is crucial to ensure the insufflator is functioning correctly before the procedure begins?
A) Ensuring the insufflator is set to the correct pressure setting.
B) Checking the insufflator tubing for kinks or obstructions.
C) Verifying the insufflator is properly connected to the CO2 tank.
D) Confirming the insufflator is sterilized.

Question 117: What is the primary purpose of using cautery during postoperative procedures?
A) To reduce the risk of infection
B) To minimize blood loss
C) To enhance wound healing
D) To remove foreign bodies

Question 118: During the preparation of an autograft, which step is crucial to ensure the viability of the graft tissue?
A) Sterilization of the graft
B) Immediate transplantation after harvesting
C) Use of chemical preservatives
D) Freezing the graft for future use

Question 119: What is the primary reason for monitoring a postoperative patient for signs of hematoma formation?
A) To ensure patient comfort.
B) To prevent infection.
C) To detect potential bleeding complications.
D) To monitor for allergic reactions.

Question 120: During a thoracic surgery on a patient named Mr. Johnson, the surgical

technologist is tasked with maintaining the retractors. The surgeon notes that the retractor is slipping and requests an adjustment. What should the surgical technologist do to ensure the retractor remains stable?
A) Tighten the retractor's screws
B) Replace the retractor with a larger one
C) Adjust the retractor's position and ensure proper tissue engagement
D) Apply more pressure manually

Question 121: Which of the following structures prevents the backflow of stomach contents into the esophagus?
A) Pyloric sphincter
B) Ileocecal valve
C) Lower esophageal sphincter
D) Hepatopancreatic sphincter

Question 122: During the preoperative preparation for a laparoscopic cholecystectomy on Mr. Smith, the surgical technologist needs to ensure proper lighting. Which of the following steps is MOST crucial in optimizing the lighting for this procedure?
A) Adjust the overhead lights to maximum brightness.
B) Position the surgical lights to eliminate shadows on the surgical field.
C) Ensure the laparoscope light source is set to a low intensity.
D) Use ambient room lighting to supplement the surgical lights.

Question 123: Which of the following steps is essential for ensuring the proper functioning of a surgical microscope before an intraoperative procedure?
A) Checking the microscope's light source intensity
B) Adjusting the microscope's ocular lenses for magnification
C) Ensuring the microscope's foot pedal is connected
D) Cleaning the microscope's external surfaces

Question 124: A 45-year-old patient named John is undergoing a thyroidectomy due to a large goiter. During the surgery, the surgeon accidentally damages the parathyroid glands. What immediate post-operative complication is John most at risk for?
A) Hypercalcemia
B) Hypocalcemia
C) Hyperkalemia
D) Hypokalemia

Question 125: During a surgical procedure, the surgical technologist, Alex, notices that a fellow team member, Dr. Smith, is not following proper sterile technique. What should Alex do to ensure ethical and legal practices in surgical patient care?
A) Ignore the breach to maintain team harmony.
B) Report the incident after the surgery is completed.

C) Immediately inform Dr. Smith about the breach.
D) Ask another team member to address the issue.

Question 126: During a laparoscopic cholecystectomy on a patient named Mr. Johnson, the surgeon uses monopolar cautery to dissect the gallbladder from the liver bed. What is the most important step the surgical technologist should take to ensure patient safety when using monopolar cautery?
A) Ensure the grounding pad is properly placed on the patient's thigh.
B) Use a bipolar cautery instead of monopolar cautery.
C) Increase the power setting on the cautery machine.
D) Apply saline to the surgical site before using the cautery.

Question 127: Which structure in the male reproductive system is responsible for the production of sperm?
A) Epididymis
B) Prostate gland
C) Seminiferous tubules
D) Vas deferens

Question 128: During a laparoscopic cholecystectomy on a patient named Mr. Smith, the surgeon requests the surgical technologist to adjust the insufflation pressure. What should the surgical technologist do to ensure optimal visualization and patient safety?
A) Increase the insufflation pressure to 25 mmHg.
B) Decrease the insufflation pressure to 5 mmHg.
C) Maintain the insufflation pressure at 15 mmHg.
D) Turn off the insufflation device.

Question 129: During a colon resection surgery on a 60-year-old patient named Mrs. Smith, the surgeon needs to identify the blood supply to the descending colon. Which artery should the surgical technologist anticipate being ligated?
A) Superior mesenteric artery
B) Inferior mesenteric artery
C) Celiac trunk
D) Renal artery

Question 130: During a total knee arthroplasty, the surgical technologist needs to apply the light handles. What is the correct procedure to ensure sterility is maintained?
A) The surgeon should apply the light handles with sterile gloves.
B) The surgical technologist should apply the light handles using a sterile light handle cover.
C) The circulating nurse should apply the light handles with clean gloves.
D) The surgical technologist should apply the light handles with clean gloves.

Question 131: During a total knee replacement surgery, the surgeon encounters diffuse oozing

from the soft tissues around the knee. Which chemical hemostatic agent would be most effective in this scenario?
A) Fibrin sealant
B) Hydrogen peroxide
C) Lidocaine
D) Sodium chloride

Question 132: During a surgical procedure, what is the correct method to pass a suture needle to the surgeon?
A) Pass the needle directly into the surgeon's hand.
B) Use a needle holder to pass the needle.
C) Hand the needle with the sharp end pointing towards the surgeon.
D) Place the needle on the instrument table for the surgeon to pick up.

Question 133: Which of the following is the primary purpose of applying a sterile dressing to a surgical wound site?
A) To prevent the wound from drying out
B) To absorb exudate and provide a barrier to infection
C) To allow for easy access to the wound
D) To reduce the need for postoperative antibiotics

Question 134: Sarah, a 45-year-old patient, is undergoing a laser-assisted cervical conization for the treatment of cervical dysplasia. Which of the following is a critical safety measure that the surgical technologist must ensure during the procedure?
A) Ensuring the laser is set to the highest power setting
B) Using a wet drape to cover surrounding tissues
C) Placing the laser directly on the tissue for maximum effect
D) Keeping the laser in standby mode when not in use

Question 135: Which of the following is the most appropriate method for labeling a specimen container in the operating room?
A) Using a pre-printed label with the patient's information.
B) Writing the patient's name and date of birth on the container.
C) Including the patient's medical record number and type of specimen.
D) Attaching a label with the surgeon's name and procedure date.

Question 136: During a surgical procedure, the surgical technologist notices that several sterile items have been opened but not used. What is the best course of action to follow proper cost containment processes?
A) Discard all unused sterile items immediately.
B) Return the unused sterile items to the sterile supply room.
C) Document the unused sterile items and return them to the sterile supply room if unopened.

D) Leave the unused sterile items on the surgical tray for the next procedure.

Question 137: Which of the following is a significant advantage of using a harmonic scalpel over traditional electrosurgery in minimally invasive procedures?
A) Higher risk of thermal injury
B) Increased blood loss
C) Reduced smoke production
D) Slower cutting speed

Question 138: Which of the following conditions is characterized by the inflammation of the appendix, often resulting in severe abdominal pain and requiring surgical intervention?
A) Cholecystitis
B) Diverticulitis
C) Appendicitis
D) Pancreatitis

Question 139: During a laparoscopic cholecystectomy, the surgical technologist notices that the patient's end-tidal CO2 levels are steadily rising. What should be the immediate course of action?
A) Increase the oxygen flow rate.
B) Inform the surgeon and anesthesiologist immediately.
C) Check for equipment malfunction.
D) Administer a muscle relaxant.

Question 140: Which of the following is the most appropriate action for a surgical technologist to take when reporting the amount of solution used during surgery?
A) Estimate the amount used based on typical usage
B) Record the amount used immediately after the procedure
C) Wait until the end of the day to report all solutions used
D) Report only the solutions that were completely used

Question 141: During a surgical procedure, Sarah, a Certified Surgical Technologist, is preparing to assist the surgeon by donning her gown and gloves. Which of the following steps should Sarah perform first to ensure sterility?
A) Don the gloves first, then the gown.
B) Don the gown first, then the gloves.
C) Wash hands, don gloves, then gown.
D) Wash hands, don gown, then gloves.

Question 142: What is the recommended temperature range for the water used in the manual cleaning of surgical instruments?
A) 50-60°F
B) 70-80°F
C) 80-110°F
D) 120-140°F

Question 143: John, a 60-year-old patient from a different cultural background, is scheduled for surgery. He has specific cultural beliefs regarding medical interventions. How should the surgical technologist ensure that John's cultural beliefs are respected during the surgical procedure?
A) Assume that John's cultural beliefs will not affect the surgical procedure.
B) Document John's cultural beliefs in his medical record and discuss them with the surgical team.
C) Tell John that his cultural beliefs will be considered only if they align with medical protocols.
D) Inform John that cultural beliefs are secondary to medical procedures and cannot be accommodated.

Question 144: Which chamber of the heart receives oxygenated blood from the lungs?
A) Right atrium
B) Left atrium
C) Right ventricle
D) Left ventricle

Question 145: During a spinal surgery on a patient named Mary, the surgeon needs to avoid damaging the structure that transmits motor signals from the brain to the spinal cord. Which structure should the surgical technologist ensure is protected?
A) Dorsal root ganglion
B) Ventral root
C) Dorsal column
D) Spinothalamic tract

Question 146: During a mastectomy, the surgeon removes a lymph node for biopsy. What is the correct method for verifying, preparing, and labeling this specimen?
A) Place the lymph node in formalin and label it with the patient's name and type of specimen.
B) Place the lymph node in a dry container and label it with the patient's name, date of surgery, and type of specimen.
C) Place the lymph node in formalin and label it with the patient's name, date of surgery, and type of specimen.
D) Place the lymph node in saline and label it with the patient's name and type of specimen.

Question 147: During an open appendectomy on a patient named Ms. Johnson, the surgeon requests a "Babcock forceps." What is the primary use of this instrument?
A) Clamping blood vessels
B) Grasping delicate tissue without causing trauma
C) Cutting sutures
D) Retracting tissue

Question 148: What is the primary advantage of using synthetic bone grafts in surgical procedures?
A) They integrate faster with the host bone.
B) They eliminate the risk of disease transmission.
C) They are more cost-effective than autografts.
D) They provide superior mechanical strength compared to natural bone.

Question 149: Which of the following is the most critical step in ensuring proper fit and function when applying a splint?
A) Choosing the correct type of splint material
B) Ensuring the limb is in the correct anatomical position
C) Wrapping the splint tightly to prevent movement
D) Applying padding only to the injured area

Question 150: Mr. Smith, a postoperative patient who underwent a knee arthroplasty, complains of calf pain, swelling, and redness. What is the most appropriate action for a Certified Surgical Technologist to take?
A) Encourage Mr. Smith to walk to relieve the pain.
B) Apply an ice pack to the affected area.
C) Report the symptoms to the medical team immediately.
D) Elevate Mr. Smith's leg and monitor for changes.

ANSWER WITH DETAILED EXPLANATION SET [5]

Question 1: Correct Answer: B) Increased swelling and pain at the surgical site
Rationale: Increased swelling and pain at the surgical site are common signs that a hematoma is expanding and may require urgent intervention. Decreased heart rate (A) is not typically associated with hematomas, improved range of motion (C) is unlikely in the presence of a hematoma, and decreased drainage (D) does not specifically indicate an expanding hematoma. Prompt recognition and intervention are critical to prevent complications.

Question 2: Correct Answer: B) The surgeon must explain the procedure, risks, benefits, and alternatives.
Rationale: Obtaining informed consent legally requires the surgeon to explain the procedure, including its risks, benefits, and alternatives, ensuring the patient fully understands before consenting. Simply signing a form without explanation, having a nurse provide the information, or accepting verbal consent without documentation does not meet legal standards, as they do not ensure the patient's comprehensive understanding and voluntary agreement.

Question 3: Correct Answer: D) Delay the procedure until the laser safety goggles are available.
Rationale: Laser safety goggles are essential to protect the eyes from laser radiation. Proceeding without them (Options A and C) or using regular safety glasses (Option B) does not provide adequate protection. Delaying the procedure until the correct goggles are available (Option D) ensures compliance with safety standards and protects all personnel from potential eye injuries.

Question 4: Correct Answer: B) Electrocautery
Rationale: Electrocautery is the most appropriate method for controlling bleeding from the cystic artery during a laparoscopic cholecystectomy due to its precision and effectiveness in coagulating blood vessels. Manual compression (A) is not feasible in a laparoscopic setting. Topical hemostatic agents (C) are less effective for arterial bleeding. Ligature (D) is challenging to apply laparoscopically and may not provide immediate hemostasis compared to electrocautery.

Question 5: Correct Answer: C) Inform the circulating nurse about the request and let them handle it.
Rationale: The correct response is to inform the circulating nurse, who is responsible for managing the operating room environment. This ensures that the task is handled promptly without disrupting the anesthesiologist's focus on the patient's vitals. Adjusting the lighting himself (A) or waiting for Dr. Smith (B) could delay the procedure, and ignoring the request (D) is unprofessional and could compromise the surgical environment.

Question 6: Correct Answer: D) Reverse Trendelenburg
Rationale: The reverse Trendelenburg position is most appropriate for a laparoscopic cholecystectomy as it allows better access to the upper abdomen and reduces the risk of aspiration. The supine position (A) does not provide optimal exposure. The prone position (B) is unsuitable for abdominal surgeries. Trendelenburg (C) may increase the risk of aspiration and does not facilitate access to the gallbladder.

Question 7: Correct Answer: A) To reduce blood loss by compressing blood vessels
Rationale: The primary purpose of a pneumatic tourniquet in orthopedic surgery is to reduce blood loss by compressing blood vessels. This allows for a bloodless field, enhancing visibility (option C) but not as its primary function. Stabilizing the bone (option B) and preventing infection (option D) are not functions of the tourniquet. The main goal is to control blood flow, which is critical for a clear surgical field and reducing intraoperative blood loss.

Question 8: Correct Answer: B) To prevent pressure ulcers and nerve damage
Rationale: The primary purpose of using protective padding during surgical procedures is to prevent pressure ulcers and nerve damage. While enhancing comfort (A) and maintaining body temperature (D) are important, they are secondary considerations. Absorbing excess fluids (C) is not a function of protective padding. Protective padding ensures that prolonged pressure on specific body parts does not lead to tissue injury or nerve compression, which are critical for patient safety.

Question 9: Correct Answer: C) Army-Navy retractor
Rationale: The Army-Navy retractor is specifically designed for retracting the abdominal wall and other tissues during surgery. Gelpi retractors are used for smaller, more precise retractions, DeBakey forceps are used for grasping delicate tissues, and Allis clamps are used for holding or grasping tissue. The Army-Navy retractor's design and application make it the most suitable choice for retracting the abdominal wall, unlike the other instruments which have different primary uses.

Question 10: Correct Answer: C) Reduced thermal spread
Rationale: The harmonic scalpel offers reduced thermal spread compared to traditional electrosurgery, which minimizes damage to adjacent tissues. Unlike options A, B, and D, which are disadvantages of traditional electrosurgery, the harmonic scalpel's reduced thermal spread enhances precision and safety, leading to better surgical outcomes and faster patient recovery.

Question 11: Correct Answer: B) Notify the surgeon immediately.
Rationale: The presence of a firm, swollen, and painful area near the incision site suggests a possible hematoma. The correct action is to notify the surgeon immediately to assess and manage the hematoma. Applying a warm compress (A) or encouraging ambulation (C) could exacerbate the condition, and administering pain medication (D) addresses symptoms but not the underlying issue.

Question 12: Correct Answer: B) Send a message through the hospital's secure messaging system.
Rationale: Sending a message through the hospital's secure messaging system ensures that the communication is immediate and secure, allowing the pathology department to act promptly. Leaving a voicemail (Option A) or sending a note via interdepartmental mail (Option C) may delay the response time. Waiting for a callback (Option D) is not proactive and could lead to critical delays in specimen analysis. Secure messaging ensures timely and effective interdepartmental communication.

Question 13: Correct Answer: C) Parathyroid gland
Rationale: The parathyroid glands, located behind the thyroid gland, secrete parathyroid hormone (PTH), which regulates calcium levels in the blood. The thyroid gland (A) produces thyroxine and calcitonin, the adrenal gland (B) secretes cortisol and adrenaline, and the pituitary gland (D) releases various hormones, but not PTH. The parathyroid gland's specific function in calcium regulation makes it the correct answer.

Question 14: Correct Answer: B) Properly maintaining and handling surgical instruments
Rationale: Proper maintenance and handling of surgical instruments extend their lifespan and reduce the need for frequent replacements, thus containing costs. Always using new instruments (A) increases expenses. Frequently changing gloves (C) without necessity leads to wastage. Disposing of all unused supplies (D) is wasteful and counterproductive to cost containment efforts.

Question 15: Correct Answer: B) To provide structural support and promote bone healing
Rationale: The primary purpose of using an allograft in bone grafting procedures is to provide structural support and promote bone healing. Unlike autografts, allografts do not require harvesting from the patient, thus reducing surgical time and morbidity. Options A, C, and D are incorrect because while allografts can reduce the need for additional surgeries and have a lower infection risk than some alternatives, their main function is to support and heal bone. Immediate weight-bearing is not typically ensured by allografts.

Question 16: Correct Answer: B) Use enzymatic cleaner followed by ultrasonic cleaning.
Rationale: Using an enzymatic cleaner followed by ultrasonic cleaning is the most effective method for decontaminating instruments. Enzymatic cleaners break down organic material, and ultrasonic cleaning removes residual debris. Option A is incorrect as alcohol swabs are insufficient for thorough cleaning. Option C is incorrect because saline can cause corrosion. Option D is incorrect as hot water alone does not effectively remove all contaminants, and air drying without prior cleaning is inadequate.

Question 17: Correct Answer: C) Pulse oximeter
Rationale: The pulse oximeter is essential for continuous assessment of oxygen saturation levels, which is crucial for patients undergoing cardiac surgery. While the blood pressure cuff (A) and ECG leads (B) are important for monitoring hemodynamic status and cardiac activity, they do not provide continuous oxygen saturation data. The temperature probe (D) monitors body temperature but does not provide information on oxygenation. Therefore, the pulse oximeter (C) is the correct choice.

Question 18: Correct Answer: C) Ensure all counts are correct and accounted for.
Rationale: The first step in removing drapes and other equipment is to ensure all counts (sponges, instruments, needles) are correct and accounted for to prevent any retained surgical items. This step is crucial for patient safety. Removing instruments (A) and drapes (B) should be done after ensuring counts are correct. Disconnecting monitoring equipment (D) is also secondary to verifying counts.

Question 19: Correct Answer: D) To avoid confusion with other medications
Rationale: Labeling the mixed solution immediately is primarily to avoid confusion with other medications, ensuring that the correct medication is administered. While compliance with hospital policy (A), preventing contamination (B), and ensuring accurate administration (C) are important, the immediate labeling specifically addresses the risk of mix-ups, which is critical in the fast-paced surgical environment.

Question 20: Correct Answer: B) Confirming he has no allergies to medications
Rationale: Confirming Jacob has no allergies to medications is crucial to prevent adverse reactions during surgery. Ensuring he understands the risks (A) is important but should be age-appropriate. Discussing the procedure with his parents only (C) excludes him from understanding what will happen. Allowing him to choose his post-operative meal (D) is comforting but secondary to his safety.

Question 21: Correct Answer: C) Verify the staple size and load the stapler.
Rationale: The first step is to verify the staple size and load the stapler to ensure it is appropriate for the tissue being resected. Handing the stapler directly to the surgeon without verification (B) can lead to complications. Loading the stapler without verification (A) may result in incorrect staple size. Test firing (D) is important but should be done after loading and verification.

Question 22: Correct Answer: A) Epidermis
Rationale: The epidermis is the outermost layer of the skin and serves as the primary barrier against pathogens and environmental damage. The dermis, hypodermis, and subcutaneous tissue play supportive roles but do not provide the primary barrier function. The dermis contains connective tissue, blood vessels, and nerves, while the hypodermis and subcutaneous tissue primarily store fat and provide insulation.

Question 23: Correct Answer: C) High precision and control
Rationale: CO2 beam coagulators offer high precision and control, making them ideal for delicate surgeries. Option A is incorrect as CO2 lasers have low penetration depth, which is beneficial for surface procedures. Option B is incorrect because CO2 lasers

are highly absorbed by water, aiding in precise cutting and coagulation. Option D is incorrect as CO2 lasers have low scatter, enhancing their precision.

Question 24: Correct Answer: B) Ovarian artery

Rationale: The ovarian artery is the primary blood supply to the ovaries. The uterine artery supplies blood to the uterus, not the ovaries. The internal iliac artery supplies the pelvic organs, and the superior mesenteric artery supplies the intestines. Understanding the correct anatomical structures ensures proper assistance during surgery.

Question 25: Correct Answer: C) SPSS

Rationale: SPSS (Statistical Package for the Social Sciences) is the most commonly used software for statistical analysis in research. Microsoft Word is primarily for word processing, Adobe Photoshop for image editing, and AutoCAD for design and drafting. SPSS provides tools for data management and statistical analysis, making it essential for research in a surgical setting where data interpretation is crucial.

Question 26: Correct Answer: B) Drop the instruments gently from a height of 6 inches.

Rationale: Dropping instruments gently from a height of 6 inches minimizes the risk of contaminating the sterile field. Dropping from 12 inches (Option A) increases the risk of contamination due to a greater distance. Placing instruments directly with hands (Option C) and sliding them (Option D) both compromise sterility by increasing the chance of contact with non-sterile surfaces.

Question 27: Correct Answer: B) The patient cart

Rationale: The patient cart, which includes the robotic arms that interact directly with the patient, must be draped to maintain sterility. The surgeon console (A) and vision cart (C) do not come into direct contact with the sterile field, and the operating room lights (D) are not part of the Da Vinci system. Draping the patient cart is essential to prevent infection and ensure a sterile surgical environment.

Question 28: Correct Answer: B) Provide emotional support and refer the patient to a palliative care specialist.

Rationale: The correct approach is to provide emotional support and refer the patient to a palliative care specialist. This ensures that the patient receives comprehensive care focused on comfort and quality of life. Option A is incorrect as it is the surgeon's role to discuss prognosis and treatment options. Option C is inappropriate as avoiding the topic can lead to mistrust. Option D, while sometimes beneficial, is not the immediate priority in providing end-of-life care.

Question 29: Correct Answer: B) Respond to the surgeon with a calm and respectful tone, acknowledging his concerns.

Rationale: Responding calmly and respectfully helps de-escalate tension, maintains professionalism, and ensures the procedure continues smoothly. Ignoring the behavior (Option A) can worsen the situation, leaving the room (Option C) is unprofessional, and asking another team member to intervene (Option D) may not address the issue directly and timely.

Question 30: Correct Answer: C) Create an open and inclusive environment by asking for everyone's input, including Alex's.

Rationale: Creating an open and inclusive environment by asking for everyone's input, including Alex's, encourages participation and makes Alex feel valued. Directly asking why they are not participating (Option A) can be confrontational. Criticizing Alex (Option B) can demoralize them. Ignoring the behavior (Option D) does not address the issue and can lead to continued disengagement.

Question 31: Correct Answer: C) To protect the wound from infection and absorb exudate

Rationale: The primary purpose of applying a sterile dressing is to protect the wound from infection and absorb any exudate. While keeping the wound dry (A) and preventing exposure to air (B) are important, they are secondary to infection control and exudate management. Promoting scab formation (D) is not a primary goal in the immediate postoperative period.

Question 32: Correct Answer: B) Check for any visible tears or holes

Rationale: The first step in checking the integrity of a sterile package is to inspect it for any visible tears or holes. This ensures that the sterile barrier has not been compromised. While verifying the expiration date, sterilization indicator, and package contents are also important, they come after confirming the physical integrity of the package. Tears or holes can immediately compromise sterility, making this the priority check.

Question 33: Correct Answer: B) Encouraging ambulation and deep breathing exercises

Rationale: Encouraging ambulation and deep breathing exercises helps to alleviate shoulder pain caused by residual carbon dioxide gas used during laparoscopic procedures. Administering a muscle relaxant (A) or increasing pain medication (D) may not address the root cause, and applying a heating pad (C) is less effective for gas-related pain. Ambulation and deep breathing promote gas absorption and relieve discomfort.

Question 34: Correct Answer: D) Report the unused instruments to the supervisor and follow the facility's policy for handling unused sterile items.

Rationale: The correct action is to report the unused instruments to the supervisor and follow the facility's policy. This ensures proper documentation and adherence to cost containment policies. Discarding (A) wastes resources, re-sterilizing (B) may not be allowed by policy, and returning to the sterile supply area (C) without proper documentation can lead to inventory discrepancies.

Question 35: Correct Answer: A) Compress the Hemovac reservoir before connecting it to the tubing.

Rationale: Compressing the Hemovac reservoir before connecting it to the tubing creates a vacuum necessary for effective suction. Option B is incorrect because compressing after connection does not create a vacuum. Option C is incorrect as filling with saline is unnecessary and could cause contamination. Option D is incorrect as a fully expanded reservoir would not create the required suction.

Question 36: Correct Answer: B) McBurney's incision
Rationale: McBurney's incision is specifically used for an appendectomy as it provides direct access to the appendix. The midline incision (A) is generally used for exploratory laparotomy, the Pfannenstiel incision (C) is used for gynecological surgeries, and the subcostal incision (D) is used for gallbladder surgeries. McBurney's incision minimizes muscle damage and provides optimal exposure for appendectomy, making it the most appropriate choice.

Question 37: Correct Answer: C) Persistent high fever
Rationale: Persistent high fever postoperatively can indicate a serious infection or other complications such as sepsis. Slight redness (A) and mild swelling (B) are common and often expected postoperative findings. A small amount of serous drainage (D) is also typically normal. However, a high fever requires immediate attention to prevent further complications.

Question 38: Correct Answer: C) Check the integrity of the power cord and connections.
Rationale: The first step in ensuring the power equipment is functioning correctly is to check the integrity of the power cord and connections. This prevents electrical hazards and ensures safe operation. Connecting the power equipment to the power source (Option A) should follow this step. Verifying the equipment settings (Option B) and testing the equipment on a sterile surface (Option D) are also important but come after ensuring the equipment is safe to use.

Question 39: Correct Answer: C) Place the drape in a designated biohazard waste container.
Rationale: Placing the blood-soaked drape in a designated biohazard waste container ensures proper containment and disposal of potentially infectious materials, adhering to Standard Precautions. Option A is incorrect as regular laundry hampers do not provide appropriate containment. Option B is impractical and not typically done in a surgical setting. Option D is incorrect because washing the drape before disposal can spread contaminants and is not compliant with Standard Precautions.

Question 40: Correct Answer: B) The phaco tip is clogged.
Rationale: The most likely cause of ineffective emulsification during phacoemulsification is a clogged phaco tip. This prevents the ultrasound energy from effectively breaking up the lens material. Warm irrigation fluid (A) and high aspiration flow rate (C) are less likely to cause this issue. Low power settings (D) could contribute but are not as common as a clogged tip.

Question 41: Correct Answer: C) Before the surgical procedure begins.
Rationale: The first instrument count should be performed before the surgical procedure begins to ensure all instruments are accounted for and to prevent any retained surgical items. Option A is incorrect as the count is not performed before the patient enters the OR. Option B is incorrect because the count should be done before any incision is made.

Option D is incorrect as the final count is done after the procedure, not the first count.

Question 42: Correct Answer: A) Make a note of the change and update the preference card after confirming with Dr. Johnson.
Rationale: The best practice is to make a note and confirm the change with Dr. Johnson before updating the preference card. This ensures accuracy and that the change is a permanent preference. Ignoring the change (Option B) or waiting for the nurse (Option D) could result in outdated information. Updating without confirmation (Option C) risks incorporating incorrect information.

Question 43: Correct Answer: B) To ensure compliance with laser safety protocols
Rationale: The primary role of a Laser Safety Officer (LSO) is to ensure compliance with laser safety protocols, which includes training staff, maintaining equipment, and enforcing safety measures. Operating the laser equipment (A) is the responsibility of the surgical team. Assisting the surgeon (C) and monitoring vital signs (D) are not the LSO's primary duties, making B the most accurate answer.

Question 44: Correct Answer: B) Report the discrepancy to the circulating nurse immediately.
Rationale: The correct action is to report the discrepancy to the circulating nurse immediately. Ignoring the discrepancy (Option A) or adjusting the recorded amount without informing anyone (Option C) can lead to serious medical errors. Waiting until the end of the shift (Option D) delays the correction and may compromise patient safety. Immediate reporting ensures accurate documentation and patient safety.

Question 45: Correct Answer: C) Great saphenous vein
Rationale: The great saphenous vein is the most commonly used vein for coronary artery bypass grafting due to its length and accessibility. The femoral vein is a deep vein and not typically used for grafting. The basilic and cephalic veins are located in the arm and are not as commonly used for CABG. Therefore, the great saphenous vein is the correct answer due to its suitability for the procedure.

Question 46: Correct Answer: C) 5 minutes
Rationale: The recommended duration for an initial surgical scrub is 5 minutes to ensure thorough removal of microorganisms. Option A is too short to be effective. Option B is insufficient for an initial scrub, though it may be acceptable for subsequent scrubs. Option D is unnecessarily long and can cause skin irritation. The 5-minute duration balances efficacy and skin health.

Question 47: Correct Answer: C) Replace the malfunctioning power drill with a reserved backup.
Rationale: The immediate next step is to replace the malfunctioning power drill with a reserved backup, ensuring the surgery can proceed as planned. Notifying the surgeon and waiting for instructions (A) could cause unnecessary delays. Using a manual drill (B) may not be feasible for a total knee arthroplasty. Canceling the surgery (D) is an extreme measure and should be avoided if a backup is available. Ensuring

all equipment is operational is vital for surgical efficiency and patient care.

Question 48: Correct Answer: C) Slide the patient using a friction-reducing device.

Rationale: Using a friction-reducing device (C) minimizes the risk of musculoskeletal injuries among the surgical team by reducing the physical effort required. While a draw sheet (A) and proper body mechanics (B) are helpful, they do not reduce friction as effectively. Asking the patient to scoot (D) may not be feasible or safe, especially if the patient is sedated or immobile.

Question 49: Correct Answer: B) Maintain composure and respond calmly to the surgeon's requests.

Rationale: Maintaining composure and responding calmly helps de-escalate tension, ensuring a focused and efficient operating environment. Responding with equal intensity (A) can escalate conflict, ignoring the behavior (C) may lead to miscommunication, and leaving the operating room (D) disrupts the procedure and compromises patient care.

Question 50: Correct Answer: C) Perform an intraoperative cholangiogram to clarify the anatomy.

Rationale: Performing an intraoperative cholangiogram is crucial to clarify the anatomy and ensure that the correct structures are identified before proceeding. This step helps avoid potential complications. Converting to an open cholecystectomy (Option B) may be necessary later, but it is not the initial step. Removing both structures (Option A) without confirmation can be dangerous. Stopping the procedure (Option D) is unnecessary if the anatomy can be clarified intraoperatively.

Question 51: Correct Answer: A) Electromagnetic field generator

Rationale: A key component of a computer navigation system is the electromagnetic field generator, which helps in tracking the position of surgical instruments in real-time. Option B, the ultrasound transducer, is used for imaging but not specifically for navigation. Option C, the fiber optic camera, is used for visualization, not navigation. Option D, the laser scalpel, is a cutting tool and not related to the navigation system.

Question 52: Correct Answer: C) Replenish the cart with supplies from the central sterile supply area

Rationale: Replenishing the cart with supplies from the central sterile supply area ensures that all items are sterile and properly accounted for. Notifying the central supply department and waiting can cause delays, using items from another room can lead to shortages elsewhere, and leaving a note for the next shift is not immediate. Proper restocking ensures readiness for the next procedure and maintains a high standard of care.

Question 53: Correct Answer: A) Ovaries and fallopian tubes

Rationale: In medical terminology, "adnexa" refers to the appendages of an organ, in this case, the ovaries and fallopian tubes associated with the uterus. Option B (Uterine lining) is incorrect as it refers to the endometrium. Option C (Cervix) and D (Vaginal canal) are parts of the female reproductive system but are not included in the term "adnexa." This distinction is crucial for accurate surgical preparation and communication.

Question 54: Correct Answer: A) Dry hands with a sterile towel

Rationale: After completing the surgical hand scrub, it is essential to dry hands with a sterile towel to prevent recontamination and maintain sterility. Applying hand lotion (B) can introduce contaminants, putting on sterile gloves directly (C) without drying can compromise glove integrity, and rinsing hands with water (D) after scrubbing can reintroduce microorganisms, making them incorrect choices.

Question 55: Correct Answer: B) Use a gel pad under the patient's elbow.

Rationale: Using a gel pad under the patient's elbow is the most appropriate action to prevent nerve damage, particularly ulnar nerve compression. A rolled towel under the wrist (Option A) and a foam pad under the shoulder (Option D) do not provide adequate protection for the elbow. Securing the arm with a strap without additional padding (Option C) could increase the risk of nerve compression.

Question 56: Correct Answer: B) Across the patient's thighs

Rationale: Placing the safety strap across the patient's thighs ensures maximum effectiveness by securing the patient firmly to the operating table without interfering with the surgical site. Placing it across the chest (Option A) or abdomen (Option C) could restrict breathing, and across the ankles (Option D) would not provide adequate stabilization.

Question 57: Correct Answer: B) To provide a scaffold for bone growth

Rationale: Allografts are primarily used to provide a scaffold for bone growth, which facilitates the integration and healing of the graft with the host bone. While reducing infection risk (A) and eliminating the need for autograft harvesting (C) are secondary benefits, they are not the primary purpose. Accelerating the healing process (D) is also a benefit but not the main reason for using an allograft.

Question 58: Correct Answer: B) To enhance communication and teamwork among a diverse surgical team.

Rationale: Understanding cultural diversity is crucial for enhancing communication and teamwork among a diverse surgical team. This knowledge helps in recognizing and respecting different cultural perspectives, which can lead to better collaboration and patient care. Option A is incorrect as uniformity in procedures is not related to cultural diversity. Option C is incorrect because interpreters may still be needed. Option D is incorrect as cultural diversity understanding does not directly reduce preoperative preparation time.

Question 59: Correct Answer: B) Shave the area and reapply the bovie pad

Rationale: Shaving the area ensures better adhesion of the bovie pad, reducing the risk of burns and ensuring effective electrical contact. Applying more adhesive (A) is not recommended as it may not improve contact. Placing the pad on a different area without shaving (C) may still result in poor adhesion. Using a different type of electrosurgical unit (D) does not address the issue of poor pad adhesion.

Question 60: Correct Answer: C) Managing surgical instrument inventory

Rationale: Managing surgical instrument inventory is the most appropriate use of computer technology in this context. Computer systems can efficiently track and manage the availability, usage, and sterilization of surgical instruments. While tracking schedules (A), monitoring vital signs (B), and documenting consent forms (D) are important, they do not directly relate to inventory management. This ensures that all necessary instruments are available and properly maintained, reducing the risk of delays or complications during surgery.

Question 61: Correct Answer: C) Inform the surgeon and replace the compromised drape.

Rationale: The correct action is to inform the surgeon and replace the compromised drape to maintain sterility. Ignoring the tear (Option A) or moving it (Option D) risks contamination. Covering the tear (Option B) does not ensure complete sterility. Replacing the drape ensures the sterile field is maintained, preventing potential infections.

Question 62: Correct Answer: B) Fallopian Tube

Rationale: The fallopian tube is the correct structure that transports ova from the ovaries to the uterus. The ureter (A) transports urine from the kidneys to the bladder, the round ligament (C) supports the uterus, and the urethra (D) is the tube that carries urine out of the body. Identifying the correct anatomical structure is crucial for the success of reproductive surgeries.

Question 63: Correct Answer: A) DeBakey clamp

Rationale: The DeBakey clamp is specifically designed for vascular surgery and is ideal for clamping large blood vessels like the femoral artery. The Satinsky clamp is used for partial occlusion of vessels, the Bulldog clamp is for smaller vessels, and the Fogarty clamp is used for embolectomies. Therefore, the DeBakey clamp is the most appropriate choice for controlling bleeding from the femoral artery during a femoral-popliteal bypass surgery.

Question 64: Correct Answer: C) Instrument counting tray

Rationale: The instrument counting tray is essential for ensuring that all surgical instruments are accounted for and no foreign objects are left in the patient. Sponge forceps are used for handling sponges, needle holders are used for suturing, and retractors are used to hold back tissue. The instrument counting tray allows for an organized and accurate count of all instruments, ensuring patient safety and compliance with surgical protocols.

Question 65: Correct Answer: B) It helps in accurately understanding and interpreting the speaker's message

Rationale: Active listening skills help in accurately understanding and interpreting the speaker's message, fostering effective communication and collaboration. Preparing a response while others are speaking (Option A) can lead to misunderstandings. Reducing meeting time (Option C) is not the primary benefit of active listening. Prioritizing the loudest team member's opinions (Option D) undermines equitable participation and can lead to biased decision-making.

Question 66: Correct Answer: B) Cholecystitis

Rationale: Cholecystitis is characterized by inflammation of the gallbladder, often presenting with severe abdominal pain, nausea, vomiting, and a positive Murphy's sign. Appendicitis typically presents with pain in the lower right quadrant, pancreatitis with epigastric pain radiating to the back, and diverticulitis with lower left quadrant pain. The positive Murphy's sign is a key indicator differentiating cholecystitis from the other conditions.

Question 67: Correct Answer: C) Turn off the oxygen supply.

Rationale: Turning off the oxygen supply is crucial to prevent the fire from intensifying. Evacuating the patient (A) and using a fire extinguisher (B) are important but secondary steps. Calling for help (D) is also necessary but should follow the immediate action of cutting off the oxygen supply to reduce the fire hazard.

Question 68: Correct Answer: C) To remove airborne contaminants

Rationale: The primary reason for using a smoke evacuator during laser surgery is to remove airborne contaminants, such as surgical smoke, which can contain harmful chemicals and pathogens. While reducing the risk of fire, maintaining a sterile field, and enhancing visibility are important, the main purpose of the smoke evacuator is to ensure the air quality and safety of the surgical team.

Question 69: Correct Answer: A) Inform the surgeon and switch to a backup smoke evacuation system.

Rationale: Informing the surgeon and switching to a backup smoke evacuation system ensures continuous removal of hazardous smoke, maintaining a safe environment. Using a handheld suction device (Option B) is less effective and may not adequately remove smoke. Adjusting the HVAC system (Option C) does not provide immediate relief. Ignoring the issue (Option D) poses health risks to the surgical team and patient.

Question 70: Correct Answer: C) Tibialis Anterior

Rationale: The tibialis anterior muscle is primarily responsible for dorsiflexion of the foot at the ankle joint. The gastrocnemius and soleus muscles are involved in plantarflexion, not dorsiflexion. The peroneus longus assists in plantarflexion and eversion of the foot. Thus, the tibialis anterior is the correct choice as it specifically performs dorsiflexion.

Question 71: Correct Answer: C) Patellar tendon from the patient

Rationale: An autograft involves using tissue from the patient's own body, making the patellar tendon from Mr. Johnson the most appropriate source. Allografts (A) and xenografts (D) involve donor tissue from other sources, and synthetic ligaments (B) are not autografts. Autografts reduce the risk of immune rejection and disease transmission, making them preferable in many surgical scenarios.

Question 72: Correct Answer: B) Report the defect and remove the instrument from the set.

Rationale: The correct action is to report the defect and remove the instrument from the set. Using a cracked instrument (Option A) can lead to breakage and patient harm. Re-sterilizing (Option C) does not address the structural defect. Using the instrument while informing the surgeon (Option D) still poses a risk. Removing the defective instrument ensures patient safety and maintains the integrity of the surgical procedure.

Question 73: Correct Answer: B) Preventing pressure on the peroneal nerve

Rationale: Preventing pressure on the peroneal nerve is crucial to avoid nerve damage, which can result in foot drop. While tucking the arms (A) and elevating the head (C) are important, they are not specific to the lithotomy position. Fully extending the legs (D) is incorrect as the legs should be flexed and supported in stirrups.

Question 74: Correct Answer: B) The patient's heels.

Rationale: Padding the patient's heels is critical to prevent pressure injuries, as they are particularly susceptible to pressure ulcers during prolonged surgeries like total knee arthroplasty. The lower back (Option A), upper arms (Option C), and neck (Option D) are less prone to pressure injuries in this context. Proper padding of the heels helps distribute pressure and prevent skin breakdown.

Question 75: Correct Answer: D) Immobilize the leg and cover the wound with a sterile dressing

Rationale: The initial management of an open fracture includes immobilizing the limb and covering the wound with a sterile dressing to prevent infection and further injury. Administering antibiotics (B) and surgical debridement (C) are important but follow initial stabilization. Applying a tourniquet (A) is not recommended unless there is life-threatening bleeding.

Question 76: Correct Answer: D) Ask another team member to take over while you scrub out and re-gown.

Rationale: The correct action is to ask another team member to take over while you scrub out and re-gown to maintain aseptic technique. Continuing with the procedure (Option A) or wiping the area with a sterile cloth (Option C) does not ensure sterility. Informing the circulating nurse (Option B) addresses the contamination but does not resolve the technologist's compromised sterility. Scrubbing out and re-gowning ensures the sterile field is maintained.

Question 77: Correct Answer: D) Check for a backup power drill

Rationale: The immediate course of action should be to check for a backup power drill to avoid any delay in the surgery. Informing the circulating nurse is important but secondary to ensuring the availability of a functioning drill. Proceeding with manual instruments or attempting to repair the drill could compromise the surgery's efficiency and safety.

Question 78: Correct Answer: B) Inform the surgeon and assist in replacing the tubing.

Rationale: Informing the surgeon and assisting in replacing the tubing is the correct action to ensure adequate pneumoperitoneum and patient safety. Simply straightening the tubing (A) may not fully resolve the issue. Increasing the insufflation pressure (C) could cause over-insufflation and harm. Ignoring the kink (D) could lead to complications such as inadequate visualization or injury. Communication and proper equipment handling are crucial for preventing harm.

Question 79: Correct Answer: B) Ensure the C-arm is draped with a sterile cover after the surgical site is prepped and draped.

Rationale: Draping the C-arm after the surgical site is prepped and draped ensures that the sterile field is maintained throughout the procedure. Option A is incorrect because draping before the patient is brought in can compromise sterility. Option C is incorrect as positioning the C-arm first can lead to contamination. Option D is incorrect because disinfectant spray alone does not ensure sterility.

Question 80: Correct Answer: C) Shut off the oxygen supply

Rationale: The most effective first step is to shut off the oxygen supply because oxygen can fuel the fire, making it spread more rapidly. Using a fire extinguisher (A) is important but secondary to removing the oxygen source. Evacuating the patient and staff (B) is crucial but should follow the initial step of shutting off the oxygen. Calling for help (D) is also necessary but not the immediate first action.

Question 81: Correct Answer: C) The surgeon

Rationale: The surgeon is primarily responsible for obtaining informed consent from the patient, as they are the one performing the procedure and must ensure the patient understands the risks, benefits, and alternatives. While the anesthesiologist, nurse, and surgical technologist play crucial roles in patient care, they do not have the primary responsibility for obtaining informed consent.

Question 82: Correct Answer: B) Wash hands and forearms up to the elbows for at least 2 minutes.

Rationale: The correct procedure for a medical hand wash includes washing hands and forearms up to the elbows for at least 2 minutes to ensure thorough removal of microorganisms. Option A is incorrect as scrubbing under the nails should be done but not limited to 15 seconds. Option C is incorrect as reusable cloth towels can harbor bacteria. Option D is incorrect because applying lotion immediately after washing can compromise the aseptic technique.

Question 83: Correct Answer: B) Refuse to falsify the record and report the request to the hospital's compliance officer.

Rationale: Sarah should refuse to falsify the record and report the request to the hospital's compliance officer to uphold ethical and legal standards. Complying with the request (Option A) or altering the record (Option C) is unethical and illegal. Discussing the situation with the patient (Option D) is inappropriate as it does not address the ethical breach. Reporting ensures accountability and maintains the integrity of patient care documentation.

Question 84: Correct Answer: B) Ensuring the grounding pad is properly placed on a well-vascularized muscle mass.

Rationale: Proper placement of the grounding pad on a well-vascularized muscle mass is crucial to prevent patient burns. Placing it on a bony prominence can increase the risk of burns. While using the lowest power setting and checking the unit's temperature are important, they do not directly address the grounding pad's placement, which is essential for patient safety.

Question 85: Correct Answer: C) Battery-powered saws eliminate the need for air hoses

Rationale: The primary reason for using a battery-powered surgical saw is that it eliminates the need for air hoses, reducing clutter and potential hazards in the operating room. While battery-powered saws might be quieter (B) and more convenient, they are not necessarily more powerful (A) or less expensive (D) than pneumatic saws.

Question 86: Correct Answer: D) 5 minutes

Rationale: The recommended duration for performing a medical hand wash before a surgical procedure is 5 minutes. This ensures thorough removal of transient microorganisms and reduces the risk of infection. Options A and B are too short to effectively eliminate pathogens, while Option C, although closer, does not meet the standard duration required for surgical asepsis.

Question 87: Correct Answer: C) Quadriceps femoris

Rationale: The quadriceps tendon is part of the quadriceps femoris muscle group, which is responsible for knee extension. The hamstrings are involved in knee flexion, the adductors in thigh adduction, and the gastrocnemius in plantar flexion of the foot. Understanding the correct muscle group is crucial for surgical access and effective procedure outcomes.

Question 88: Correct Answer: C) Use of an anaerobic chamber

Rationale: Anaerobic bacteria require an oxygen-free environment to grow, which is provided by an anaerobic chamber (C). Exposure to room air (A) would kill anaerobic bacteria, making it incorrect. A CO_2 incubator (B) is used for microaerophilic bacteria, not anaerobes. Immediate freezing (D) is not suitable for anaerobic cultures as it does not provide the necessary conditions for their growth. Therefore, using an anaerobic chamber is essential for accurate growth.

Question 89: Correct Answer: C) To maintain traceability and ensure compatibility

Rationale: Maintaining traceability and ensuring compatibility are crucial in tissue procurement to prevent any mix-ups and ensure the recipient receives compatible tissue. While preventing legal issues (B) and expediting the process (D) are important, they are secondary to the primary goal of traceability and compatibility. Ensuring the tissue is used within the same hospital (A) is not a primary concern, as tissues can be transported to different locations. Proper labeling and documentation help in tracking the tissue from donor to recipient, ensuring safety and efficacy.

Question 90: Correct Answer: B) Ventricular systole

Rationale: Ventricular systole is the phase of the cardiac cycle during which the ventricles contract and eject blood into the aorta and pulmonary arteries. Atrial systole refers to the contraction of the atria, pushing blood into the ventricles. Atrial diastole is the relaxation of the atria, while ventricular diastole is the relaxation of the ventricles, allowing them to fill with blood. Ventricular systole is the only phase where the ventricles are actively ejecting blood into the arteries.

Question 91: Correct Answer: A) Cutting and coagulating tissue

Rationale: The Bovie electrosurgical pencil is designed to cut and coagulate tissue using electrical current. This is in contrast to holding sutures (B), which is typically done with needle holders, retracting tissue (C), which is the function of retractors, and suctioning fluids (D), which is done with suction tips. Therefore, the primary function of the Bovie electrosurgical pencil is cutting and coagulating tissue.

Question 92: Correct Answer: B) Immediately change gloves and continue assisting.

Rationale: The correct action is to immediately change gloves and continue assisting. This minimizes the risk of cross-contamination and maintains a sterile field. Option A is incorrect because it disregards the need for changing contaminated gloves. Option C is partially correct but does not prioritize immediate glove change. Option D is unnecessary and delays patient care.

Question 93: Correct Answer: A) Apply a new sterile dressing and notify the surgeon.

Rationale: The most appropriate initial action is to apply a new sterile dressing and notify the surgeon. This ensures the wound is protected from infection and the surgeon is aware of potential complications. Increasing IV fluids (B) and administering pain medication (C) do not address the drainage issue. Encouraging ambulation (D) is not appropriate until the drainage is assessed and controlled.

Question 94: Correct Answer: A) Epinephrine

Rationale: Epinephrine is commonly used to achieve hemostasis through vasoconstriction, reducing blood flow to the surgical site. It is often combined with local anesthetics to prolong their effect and minimize bleeding. Protamine Sulfate neutralizes heparin, Fibrin Sealant is used for tissue adhesion, and Vitamin K is essential for clotting factor synthesis but not for immediate hemostasis. Therefore, Epinephrine is the correct choice for vasoconstriction-induced hemostasis.

Question 95: Correct Answer: D) Compress the bulb after insertion to create suction

Rationale: Compressing the bulb after insertion to create suction is critical for the proper function of a Jackson-Pratt drain. Attaching the bulb to the tubing before insertion (A) and ensuring the tubing is clamped before insertion (B) are preparatory steps but do not ensure functionality. Priming the tubing with saline (C) is unnecessary and incorrect. The suction created by compressing the bulb facilitates effective drainage of fluids from the surgical site.

Question 96: Correct Answer: A) Anterior to the scalene muscle

Rationale: The phrenic nerve runs anterior to the scalene muscle, making it a reliable landmark during surgery. Options B, C, and D are incorrect as they do not accurately describe the phrenic nerve's anatomical pathway. The sternocleidomastoid muscle is posterior to the nerve, the trachea is medial, and the carotid artery is lateral but not a direct landmark for the phrenic nerve.

Question 97: Correct Answer: B) To improve access to the upper abdomen

Rationale: The reverse Trendelenburg position is used in laparoscopic cholecystectomy to improve access to the upper abdomen by using gravity to shift the abdominal contents downward. This position helps in better visualization and access to the gallbladder. Options A and C are not relevant to the surgical access, while D is incorrect as it pertains to pelvic organs, not the upper abdomen.

Question 98: Correct Answer: B) Confirming the allograft is free from infectious agents

Rationale: The primary consideration when preparing an allograft for implantation is to confirm it is free from infectious agents to prevent postoperative infections. While matching the size (Option C) and cryopreservation (Option D) are important, they are secondary to ensuring the allograft is safe from infections. Sourcing from a living donor (Option A) is less common and not a primary consideration.

Question 99: Correct Answer: B) Small intestine

Rationale: The small intestine is primarily responsible for nutrient absorption due to its extensive surface area provided by villi and microvilli. The stomach mainly aids in digestion through acid and enzymes, the large intestine absorbs water and electrolytes, and the esophagus is a conduit for food passage. Therefore, the small intestine is the correct answer.

Question 100: Correct Answer: B) Thyroxine

Rationale: Thyroxine, produced by the thyroid gland, is primarily responsible for regulating metabolism and energy production in the body. Insulin (A) regulates blood glucose levels, cortisol (C) is involved in stress response and metabolism, and glucagon (D) raises blood glucose levels. Thyroxine's role in controlling the rate of metabolic processes makes it the correct answer.

Question 101: Correct Answer: B) Electrocautery

Rationale: Electrocautery is the most commonly used thermal method for achieving hemostasis during laparoscopic surgery due to its effectiveness in coagulating blood vessels. Cryotherapy is less commonly used for hemostasis, ultrasonic scalpels are primarily used for cutting and coagulating simultaneously, and laser coagulation, while effective, is less frequently used in laparoscopic procedures. Electrocautery provides a reliable and controlled

means of achieving hemostasis, making it the preferred choice.

Question 102: Correct Answer: B) The cessation of bleeding

Rationale: Hemostasis is the process of stopping bleeding, which is crucial during surgical procedures to prevent excessive blood loss. This involves the coagulation cascade and other mechanisms. Option A refers to hematopoiesis, C refers to vasculitis, and D refers to hemolysis. These terms are related to blood but do not accurately describe the process of stopping bleeding.

Question 103: Correct Answer: B) Allis forceps

Rationale: Allis forceps are designed specifically for grasping and holding tissues, making them ideal for this purpose. Metzenbaum and Mayo scissors are primarily used for cutting tissues, while Babcock forceps are used for grasping delicate structures without causing damage. The Allis forceps have teeth that provide a firm grip, making them the best choice for securely holding tissues during surgery.

Question 104: Correct Answer: A) Load instruments loosely, use a high temperature, and ensure adequate drying time

Rationale: For effective sterilization using a short cycle, instruments should be loaded loosely to ensure steam penetration, a high temperature should be used to kill microorganisms quickly, and adequate drying time is essential to prevent contamination. Packing instruments tightly or skipping drying time can lead to ineffective sterilization and increased risk of infection.

Question 105: Correct Answer: B) Keeping the drainage system below chest level

Rationale: Keeping the drainage system below chest level ensures proper drainage and prevents backflow, which could lead to complications. Clamping the chest tube can cause tension pneumothorax, removing the chest tube is inappropriate, and placing the patient in a prone position can compromise breathing and tube function.

Question 106: Correct Answer: B) Hypocalcemia

Rationale: The parathyroid glands regulate calcium levels in the blood. Damage to these glands can lead to hypocalcemia, characterized by low calcium levels, which can cause muscle cramps and cardiac issues. Hypercalcemia (A) is an excess of calcium, hyperthyroidism (C) is an overactive thyroid, and hypothyroidism (D) is an underactive thyroid, none of which are immediate concerns post-parathyroid gland damage.

Question 107: Correct Answer: B) It helps in tailoring patient care to meet the specific cultural needs of each patient.

Rationale: Cultural competence in patient care involves tailoring care to meet the specific cultural needs of each patient, ensuring more personalized and effective treatment. Option A is incorrect as identical treatment does not account for individual cultural needs. Option C is incorrect because cultural sensitivity training is still necessary. Option D is incorrect as cultural competence encompasses more than just language barriers, including beliefs, values, and practices.

Question 108: Correct Answer: B) Disposing of all sharps and biohazard materials

Rationale: Disposing of all sharps and biohazard materials is the most critical step to ensure proper room turnover because it directly addresses the immediate safety hazards. While wiping down surfaces, restocking supplies, and mopping the floor are important, they do not mitigate the risk of injury or infection as effectively as disposing of sharps and biohazard materials. Ensuring these items are properly handled prevents potential harm to staff and patients.

Question 109: Correct Answer: B) Place the four towels first, followed by the fenestrated drape.

Rationale: The correct sequence for draping involves placing the four towels first to outline the surgical site, followed by the fenestrated drape to cover the area and create a sterile field. Option A is incorrect because the fenestrated drape should not be placed first. Option C and D are incorrect as they do not follow the standard draping procedure for abdominal surgeries.

Question 110: Correct Answer: C) Send an email with the schedule to all team members.

Rationale: Sending an email with the schedule ensures that all team members receive the information directly and can refer back to it as needed. While posting on the bulletin board (B) and using the electronic scheduling system (D) are useful, they rely on team members actively checking these sources. Verbal communication (A) can lead to misunderstandings and omissions. Email provides a clear, direct, and documented method of communication.

Question 111: Correct Answer: D) Endoscopic clip applier

Rationale: An endoscopic clip applier is specifically designed for laparoscopic procedures to secure structures like the cystic duct. A linear stapler (Option A) is used for transecting and anastomosing tissues, not for securing ducts. A circular stapler (Option B) is used for end-to-end anastomosis in gastrointestinal surgery. A skin stapler (Option C) is used for closing skin incisions and is not suitable for internal structures like the cystic duct.

Question 112: Correct Answer: C) Enrolling in accredited online courses and webinars

Rationale: Enrolling in accredited online courses and webinars ensures that Sarah receives valid continuing education credits recognized by the NBSTSA. Unlike watching YouTube videos (B), which may not be accredited, or reading journals (D), which may not provide credits, accredited online courses offer structured, recognized education. In-person workshops (A) are beneficial but do not utilize computer technology.

Question 113: Correct Answer: B) Notify the surgeon immediately

Rationale: Notifying the surgeon immediately is crucial as the rash and itching could indicate a developing infection or allergic reaction to surgical

materials. Applying a topical antibiotic or cleaning with antiseptic might be part of the treatment but should only be done under the surgeon's direction. Advising antihistamines without a proper diagnosis could mask symptoms and delay appropriate treatment. Immediate reporting ensures timely and accurate intervention.

Question 114: Correct Answer: B) Verifying the correct drill bit is securely attached

Rationale: Verifying the correct drill bit is securely attached is a critical step when assembling a powered surgical drill. This ensures precision and safety during the procedure. While ensuring the drill is charged (option A) and testing on a sample material (option D) are important, they are secondary to secure attachment. Applying lubricant to the drill motor (option C) is generally unnecessary and could damage the equipment. Proper assembly is crucial for effective and safe operation.

Question 115: Correct Answer: A) Deltoid

Rationale: The deltoid muscle is primarily responsible for the abduction of the shoulder joint. The biceps brachii primarily flexes the elbow, the trapezius elevates and retracts the scapula, and the pectoralis major is involved in the adduction and internal rotation of the shoulder. Thus, while the other muscles play significant roles in shoulder movement, the deltoid is the key muscle for abduction.

Question 116: Correct Answer: C) Verifying the insufflator is properly connected to the CO2 tank.

Rationale: Verifying the insufflator is properly connected to the CO2 tank is crucial as it ensures the device can deliver the necessary gas to create pneumoperitoneum. While ensuring the correct pressure setting (A) and checking for kinks (B) are important, they are secondary to establishing a proper connection. Sterilization (D) is essential but not specific to the function of the insufflator.

Question 117: Correct Answer: B) To minimize blood loss

Rationale: The primary purpose of using cautery during postoperative procedures is to minimize blood loss by coagulating blood vessels. While reducing infection risk (A) and enhancing wound healing (C) are important, they are secondary benefits. Removing foreign bodies (D) is not a function of cautery. Therefore, B is the correct answer as it directly addresses the main purpose of cautery.

Question 118: Correct Answer: B) Immediate transplantation after harvesting

Rationale: Immediate transplantation after harvesting is crucial to maintain the viability of the autograft tissue. Delays can lead to cell death and reduced effectiveness of the graft. Sterilization (A) is not applicable as it can damage living cells. Chemical preservatives (C) and freezing (D) are more relevant to allografts or xenografts, not autografts, as they can compromise the viability of the tissue.

Question 119: Correct Answer: C) To detect potential bleeding complications.

Rationale: Monitoring for signs of hematoma formation is crucial to detect potential bleeding complications, which can be life-threatening if not addressed promptly. Ensuring patient comfort (A) and preventing infection (B) are important but are not the primary reasons for monitoring hematoma formation. Monitoring for allergic reactions (D) is unrelated to hematoma formation.

Question 120: Correct Answer: C) Adjust the retractor's position and ensure proper tissue engagement

Rationale: Adjusting the retractor's position and ensuring proper tissue engagement is essential for maintaining stability. Tightening screws or replacing the retractor may not address the underlying issue of improper placement. Applying more pressure manually is not a sustainable solution and could cause tissue damage. Proper adjustment ensures the retractor remains stable and the surgical field remains clear, enhancing the procedure's efficiency and safety.

Question 121: Correct Answer: C) Lower esophageal sphincter

Rationale: The lower esophageal sphincter (LES) prevents the backflow of stomach contents into the esophagus. The pyloric sphincter regulates the passage of chyme from the stomach to the duodenum, the ileocecal valve controls the flow from the small intestine to the large intestine, and the hepatopancreatic sphincter regulates the flow of bile and pancreatic juice. Therefore, the LES is the correct answer as it specifically prevents gastroesophageal reflux.

Question 122: Correct Answer: B) Position the surgical lights to eliminate shadows on the surgical field.

Rationale: Proper positioning of surgical lights to eliminate shadows is crucial for optimal visibility during laparoscopic procedures. Adjusting overhead lights to maximum brightness (A) can cause glare, while setting the laparoscope light source to low intensity (C) would reduce visibility. Ambient room lighting (D) is insufficient for detailed surgical work. Therefore, positioning the surgical lights correctly ensures a clear and shadow-free view of the surgical field, which is essential for the precision required in laparoscopic surgery.

Question 123: Correct Answer: A) Checking the microscope's light source intensity

Rationale: Ensuring the microscope's light source intensity is essential for proper visualization during surgery. Without adequate light, the surgeon's ability to see fine details is compromised. While adjusting ocular lenses (B) and ensuring the foot pedal is connected (C) are important, they are secondary to light source functionality. Cleaning external surfaces (D) is necessary for hygiene but does not directly impact the microscope's operational readiness.

Question 124: Correct Answer: B) Hypocalcemia

Rationale: Damage to the parathyroid glands can lead to a decrease in parathyroid hormone (PTH) production, causing hypocalcemia. This is because PTH is crucial for regulating calcium levels in the blood. Hypercalcemia (A) is incorrect as it results from excessive PTH. Hyperkalemia (C) and hypokalemia (D) are related to potassium imbalances, not calcium, and are not directly affected by parathyroid damage.

Question 125: Correct Answer: C) Immediately inform Dr. Smith about the breach.

Rationale: Alex should immediately inform Dr. Smith about the breach to prevent potential harm to the patient and maintain sterile conditions. Ignoring the breach (Option A) or reporting it after surgery (Option B) could compromise patient safety. Asking another team member (Option D) might delay corrective action. Immediate intervention is crucial for patient safety and adherence to ethical and legal standards.

Question 126: Correct Answer: A) Ensure the grounding pad is properly placed on the patient's thigh.

Rationale: Proper placement of the grounding pad is crucial to prevent burns and ensure the electrical circuit is complete. Option B is incorrect because the question specifies the use of monopolar cautery. Option C is incorrect as increasing power may cause tissue damage. Option D is incorrect because saline can conduct electricity and increase the risk of burns.

Question 127: Correct Answer: C) Seminiferous tubules

Rationale: The seminiferous tubules, located within the testes, are the specific sites where spermatogenesis occurs, leading to the production of sperm. The epididymis (A) stores and matures sperm, the prostate gland (B) produces seminal fluid, and the vas deferens (D) transports mature sperm to the urethra. Therefore, the seminiferous tubules are the correct answer as they directly produce sperm.

Question 128: Correct Answer: C) Maintain the insufflation pressure at 15 mmHg.

Rationale: The optimal insufflation pressure for a laparoscopic cholecystectomy is typically around 12-15 mmHg to ensure adequate visualization while minimizing the risk of complications. Increasing the pressure to 25 mmHg (Option A) can lead to cardiovascular and respiratory issues, while decreasing it to 5 mmHg (Option B) may not provide sufficient visualization. Turning off the insufflation device (Option D) would collapse the operative field, making the procedure impossible to continue.

Question 129: Correct Answer: B) Inferior mesenteric artery

Rationale: The inferior mesenteric artery supplies blood to the descending colon and is typically ligated during a colon resection. The superior mesenteric artery supplies the small intestine and part of the large intestine, but not the descending colon. The celiac trunk supplies the stomach, liver, and spleen, while the renal artery supplies the kidneys. Therefore, the inferior mesenteric artery is the correct answer, as it directly relates to the descending colon.

Question 130: Correct Answer: B) The surgical technologist should apply the light handles using a sterile light handle cover.

Rationale: Using a sterile light handle cover ensures that the light handles remain sterile when adjusted during surgery. Having the surgeon apply the handles

(A) is unnecessary and inefficient. The circulating nurse (C) and using clean gloves (D) do not maintain sterility, as they are not part of the sterile field.

Question 131: Correct Answer: A) Fibrin sealant
Rationale: Fibrin sealant is effective for controlling diffuse oozing as it mimics the final stages of the coagulation cascade, forming a stable fibrin clot. Hydrogen peroxide is an antiseptic, lidocaine is a local anesthetic, and sodium chloride is a saline solution. These alternatives do not provide the hemostatic properties required for controlling surgical bleeding, making fibrin sealant the correct choice.

Question 132: Correct Answer: B) Use a needle holder to pass the needle.
Rationale: Using a needle holder to pass the needle ensures safety and precision, reducing the risk of accidental injury. Passing the needle directly into the surgeon's hand (Option A) or with the sharp end pointing towards the surgeon (Option C) increases the risk of injury. Placing the needle on the instrument table (Option D) is inefficient and can disrupt the surgical flow. Thus, Option B is the correct and safest method.

Question 133: Correct Answer: B) To absorb exudate and provide a barrier to infection
Rationale: The primary purpose of a sterile dressing is to absorb exudate and provide a barrier to infection, ensuring the wound remains clean and protected. Option A is incorrect because while preventing the wound from drying out is important, it is not the primary purpose. Option C is incorrect as easy access is not a priority over sterility. Option D is incorrect because dressings do not reduce the need for antibiotics; they are used to prevent infection, not treat it.

Question 134: Correct Answer: D) Keeping the laser in standby mode when not in use
Rationale: A critical safety measure is keeping the laser in standby mode when not in use to prevent accidental burns or injuries. Using a wet drape (B) is important but secondary. Setting the laser to the highest power (A) and placing it directly on tissue (C) are incorrect and could cause excessive damage.

Question 135: Correct Answer: C) Including the patient's medical record number and type of specimen.
Rationale: The most appropriate method for labeling a specimen container is to include the patient's medical record number and type of specimen. This ensures precise identification and tracking. Using a pre-printed label (Option A) or just the patient's name and date of birth (Option B) may not provide enough detail. Attaching a label with the surgeon's name and procedure date (Option D) is insufficient for accurate specimen identification.

Question 136: Correct Answer: C) Document the unused sterile items and return them to the sterile supply room if unopened.
Rationale: Proper cost containment involves documenting and returning unused, unopened sterile items to the supply room to avoid unnecessary waste and reduce costs. Discarding items (A) leads to

waste, returning without documentation (B) lacks accountability, and leaving items on the tray (D) risks contamination and mismanagement.

Question 137: Correct Answer: C) Reduced smoke production
Rationale: The harmonic scalpel produces less smoke compared to traditional electrosurgery, which is a significant advantage in minimally invasive procedures. This reduction in smoke improves visibility for the surgeon and reduces the need for smoke evacuation systems. Options A) Higher risk of thermal injury and B) Increased blood loss are incorrect as the harmonic scalpel minimizes thermal damage and blood loss. D) Slower cutting speed is also incorrect; the harmonic scalpel offers efficient cutting speeds suitable for various surgical applications.

Question 138: Correct Answer: C) Appendicitis
Rationale: Appendicitis is the inflammation of the appendix, presenting with severe abdominal pain, typically in the lower right quadrant, and often necessitates surgical removal. Cholecystitis involves inflammation of the gallbladder, diverticulitis is the inflammation of diverticula in the colon, and pancreatitis is the inflammation of the pancreas. These conditions, while involving inflammation, affect different organs and have distinct clinical presentations.

Question 139: Correct Answer: B) Inform the surgeon and anesthesiologist immediately.
Rationale: Rising end-tidal CO_2 levels can indicate hypoventilation or CO_2 insufflation issues, which are critical intraoperative concerns. Informing the surgeon and anesthesiologist immediately ensures timely intervention. Increasing oxygen flow (Option A) or checking for equipment malfunction (Option C) are secondary steps. Administering a muscle relaxant (Option D) is inappropriate without further assessment.

Question 140: Correct Answer: B) Record the amount used immediately after the procedure
Rationale: The most appropriate action is to record the amount used immediately after the procedure to ensure accuracy and completeness. Estimating (A) can lead to errors, waiting until the end of the day (C) risks forgetting details, and reporting only completely used solutions (D) omits partial amounts, all of which compromise the integrity of patient records and postoperative care.

Question 141: Correct Answer: D) Wash hands, don gown, then gloves.
Rationale: The correct sequence is to wash hands thoroughly, don the sterile gown first, and then don the sterile gloves. This ensures that the gloves remain sterile as they are put on after the gown. Option A is incorrect because gloves should not be donned before the gown. Option B is partially correct but misses the critical handwashing step. Option C is incorrect because gloves should not be donned before the gown.

Question 142: Correct Answer: C) 80-110°F
Rationale: The recommended temperature range for

water used in the manual cleaning of surgical instruments is 80-110°F. This temperature range is optimal for the effectiveness of enzymatic and detergent solutions. Water that is too cold (A, B) will not activate the cleaning agents effectively, and water that is too hot (D) can cause protein coagulation, making contaminants more difficult to remove.

Question 143: Correct Answer: B) Document John's cultural beliefs in his medical record and discuss them with the surgical team.

Rationale: Documenting John's cultural beliefs and discussing them with the surgical team ensures that his beliefs are respected and integrated into his care plan. Assuming his beliefs are irrelevant (Option A) or secondary (Option D) is dismissive and can lead to patient distress. Only considering beliefs that align with protocols (Option C) is not culturally competent. Proper documentation and communication promote respect and understanding of cultural diversity in healthcare.

Question 144: Correct Answer: B) Left atrium

Rationale: The left atrium receives oxygenated blood from the lungs via the pulmonary veins. The right atrium receives deoxygenated blood from the body, the right ventricle pumps deoxygenated blood to the lungs, and the left ventricle pumps oxygenated blood to the body. This distinction is crucial for understanding the flow of blood through the heart and the systemic and pulmonary circuits.

Question 145: Correct Answer: B) Ventral root

Rationale: The ventral root transmits motor signals from the brain to the spinal cord. The dorsal root ganglion contains sensory neuron cell bodies, the dorsal column transmits sensory information, and the spinothalamic tract carries pain and temperature sensations. Protecting the ventral root is essential to preserve motor function, making option B the correct answer.

Question 146: Correct Answer: C) Place the lymph node in formalin and label it with the patient's name, date of surgery, and type of specimen.

Rationale: For a lymph node biopsy, the specimen should be placed in formalin to preserve the tissue for pathological examination. It must be labeled with the patient's name, date of surgery, and type of specimen to ensure accurate identification and processing. Incorrect options include placing the specimen in a dry container (B) or saline (D), which are not appropriate for preserving lymph node tissue. Option A lacks the date of surgery, which is necessary for proper documentation.

Question 147: Correct Answer: B) Grasping delicate tissue without causing trauma

Rationale: Babcock forceps are designed to grasp delicate tissues, such as the appendix, without causing trauma. Clamping blood vessels (A) is typically done with hemostats. Cutting sutures (C) requires scissors, and retracting tissue (D) is performed with retractors. Therefore, the primary use of Babcock forceps is to grasp delicate tissue without causing trauma (B).

Question 148: Correct Answer: B) They eliminate the risk of disease transmission.

Rationale: Synthetic bone grafts eliminate the risk of disease transmission, which is a significant concern with autografts and allografts. While options A, C, and D present plausible benefits, they are not the primary advantage. Synthetic grafts do not necessarily integrate faster (A), can be more expensive (C), and do not always provide superior mechanical strength (D). The elimination of disease transmission is the most definitive benefit, making option B the correct answer.

Question 149: Correct Answer: B) Ensuring the limb is in the correct anatomical position

Rationale: Ensuring the limb is in the correct anatomical position is crucial for proper healing and function. Incorrect positioning can lead to improper healing and complications. While choosing the correct type of splint material (A) and applying padding (D) are important, they are secondary to positioning. Wrapping the splint tightly (C) can cause circulation issues and is not recommended.

Question 150: Correct Answer: C) Report the symptoms to the medical team immediately.

Rationale: Calf pain, swelling, and redness are indicative of a possible deep vein thrombosis (DVT), a serious postoperative complication. Immediate reporting to the medical team is crucial for prompt diagnosis and treatment. Option A is incorrect as walking could dislodge a clot. Option B and D are partial measures that do not address the potential severity of DVT. Immediate reporting ensures appropriate and potentially life-saving intervention.

CST Exam Practice Questions [SET 6]

Question 1: When a surgical technologist notices a team member struggling with a task, what is the most appropriate initial response to ensure effective team dynamics and patient safety?
A) Ignore the situation to avoid embarrassing the team member.
B) Offer immediate assistance and communicate supportively.
C) Report the situation to the supervisor without intervening.
D) Wait until the task is completed to discuss the issue privately.

Question 2: During a preoperative staff meeting, the surgical team discusses the importance of maintaining accurate and up-to-date surgical logs. Which of the following is the primary reason for keeping detailed surgical logs?
A) To ensure compliance with hospital policies
B) To facilitate future surgical research
C) To provide legal documentation in case of litigation
D) To improve patient care and safety

Question 3: During the postoperative cleanup after Mrs. Smith's surgery, the surgical technologist encounters a used scalpel blade. What is the appropriate action to take in compliance with Standard Precautions?
A) Recap the scalpel blade before disposal.
B) Use forceps to place the scalpel blade in a sharps container.
C) Dispose of the scalpel blade in the regular trash.
D) Place the scalpel blade on a tray for later disposal.

Question 4: What is the primary reason for wiping down the room and furniture in the operating room before a surgical procedure?
A) To reduce the risk of surgical site infections
B) To make the room look clean for the surgical team
C) To comply with hospital housekeeping policies
D) To remove visible dust and debris only

Question 5: During a total knee arthroplasty on a patient named Sarah, the surgeon decides to use a chemical hemostatic agent to control bleeding from the bone surface. Which agent is most suitable for this purpose?
A) Collagen
B) Epinephrine
C) Fibrin sealant
D) Warfarin

Question 6: What is the primary role of the surgical technologist during the transfer of a patient from the operating table to the stretcher?
A) Administering postoperative medications
B) Monitoring the patient's vital signs
C) Assisting with the physical transfer of the patient
D) Documenting the procedure in the patient's medical record

Question 7: During an open appendectomy on a patient named John, the surgeon asks the surgical technologist to pass a suture for closing the fascia. Which of the following sutures should the surgical technologist pass?
A) 1-0 non-absorbable suture.
B) 2-0 absorbable suture.
C) 0 absorbable suture.
D) 3-0 non-absorbable suture.

Question 8: When a surgical technologist notices a colleague consistently making minor errors, which diplomatic approach should they take to address the issue?
A) Publicly correct the colleague during the procedure
B) Discuss the errors with the colleague privately
C) Report the errors to the supervisor immediately
D) Ignore the errors as they are minor

Question 9: After a cholecystectomy, Mr. Smith begins to exhibit signs of excessive bleeding at the surgical site. As a Certified Surgical Technologist, what is the most appropriate immediate action to take?
A) Apply a cold compress to the area.
B) Elevate the affected limb.
C) Apply direct pressure to the site.
D) Administer pain medication.

Question 10: How can computer technology enhance the management of surgeon's preference cards?
A) By automatically updating patient vital signs
B) By providing real-time inventory management
C) By enabling electronic updates and easy access
D) By scheduling operating room times

Question 11: During an orthopedic surgery on Mr. Thompson, the surgeon needs an instrument to cut through bone. Which instrument should the surgical technologist provide?
A) Mayo Scissors
B) Osteotome
C) DeBakey Forceps
D) Metzenbaum Scissors

Question 12: Which chemical hemostatic agent is used topically to control bleeding and is derived from bovine sources?
A) Fibrin glue
B) Oxidized cellulose
C) Absorbable gelatin sponge
D) Microfibrillar collagen

Question 13: Which type of cells in the epidermis are responsible for producing melanin, the pigment that gives skin its color?

A) Keratinocytes
B) Melanocytes
C) Langerhans cells
D) Merkel cells

Question 14: During a laparoscopic cholecystectomy on Ms. Johnson, the surgical technologist is responsible for ensuring the equipment functions properly. Which of the following actions is essential before the procedure begins?
A) Calibrating the insufflator
B) Sterilizing the endoscope
C) Testing the light source
D) Ensuring adequate CO2 supply

Question 15: What is the primary reason for ensuring that a Foley catheter is properly lubricated before insertion?
A) To prevent infection
B) To reduce patient discomfort
C) To ensure proper drainage
D) To maintain catheter sterility

Question 16: During a parotidectomy on a patient named Mr. Johnson, the surgeon must carefully avoid injuring a specific cranial nerve that runs through the parotid gland. Which cranial nerve is this?
A) Trigeminal nerve (CN V)
B) Facial nerve (CN VII)
C) Glossopharyngeal nerve (CN IX)
D) Vagus nerve (CN X)

Question 17: During the preoperative preparation for Ms. Smith's total hip arthroplasty, the surgical technologist must gather the necessary instruments and supplies. Which of the following items is crucial for this type of surgery?
A) Arthroscope
B) Hip retractor set
C) Laparotomy sponge
D) Bronchoscope

Question 18: During the postoperative assessment of Mr. Johnson, a patient who underwent abdominal surgery, you notice a red, itchy rash around the surgical site. Which of the following is the most appropriate immediate action?
A) Apply a topical antibiotic ointment to the rash.
B) Notify the surgeon and document the findings.
C) Administer an antihistamine to the patient.
D) Clean the area with an antiseptic solution.

Question 19: Which of the following nondisposable items should be immediately removed from the sterile field and properly decontaminated after surgery?
A) Surgical drapes
B) Surgical instruments
C) Surgical gloves

D) Surgical sponges

Question 20: What type of joint is the hip joint classified as?
A) Hinge joint
B) Ball-and-socket joint
C) Pivot joint
D) Saddle joint

Question 21: When reviewing preoperative documentation, which of the following is essential to confirm regarding the patient's medical history?
A) Patient's employment history
B) Patient's past surgical procedures
C) Patient's travel history
D) Patient's educational background

Question 22: During a surgical procedure involving the use of a laser, the surgical technologist notices that the laser warning sign is not posted outside the operating room. What should be the immediate course of action?
A) Continue with the procedure and post the sign later.
B) Inform the surgeon and continue with the procedure.
C) Stop the procedure and post the laser warning sign immediately.
D) Ignore the missing sign as it is not critical.

Question 23: Which muscle plays a crucial role in the process of inhalation by contracting and increasing the thoracic cavity volume?
A) Diaphragm
B) Intercostal muscles
C) Abdominal muscles
D) Pectoralis major

Question 24: During a laparoscopic cholecystectomy on Mr. Johnson, the surgeon requests a grasper to manipulate the gallbladder. Which instrument should the surgical technologist hand to the surgeon?
A) Babcock forceps
B) Kelly clamp
C) Maryland dissector
D) Allis forceps

Question 25: During an abdominal surgery, the surgical technologist is responsible for assembling and maintaining the retractors. The surgeon requests a self-retaining retractor to keep the incision open. Which of the following retractors should the surgical technologist prepare?
A) Army-Navy retractor
B) Balfour retractor
C) Deaver retractor
D) Richardson retractor

Question 26: What is the primary purpose of

applying a splint during the intraoperative phase?
A) To completely immobilize the limb
B) To provide temporary support and stabilization
C) To reduce swelling by compression
D) To serve as a permanent fixation device

Question 27: What is the primary function of the aqueous humor in the eye?
A) To maintain intraocular pressure
B) To provide nutrients to the retina
C) To transmit visual information to the brain
D) To control the amount of light entering the eye

Question 28: Which disinfectant is most commonly recommended for wiping down operating room furniture and surfaces?
A) Alcohol-based disinfectants
B) Chlorine bleach solutions
C) Phenolic disinfectants
D) Quaternary ammonium compounds

Question 29: During a coronary artery bypass graft (CABG) surgery on a 58-year-old patient named Mr. Smith, the surgeon needs to identify the vessel that supplies oxygenated blood to the left atrium and the left ventricle. Which vessel is the surgeon referring to?
A) Right Coronary Artery
B) Left Anterior Descending Artery
C) Circumflex Artery
D) Pulmonary Artery

Question 30: Sarah, a Certified Surgical Technologist, is assigned to assist in a complex surgery. During the procedure, the surgeon gives a series of rapid instructions. What should Sarah do to ensure she correctly follows the surgeon's directives?
A) Wait until the surgeon finishes speaking to ask for clarification.
B) Interrupt the surgeon to ask questions immediately.
C) Acknowledge each instruction verbally as it is given.
D) Write down the instructions to review later.

Question 31: During a surgical procedure, Dr. Smith and Nurse Jane have a disagreement about the correct instrument to use. As the Certified Surgical Technologist (CST) in the room, how should you handle this situation to maintain diplomacy and ensure the procedure continues smoothly?
A) Side with Dr. Smith because he is the lead surgeon.
B) Side with Nurse Jane because she has more experience.
C) Suggest a brief pause to review the surgical plan and discuss the options.
D) Ignore the disagreement and continue with the procedure.

Question 32: Which positioning device is most

appropriate for maintaining a patient's airway during a thyroidectomy?
A) Shoulder Roll
B) Bean Bag
C) Bolster
D) Wilson Frame

Question 33: Dr. Smith has recently started using a new type of suture material for her surgeries. As a Certified Surgical Technologist, what is the most appropriate action to take regarding the surgeon's preference card?
A) Wait until the end of the month to revise the preference card.
B) Immediately update the preference card to include the new suture material.
C) Discuss the change with the surgical team before updating the preference card.
D) Only update the preference card if the surgeon requests it.

Question 34: 7 During a surgical procedure, a patient named Mr. Johnson develops a sudden fever. The surgical team suspects a bacterial infection. Which of the following classifications best describes the bacteria most likely responsible for a rapid onset infection?
A) Gram-positive cocci
B) Gram-negative bacilli
C) Acid-fast bacilli
D) Spirochetes

Question 35: How can a Certified Surgical Technologist (CST) utilize computer technology to enhance communication within the surgical team?
A) Sending emails to team members
B) Playing team-building games online
C) Browsing social media platforms
D) Using surgical simulation software

Question 36: What is the most important consideration when preparing a pediatric patient for surgery?
A) Ensuring the child has fasted for at least 12 hours
B) Explaining the procedure in medical terms to the child
C) Involving the parents in the preoperative preparation
D) Administering preoperative antibiotics

Question 37: Which of the following is the most appropriate action for a surgical technologist to take when encountering a discrepancy in the surgical count?
A) Ignore the discrepancy and continue with the procedure.
B) Report the discrepancy to the surgeon immediately.
C) Attempt to resolve the discrepancy independently.
D) Wait until the end of the procedure to address the discrepancy.

Question 38: During a preoperative assessment, the surgical technologist notices that the operating room temperature is set to 65°F. The patient, Mr. Johnson, is scheduled for a lengthy abdominal surgery. What should the surgical technologist do to ensure an optimal environment for the patient?
A) Increase the room temperature to 75°F.
B) Maintain the current room temperature.
C) Increase the room temperature to 68°F.
D) Decrease the room temperature to 60°F.

Question 39: A postoperative patient develops a rash that is red, raised, and itchy. Which of the following is the least likely cause of this rash?
A) Allergic reaction to medication
B) Surgical site infection
C) Contact dermatitis from adhesive
D) Deep vein thrombosis (DVT)

Question 40: 9 Which of the following microorganisms is classified as a Gram-positive cocci and is a common cause of surgical site infections?
A) Escherichia coli
B) Staphylococcus aureus
C) Pseudomonas aeruginosa
D) Candida albicans

Question 41: Which of the following actions is most critical in maintaining a sterile field during an intraoperative procedure?
A) Wearing double gloves
B) Keeping hands above waist level
C) Using sterile drapes
D) Wearing a surgical mask

Question 42: What is the first step a Certified Surgical Technologist should take in the event of a chemical spill in the operating room?
A) Evacuate the operating room immediately.
B) Notify the supervisor and follow the facility's spill response protocol.
C) Attempt to clean the spill using available cleaning supplies.
D) Ignore the spill if it is small and continue with the procedure.

Question 43: Which gland secretes the hormone responsible for regulating the body's metabolic rate?
A) Adrenal gland
B) Thyroid gland
C) Pancreas
D) Parathyroid gland

Question 44: Ms. Smith, a 45-year-old patient, is being prepared for an abdominal surgery. Which patient safety device should be applied to ensure proper positioning and avoid nerve damage during the procedure?
A) Anti-embolism stockings

B) Safety straps
C) Electrocardiogram (ECG) leads
D) Thermal blanket

Question 45: Which part of the brain is primarily responsible for coordinating voluntary movements and maintaining balance?
A) Cerebrum
B) Cerebellum
C) Medulla Oblongata
D) Thalamus

Question 46: Mrs. Smith, a diabetic patient, is scheduled for a total knee replacement. During the preoperative preparation, she mentions that she has not taken her insulin today. What should the surgical technologist do?
A) Advise Mrs. Smith to take her insulin immediately.
B) Inform the anesthesiologist and the surgical team about Mrs. Smith's insulin status.
C) Reassure Mrs. Smith that missing one dose of insulin is not critical.
D) Proceed with the preoperative preparation without addressing the insulin issue.

Question 47: Which of the following is the most appropriate action to take if a patient has not adhered to the preoperative fasting guidelines?
A) Proceed with the surgery as planned
B) Administer a laxative to clear the digestive tract
C) Inform the surgical team and potentially reschedule the surgery
D) Allow the patient to drink clear fluids before surgery

Question 48: When preparing suture material for a surgical procedure, which of the following is the most important consideration to ensure sterility?
A) Using non-sterile gloves to handle the suture material
B) Ensuring the suture material is within its expiration date
C) Cutting the suture material with non-sterile scissors
D) Storing the suture material in a non-sterile environment

Question 49: During the preoperative preparation for a laparoscopic cholecystectomy, you notice that Dr. Johnson's preference card indicates the use of a specific insufflation gas. Which gas should you ensure is available?
A) Nitrous oxide
B) Oxygen
C) Carbon dioxide
D) Helium

Question 50: Which of the following preoperative considerations is most crucial for a bariatric patient undergoing surgery?
A) Ensuring the patient has fasted for at least 12 hours
B) Assessing the patient's nutritional deficiencies
C) Confirming the patient's weight loss history

D) Evaluating the patient's psychological readiness

Question 51: What is the best practice for documenting a patient's allergy to antibiotics in the preoperative phase?
A) Noting it in the patient's chart only
B) Informing the surgeon verbally
C) Applying an allergy alert bracelet to the patient
D) Documenting it in the patient's chart and applying an allergy alert bracelet

Question 52: Which structure in the female reproductive system is responsible for the production of estrogen and progesterone?
A) Fallopian tubes
B) Ovaries
C) Uterus
D) Cervix

Question 53: During an orthopedic surgery, Mr. Smith requires the use of an arthroscopic shaver. What is the most important step the surgical technologist should take when assembling the shaver system?
A) Ensuring the shaver blade is securely attached.
B) Verifying the shaver handpiece is properly connected to the power source.
C) Testing the shaver's suction function.
D) Confirming the shaver's irrigation system is working.

Question 54: During a laparoscopic cholecystectomy on a patient named Mr. Johnson, the surgeon requests a Maryland dissector. Which of the following is the most appropriate way for the surgical technologist to pass this instrument?
A) Pass the instrument with the tips pointing upwards.
B) Pass the instrument with the tips pointing downwards.
C) Pass the instrument with the tips pointing towards the surgeon.
D) Pass the instrument with the tips pointing away from the surgeon.

Question 55: Which of the following is the most appropriate initial action for a surgical technologist to take upon identifying a postoperative hematoma at the surgical site?
A) Apply a warm compress to the area
B) Notify the surgeon immediately
C) Massage the hematoma to disperse the blood
D) Increase the patient's intravenous fluid rate

Question 56: During a thoracotomy procedure on Mr. Johnson, the surgeon asks the surgical technologist to identify the structure that separates the right and left pleural cavities. Which structure should the technologist identify?
A) Diaphragm
B) Mediastinum
C) Pleural effusion
D) Pericardium

Question 57: During a laparoscopic cholecystectomy, the surgeon requests a chemical hemostatic agent to control minor bleeding from the liver bed. Which of the following agents is most appropriate for this situation?
A) Epinephrine
B) Thrombin
C) Silver nitrate
D) Acetic acid

Question 58: Sarah, a Certified Surgical Technologist, is responsible for managing the inventory of surgical instruments. What is the most critical step she should take to ensure the availability of necessary instruments for upcoming surgeries?
A) Conducting a weekly inventory check
B) Relying on previous usage patterns
C) Communicating with the surgical team about upcoming procedures
D) Ordering extra instruments to avoid shortages

Question 59: How can computer technology be utilized to enhance communication within a surgical team?
A) By automating surgical procedures
B) By providing real-time updates on patient status
C) By replacing face-to-face meetings with emails
D) By scheduling surgeries without human intervention

Question 60: Which structure is primarily responsible for gas exchange in the lungs?
A) Bronchi
B) Alveoli
C) Trachea
D) Pleura

Question 61: What is the most appropriate method for a surgical technologist to pass a scalpel to the surgeon during a procedure?
A) Hand the scalpel directly into the surgeon's hand
B) Place the scalpel on the sterile field for the surgeon to pick up
C) Pass the scalpel handle-first into the surgeon's hand
D) Pass the scalpel blade-first into the surgeon's hand

Question 62: Which vein is commonly harvested for use in coronary artery bypass grafting (CABG)?
A) Femoral vein
B) Cephalic vein
C) Saphenous vein
D) Jugular vein

Question 63: During the preoperative assessment, a patient named Mr. Smith mentions that he has a known allergy to latex. Which of the following actions should the surgical technologist take to ensure Mr. Smith's safety during the procedure?

A) Use latex-free gloves and equipment.
B) Administer antihistamines preoperatively.
C) Schedule the surgery in a latex-free operating room.
D) Inform the anesthesiologist of the latex allergy.

Question 64: During a surgical procedure, what is the primary purpose of using irrigation on the operative site?
A) To cool down the surgical instruments
B) To keep the surgical field clear of debris and blood
C) To sterilize the surgical site
D) To provide nutrients to the tissue

Question 65: When using interpersonal skills to manage group dynamics in a surgical setting, which of the following actions best demonstrates effective diplomacy?
A) Dominating the conversation to ensure your point is heard.
B) Actively listening to all team members and acknowledging their input.
C) Avoiding difficult conversations to maintain harmony.
D) Making decisions independently without consulting the team.

Question 66: During a spinal fusion surgery, the surgical technologist is tasked with preparing an allograft for implantation in a patient named Sarah. Which of the following is the best practice for handling the allograft to maintain its viability?
A) Keeping the allograft at room temperature until use
B) Using a dry heat sterilizer to prepare the allograft
C) Maintaining the allograft in a sterile, cold saline solution
D) Exposing the allograft to ambient air for 10 minutes before use

Question 67: Which of the following is a key benefit of using electronic health records (EHRs) in surgical research?
A) Increased patient wait times
B) Improved accuracy of patient data
C) Higher costs of data storage
D) Reduced need for surgical instruments

Question 68: Sarah, a surgical technologist, notices that a new team member, John, is struggling to keep up with the pace of the operation. The surgeon has just asked for a specific instrument. How should Sarah respond to ensure the team maintains efficiency and patient safety?
A) Hand the instrument to the surgeon herself and then assist John.
B) Ignore John's struggle and focus solely on her own tasks.
C) Ask John to hurry up and find the instrument quickly.
D) Inform the surgeon about John's inexperience and suggest a break.

Question 69: During the draping process, which of the following actions should be avoided to maintain a sterile field?
A) Handling the drape with sterile gloves
B) Allowing the drape to touch non-sterile surfaces
C) Using a drape with adhesive edges
D) Covering the entire surgical site with the drape

Question 70: Which of the following is a common site for harvesting autografts for bone grafting procedures?
A) Tibia
B) Femur
C) Iliac crest
D) Scapula

Question 71: What is the primary reason for using a biological indicator in the sterilization process?
A) To measure the temperature inside the sterilizer
B) To verify the effectiveness of the sterilization process
C) To ensure the sterilizer is not overloaded
D) To monitor the humidity levels inside the sterilizer

Question 72: Which of the following is the best practice for ensuring sterility while donning gloves after gowning?
A) Use the open glove technique
B) Use the closed glove technique
C) Use the assisted glove technique
D) Use the bare hand technique

Question 73: During a surgical procedure, the surgeon requests the identification of the primary lymphatic drainage site for the right breast. Which lymph node group should the surgical technologist identify?
A) Axillary lymph nodes
B) Inguinal lymph nodes
C) Cervical lymph nodes
D) Popliteal lymph nodes

Question 74: Which of the following methods is most effective for achieving hemostasis during a laparoscopic cholecystectomy?
A) Application of topical thrombin
B) Use of bipolar electrosurgery
C) Application of bone wax
D) Use of a tourniquet

Question 75: During a laparoscopic cholecystectomy on a 45-year-old patient named Mr. Johnson, the surgeon encounters difficulty due to the presence of dense adhesions around the gallbladder. Which anatomical structure is most at risk of injury during the dissection of these adhesions?
A) Common bile duct
B) Hepatic artery
C) Portal vein
D) Cystic duct

Question 76: During a laparoscopic cholecystectomy, the surgeon asks you to prepare a 3-0 Vicryl suture for closing the port sites. Which of the following steps should you take first?
A) Pass the suture directly to the surgeon.
B) Open the suture package and place it on the sterile field.
C) Cut the suture to the desired length before passing.
D) Ensure the suture is threaded onto a needle holder.

Question 77: During a laparoscopic cholecystectomy, the surgeon requests the use of a CO2 beam coagulator to achieve hemostasis. What is the primary advantage of using a CO2 beam coagulator in this scenario?
A) It provides deep tissue penetration.
B) It minimizes thermal damage to surrounding tissues.
C) It is more cost-effective than other coagulation methods.
D) It reduces the risk of postoperative infection.

Question 78: During a laparoscopic cholecystectomy, the patient, Mr. Johnson, suddenly exhibits signs of a severe allergic reaction, including hypotension and bronchospasm. What should be the immediate action taken by the surgical technologist?
A) Administer epinephrine and continue the procedure.
B) Notify the surgeon and prepare emergency medications.
C) Increase the oxygen flow and monitor the patient.
D) Stop the procedure and call for an anesthesiologist.

Question 79: Which hemostatic method is primarily used to control diffuse oozing from capillaries and small vessels?
A) Suturing
B) Hemostatic clips
C) Topical hemostatic agents
D) Ligation

Question 80: What is the recommended temperature range for steam sterilization of surgical instruments in an autoclave?
A) 100-120°F
B) 121-134°C
C) 150-170°C
D) 200-220°F

Question 81: When passing a needle holder to the surgeon, which of the following techniques should a surgical technologist use?
A) Pass the needle holder with the needle pointing towards the surgeon
B) Pass the needle holder with the needle pointing away from the surgeon
C) Place the needle holder on the sterile field
D) Hand the needle holder directly to the surgeon without regard to needle orientation

Question 82: During a total knee arthroplasty, the surgical team is preparing to use a synthetic bone graft. What is the primary advantage of using synthetic bone grafts over autografts or allografts?
A) Lower risk of disease transmission
B) Higher osteogenic potential
C) Faster integration with host bone
D) Reduced surgical time

Question 83: Which of the following is a critical step to ensure the effectiveness of flash sterilization for immediate use?
A) Using a high concentration of sterilizing agent
B) Ensuring instruments are wrapped tightly
C) Pre-cleaning instruments thoroughly before sterilization
D) Placing instruments in a dry container

Question 84: Which personal protective equipment (PPE) is most critical when dealing with a chemical spill in the operating room?
A) Surgical mask
B) Sterile gloves
C) Chemical-resistant gloves
D) Lead apron

Question 85: What is the primary purpose of using sequential compression devices (SCDs) in the postoperative period?
A) To prevent deep vein thrombosis (DVT)
B) To reduce postoperative pain
C) To enhance wound healing
D) To maintain body temperature

Question 86: What is the primary purpose of applying a safety strap to a patient during preoperative preparation?
A) To prevent the patient from falling off the operating table
B) To keep the surgical site sterile
C) To monitor the patient's vital signs
D) To provide comfort to the patient

Question 87: During an abdominal surgery on Mr. Johnson, the surgical technologist notices that the cautery machine is not properly grounded. What is the most appropriate action to take to prevent potential harm?
A) Continue the surgery and inform the surgeon after the procedure.
B) Immediately inform the surgeon and halt the procedure until the issue is resolved.
C) Adjust the grounding pad without informing the surgeon.
D) Ignore the issue as it is unlikely to cause any harm.

Question 88: What is the primary reason for accurately reporting the amount of medication and solution used during a surgical procedure?
A) To ensure proper billing and reimbursement
B) To maintain an accurate patient medical record
C) To comply with hospital inventory management
D) To prevent medication theft and misuse

Question 89: Which structure is primarily responsible for gas exchange in the lungs?
A) Bronchi
B) Alveoli
C) Trachea
D) Bronchioles

Question 90: During a laparoscopic cholecystectomy on a patient named John, the surgeon encounters a bleeding cystic artery. Which thermal method is most appropriate for achieving hemostasis in this scenario?
A) Cryotherapy
B) Electrocautery
C) Laser coagulation
D) Ultrasonic scalpel

Question 91: Which patient position is most commonly used for abdominal surgeries to provide optimal access to the abdominal cavity?
A) Lithotomy
B) Prone
C) Supine
D) Trendelenburg

Question 92: During a laparoscopic cholecystectomy, the surgical technologist notices that the label on a vial of medication being prepared for administration is partially obscured. What should the surgical technologist do next?
A) Administer the medication based on the visible part of the label.
B) Ask the surgeon to verify the medication before administration.
C) Discard the vial and obtain a new one with a clear label.
D) Consult the circulating nurse for verification of the medication.

Question 93: Which of the following is the primary responsibility of a surgical technologist when assisting with a skin stapler during a procedure?
A) Loading the stapler with staples
B) Ensuring the stapler is properly aligned with the incision
C) Handing the stapler to the surgeon without checking its functionality
D) Removing the staples post-operatively

Question 94: Which of the following malignancies is most commonly associated with the mutation of the BRCA1 and BRCA2 genes?
A) Lung cancer
B) Breast cancer

C) Prostate cancer
D) Colon cancer

Question 95: Which of the following is the most critical consideration when preparing an immunocompromised patient for surgery?
A) Ensuring the patient is well-hydrated
B) Administering prophylactic antibiotics
C) Scheduling surgery early in the day
D) Providing a high-protein diet

Question 96: During a surgical procedure, the electrosurgical unit (ESU) suddenly stops working. What should the Certified Surgical Technologist check first?
A) The grounding pad placement.
B) The power cord connection.
C) The ESU settings.
D) The patient's vital signs.

Question 97: During a hysterectomy procedure, the surgeon needs to ligate the blood supply to the uterus. Which artery should the surgical technologist prepare to clamp?
A) Renal Artery
B) Pulmonary Artery
C) Uterine Artery
D) Femoral Artery

Question 98: 4 What is the primary purpose of using a selective culture medium in microbiology?
A) To enhance the growth of all microorganisms
B) To differentiate between types of microorganisms
C) To inhibit the growth of certain microorganisms while allowing others to grow
D) To provide a nutrient-rich environment for fastidious organisms

Question 99: While preparing the operating room for an orthopedic surgery on Ms. Johnson, the surgical technologist notices that one of the surgical lights is flickering. What is the MOST appropriate action to take?
A) Ignore the flickering light and proceed with the surgery.
B) Attempt to fix the flickering light after the surgery has started.
C) Replace the flickering light before the surgery begins.
D) Use a flashlight as a temporary light source.

Question 100: During a laparoscopic cholecystectomy on a patient named John, the surgeon encounters significant bleeding from the cystic artery. Which mechanical method should be used to achieve hemostasis?
A) Electrocautery
B) Hemostatic clips
C) Topical thrombin
D) Fibrin sealant

Question 101: Which preoperative intervention is most important for reducing the risk of postoperative delirium in elderly patients?
A) Administering high doses of sedatives
B) Ensuring adequate hydration
C) Increasing physical activity
D) Providing detailed surgical information

Question 102: Which of the following steps is crucial when connecting a Jackson-Pratt drain to a suction apparatus?
A) Ensure the drain is fully extended before connecting.
B) Prime the suction apparatus with saline before attaching the drain.
C) Compress the bulb of the Jackson-Pratt drain before securing the cap.
D) Attach the drain to the suction apparatus without compressing the bulb.

Question 103: During an endoscopic cholecystectomy on a patient named Mr. Johnson, the surgical technologist is responsible for ensuring the laparoscopic camera is functioning correctly. Which of the following steps is crucial to verify the camera's functionality before the procedure begins?
A) Ensuring the camera is properly sterilized.
B) Checking the camera's white balance and focus.
C) Confirming the camera's battery is fully charged.
D) Verifying the camera's cable is securely connected.

Question 104: Which hormone is primarily responsible for regulating calcium levels in the blood?
A) Insulin
B) Cortisol
C) Parathyroid hormone (PTH)
D) Thyroxine

Question 105: During the postoperative phase, the surgical technologist must remove the drapes from Mrs. Smith. Which of the following actions should be taken to prevent contamination?
A) Remove the drapes slowly to avoid disturbing the sterile field.
B) Fold the drapes inward to contain any contaminants.
C) Remove the drapes and place them directly on the floor.
D) Shake the drapes to ensure all instruments are removed.

Question 106: During an open appendectomy on a patient named Sarah, the surgeon requests a hemostat. What is the most appropriate way for the surgical technologist to pass this instrument?
A) Pass the hemostat with the ratchets closed.
B) Pass the hemostat with the ratchets open.
C) Pass the hemostat with the tips pointing towards the technologist.

D) Pass the hemostat with the tips pointing towards the patient.

Question 107: During a laparotomy procedure on a patient named Mr. Johnson, the surgical technologist is responsible for assembling and maintaining the retractors. Which of the following steps is essential to ensure the retractors are functioning correctly throughout the procedure?
A) Periodically check the retractor's tension and adjust as needed.
B) Leave the retractors in place once initially positioned.
C) Use the same retractor for all types of tissue.
D) Allow the surgeon to handle retractor adjustments exclusively.

Question 108: During the preoperative preparation for a laparoscopic cholecystectomy, the surgical technologist, Alex, notices that the insufflator has not been tested. What should Alex do to ensure the operating room environment is properly prepared?
A) Ignore it and proceed with the surgery.
B) Inform the circulating nurse and test the insufflator.
C) Wait for the surgeon to arrive and ask for instructions.
D) Use a different insufflator without testing.

Question 109: During a surgical procedure, a patient named Mr. Smith requires an autograft for bone repair. Which of the following steps is essential to ensure the viability of the autograft?
A) Sterilizing the autograft using high heat
B) Keeping the autograft moist with saline solution
C) Using an autoclave to sterilize the autograft
D) Freezing the autograft before implantation

Question 110: Which muscle is primarily responsible for the abduction of the arm at the shoulder joint?
A) Deltoid
B) Biceps Brachii
C) Triceps Brachii
D) Latissimus Dorsi

Question 111: What is the primary advantage of using CO2 beam coagulators in surgical procedures?
A) Reduced thermal damage to surrounding tissues
B) Increased risk of infection
C) Higher blood loss during surgery
D) Longer recovery time for patients

Question 112: Which of the following is the most important step in ensuring that all necessary supplies are available for a surgical procedure?
A) Conducting a preoperative checklist
B) Consulting with the anesthesiologist
C) Reviewing the patient's chart
D) Sterilizing the instruments

Question 113: Which of the following conditions is characterized by the abnormal protrusion of an organ or tissue through the structure that usually contains it?
A) Hernia
B) Adhesion
C) Fistula
D) Abscess

Question 114: What is the primary reason for verifying the type and size of an implantable item with the surgeon before the procedure begins?
A) To ensure the implant matches the patient's insurance coverage
B) To confirm the implant is the correct one for the specific surgical procedure
C) To verify the implant is available in the operating room
D) To ensure the implant is sterilized properly

Question 115: During a laparoscopic cholecystectomy on Mr. Smith, the surgical team notices smoke accumulating in the abdominal cavity. What is the most appropriate immediate action to ensure safety and visibility?
A) Increase the insufflation pressure
B) Use a smoke evacuation system
C) Open the operating room doors
D) Ask the anesthesiologist to increase the oxygen flow

Question 116: During a surgical procedure, how should a surgical technologist maintain a retractor to ensure optimal visibility for the surgeon?
A) Frequently adjust the retractor's position
B) Clean the retractor with saline solution
C) Ensure the retractor is not under excessive tension
D) Replace the retractor every 30 minutes

Question 117: Sarah, a surgical technologist, is responsible for preparing the operating room for the next procedure. Which of the following is the most critical step she should take to ensure proper room turnover?
A) Quickly wipe down surfaces and arrange instruments.
B) Thoroughly clean and disinfect all surfaces and equipment.
C) Leave the cleaning to the housekeeping staff and focus on instrument setup.
D) Ensure that the previous patient's records are properly filed before cleaning.

Question 118: Which artery is primarily responsible for supplying blood to the lower extremities?
A) Brachial artery
B) Femoral artery
C) Radial artery
D) Carotid artery

Question 119: Which structure in the male genitourinary system is responsible for the production of sperm?
A) Epididymis
B) Seminal vesicle
C) Prostate gland
D) Testes

Question 120: Which of the following is the best practice for maintaining confidentiality while utilizing computer technology for interdepartmental communication?
A) Using shared login credentials for quick access
B) Encrypting sensitive information before transmission
C) Posting updates on a public forum for transparency
D) Relying solely on verbal communication to avoid digital breaches

Question 121: Sarah, a surgical technologist, is preparing to sterilize a set of laparoscopic instruments. Which of the following is the most appropriate method for ensuring these instruments are properly sterilized?
A) Soaking the instruments in a disinfectant solution for 30 minutes.
B) Using a steam autoclave cycle specifically designed for delicate instruments.
C) Wiping the instruments with alcohol and allowing them to air dry.
D) Placing the instruments in a dry heat sterilizer for 2 hours.

Question 122: What does bright red blood typically indicate during an intraoperative procedure?
A) Arterial bleeding
B) Venous bleeding
C) Capillary bleeding
D) Coagulated blood

Question 123: During a routine appendectomy on a 30-year-old female patient named Ms. Johnson, the surgeon encounters a rare congenital anomaly known as a "retrocecal appendix." What is the most appropriate action for the surgical technologist to take to assist the surgeon?
A) Suggest extending the incision for better access.
B) Recommend converting to a laparoscopic approach.
C) Provide the surgeon with a longer instrument set.
D) Advise the surgeon to stop and refer the patient for further evaluation.

Question 124: After completing a laparoscopic cholecystectomy on Mr. Smith, the surgical technologist is responsible for removing nondisposable items from the sterile field. Which of the following steps should be performed first?
A) Remove the drapes from the patient.
B) Dispose of sharps in the sharps container.
C) Remove and segregate nondisposable

instruments.
D) Wipe down the surgical lights.

Question 125: Which thermal method is most commonly used for achieving hemostasis during laparoscopic surgery?
A) Cryotherapy
B) Electrocautery
C) Laser coagulation
D) Ultrasonic scalpel

Question 126: When performing a bowel anastomosis, which stapling device is most appropriate to use?
A) Linear cutter stapler
B) Skin stapler
C) Ligating clip applier
D) Hemorrhoidal stapler

Question 127: What is the first step a surgical technologist should take when handling a specimen for pathology during an intraoperative procedure?
A) Label the specimen container immediately.
B) Verify the specimen with the surgeon.
C) Place the specimen in formalin.
D) Document the specimen in the patient's chart.

Question 128: During a preoperative team meeting, the surgeon, Dr. Smith, is explaining the surgical plan for Mr. Johnson, a patient scheduled for a complex abdominal surgery. As a Certified Surgical Technologist, how should you demonstrate effective listening skills to ensure you understand the surgical plan fully?
A) Nod occasionally and make eye contact with Dr. Smith.
B) Interrupt Dr. Smith to ask questions as soon as they arise.
C) Wait until the end of the explanation to ask clarifying questions.
D) Take detailed notes without making eye contact.

Question 129: During a surgical procedure, the surgical technologist needs to quickly access the patient's electronic health records (EHR) to verify the patient's allergy information. Which of the following steps should be taken to ensure the correct information is retrieved efficiently?
A) Ask the circulating nurse to verbally confirm the allergy information.
B) Use the computer in the operating room to access the EHR directly.
C) Wait until the surgeon has a break to check the patient's paper chart.
D) Call the hospital's medical records department for the information.

Question 130: Emily, a surgical technologist, needs to schedule a follow-up appointment for a patient post-surgery. Which of the following actions should she take using the hospital's computer system?
A) Write a note in the patient's paper chart and inform the front desk.
B) Directly enter the follow-up appointment into the hospital's scheduling software.
C) Call the patient to schedule the appointment and then update the system later.
D) Ask the surgeon to schedule the appointment and update the system.

Question 131: What is the primary purpose of using irrigation during a surgical procedure?
A) To maintain a clear view of the surgical site
B) To increase the temperature of the surgical site
C) To introduce antibiotics into the surgical site
D) To reduce the risk of air embolism

Question 132: Which muscle group is primarily involved in the extension of the knee joint?
A) Hamstrings
B) Quadriceps
C) Gastrocnemius
D) Gluteus Maximus

Question 133: John, a surgical technologist, is preparing for surgery and needs to perform a medical hand wash. Which of the following actions should he avoid to maintain proper aseptic technique?
A) Using an antimicrobial soap.
B) Keeping hands above elbows while rinsing.
C) Turning off the faucet with a clean paper towel.
D) Wearing jewelry during the wash.

Question 134: Which patient safety device is most appropriate for preventing pressure ulcers during lengthy surgical procedures?
A) Sequential compression device (SCD)
B) Anti-embolism stockings
C) Gel pads and positioning devices
D) Pulse oximeter

Question 135: During a thoracotomy procedure on Mr. Johnson, the surgeon asks you to identify the structure that separates the right and left pleural cavities. Which structure should you identify?
A) Diaphragm
B) Mediastinum
C) Pleural effusion
D) Pulmonary ligament

Question 136: During the disassembly of a surgical microscope post-procedure, which component should be handled with the utmost care to avoid damage?
A) The microscope's light bulb
B) The microscope's base
C) The microscope's objective lenses
D) The microscope's arm

Question 137: During a laparoscopic cholecystectomy on a 45-year-old patient named

Mr. Smith, the surgical team notices an unexpected increase in blood loss. What is the most appropriate initial action for the surgical technologist to take?
A) Increase the suction power to clear the surgical field.
B) Inform the surgeon and prepare for potential conversion to an open procedure.
C) Administer intravenous fluids to the patient.
D) Apply pressure to the bleeding site with a laparoscopic instrument.

Question 138: Emily, a surgical technologist, is preparing for a procedure and notices that the surgical drapes are nearing their expiration date. What should she do to follow proper cost containment processes?
A) Use the drapes immediately to avoid waste.
B) Discard the drapes and open new ones.
C) Notify the supervisor and follow the facility's protocol for near-expiration items.
D) Store the drapes for future use in non-critical procedures.

Question 139: Mrs. Smith has just undergone a total knee replacement and is now in the postoperative recovery room. What is the most important immediate postoperative care action to prevent complications?
A) Applying ice packs to the surgical site
B) Administering anticoagulants as prescribed
C) Encouraging early mobilization and physical therapy
D) Monitoring the surgical site for signs of infection

Question 140: During a neurosurgical procedure on Mr. Johnson, the surgical technologist is responsible for setting up the operating microscope. Which of the following steps is crucial to ensure the microscope remains sterile throughout the procedure?
A) Position the microscope before draping the patient.
B) Drape the microscope with a sterile cover before positioning it.
C) Adjust the microscope's focus before draping it.
D) Clean the microscope with a disinfectant before draping it.

Question 141: What is the primary purpose of using a pneumatic tourniquet during a surgical procedure?
A) To reduce blood loss by constricting blood flow to the surgical site
B) To enhance the visibility of the surgical site by expanding the blood vessels
C) To maintain a sterile field by isolating the surgical area
D) To prevent deep vein thrombosis by promoting blood circulation

Question 142: During a laparoscopic cholecystectomy, the patient, Mr. Johnson, needs to be positioned to allow optimal access to the surgical site. Which positioning device is most appropriate for maintaining the patient's position and ensuring safety?
A) Arm boards
B) Shoulder braces
C) Bean bag positioner
D) Stirrups

Question 143: 6 Which of the following best describes the mechanism by which Clostridium perfringens causes gas gangrene?
A) Production of endotoxins
B) Production of exotoxins
C) Production of biofilm
D) Production of spores

Question 144: Which document specifies a patient's wishes regarding medical treatment in situations where they are unable to communicate their decisions?
A) Living Will
B) Informed Consent
C) Surgical Consent
D) Discharge Summary

Question 145: A 45-year-old immunocompromised patient named John is scheduled for a laparoscopic cholecystectomy. Which of the following preoperative preparations is most critical to minimize the risk of infection?
A) Administering a broad-spectrum antibiotic immediately before the surgery.
B) Ensuring the patient has fasted for at least 8 hours before surgery.
C) Providing the patient with a high-protein diet the day before surgery.
D) Administering a vitamin C supplement to boost the immune system.

Question 146: A patient develops a rash around the surgical site 24 hours postoperatively. Which of the following is the most likely cause?
A) Allergic reaction to surgical drapes
B) Infection at the surgical site
C) Reaction to postoperative antibiotics
D) Contact dermatitis from adhesive dressings

Question 147: Which of the following is the most appropriate method for handling nondisposable surgical instruments immediately after a procedure?
A) Soak in saline solution
B) Rinse with sterile water
C) Place in a designated container for transport to decontamination
D) Wipe with a dry cloth

Question 148: Which of the following actions best demonstrates adherence to the Health Insurance Portability and Accountability Act (HIPAA) in a surgical setting?

A) Sharing patient information with a colleague who is not involved in the patient's care.
B) Discussing patient details in a public area of the hospital.
C) Accessing patient records only when necessary for patient care.
D) Leaving patient records unattended in a common area.

Question 149: A patient named Mary is undergoing a transsphenoidal hypophysectomy to remove a pituitary adenoma. Which hormone imbalance is the surgical technologist most likely to monitor for postoperatively?
A) Insulin
B) Cortisol
C) Thyroxine
D) Glucagon

Question 150: Which type of suture material is most appropriate for closing a contaminated wound to minimize the risk of infection?
A) Silk
B) Polypropylene
C) Chromic gut
D) Polyglycolic acid

ANSWER WITH DETAILED EXPLANATION SET [6]

Question 1: Correct Answer: B) Offer immediate assistance and communicate supportively.
Rationale: Offering immediate assistance and communicating supportively ensures the task is completed correctly and safely, fostering a collaborative environment. Ignoring the situation (A) can lead to errors, while reporting without intervening (C) delays resolution. Waiting to discuss privately (D) does not address the immediate need for assistance, potentially compromising patient safety.

Question 2: Correct Answer: D) To improve patient care and safety
Rationale: The primary reason for maintaining detailed surgical logs is to improve patient care and safety. Accurate logs ensure that all procedures are documented, which helps in tracking patient outcomes and identifying areas for improvement. While compliance with hospital policies (A), facilitating research (B), and legal documentation (C) are also important, the main focus is on enhancing patient care and safety.

Question 3: Correct Answer: B) Use forceps to place the scalpel blade in a sharps container.
Rationale: The appropriate action is to use forceps to place the scalpel blade in a sharps container, ensuring safe handling and disposal. Recapping the blade (Option A) increases the risk of needlestick injuries. Disposing of the blade in regular trash (Option C) is unsafe and non-compliant with Standard Precautions. Placing it on a tray for later disposal (Option D) increases the risk of accidental injury and contamination.

Question 4: Correct Answer: A) To reduce the risk of surgical site infections
Rationale: The primary reason for wiping down the room and furniture in the operating room is to reduce the risk of surgical site infections. This practice ensures that surfaces are free from pathogens that could potentially infect the surgical site. While making the room look clean (B) and complying with policies (C) are important, they are secondary to infection control. Removing visible dust and debris (D) is also necessary but does not address the primary goal of reducing microbial contamination.

Question 5: Correct Answer: C) Fibrin sealant
Rationale: Fibrin sealant is highly effective in achieving hemostasis on bone surfaces by mimicking the final stages of the coagulation cascade. Collagen (A) is also a hemostatic agent but is more effective on soft tissues rather than bone. Epinephrine (B) is a vasoconstrictor and not a hemostatic agent. Warfarin (D) is an anticoagulant and would exacerbate bleeding rather than control it. Therefore, fibrin sealant is the most suitable choice for controlling bleeding from the bone surface.

Question 6: Correct Answer: C) Assisting with the physical transfer of the patient
Rationale: The primary role of the surgical technologist during the transfer is to assist with the physical transfer of the patient, ensuring it is done safely and efficiently. Administering postoperative medications (A) and monitoring vital signs (B) are typically the responsibilities of the anesthesia provider or nurse. Documenting the procedure (D) is important but secondary to the immediate task of safely transferring the patient.

Question 7: Correct Answer: C) 0 absorbable suture.
Rationale: For closing the fascia, a 0 absorbable suture is typically used due to its strength and ability to be absorbed by the body over time. Option A and D are incorrect because non-absorbable sutures are not ideal for fascia closure. Option B is incorrect because a 2-0 suture is too small for this purpose. Therefore, Option C is the correct choice.

Question 8: Correct Answer: B) Discuss the errors with the colleague privately
Rationale: Discussing the errors privately with the colleague (Option B) is the most diplomatic approach, as it maintains professionalism and respects the colleague's dignity. Publicly correcting the colleague (Option A) can cause embarrassment and tension. Reporting the errors immediately (Option C) may be necessary if they pose a risk, but for minor errors, a private discussion is more appropriate. Ignoring the errors (Option D) does not address the issue and can lead to larger problems.

Question 9: Correct Answer: C) Apply direct pressure to the site.
Rationale: Applying direct pressure to the site is the most effective immediate action to control bleeding. Cold compresses (A) and elevating the limb (B) may help but are not as immediately effective. Administering pain medication (D) addresses discomfort but does not control bleeding. Direct pressure helps to reduce blood flow and allows clot formation, making it the most appropriate initial response.

Question 10: Correct Answer: C) By enabling electronic updates and easy access
Rationale: Computer technology enhances the management of surgeon's preference cards by allowing for electronic updates and easy access. This ensures that any changes in the surgeon's preferences are promptly reflected and accessible to the surgical team. Options A, B, and D are incorrect because they relate to other aspects of surgical management, such as patient monitoring, inventory control, and scheduling, rather than directly improving the efficiency of managing preference cards.

Question 11: Correct Answer: B) Osteotome
Rationale: An Osteotome is specifically designed for cutting or shaping bone, making it the correct choice. Mayo Scissors and Metzenbaum Scissors are used for cutting tissues, not bone. DeBakey Forceps are used for grasping delicate tissues and are not suitable for cutting bone. The Osteotome is the appropriate instrument for this intraoperative requirement.

Question 12: Correct Answer: D) Microfibrillar collagen
Rationale: Microfibrillar collagen, derived from bovine

sources, is used topically to control bleeding by promoting platelet aggregation. Fibrin glue is a synthetic adhesive, oxidized cellulose is a plant-based hemostatic agent, and absorbable gelatin sponge is derived from porcine sources. Thus, microfibrillar collagen is the correct answer.

Question 13: Correct Answer: B) Melanocytes
Rationale: Melanocytes are specialized cells in the epidermis responsible for producing melanin, the pigment that gives skin its color. Keratinocytes are the most abundant cells in the epidermis and produce keratin. Langerhans cells are involved in immune responses, and Merkel cells are associated with sensory reception. Only melanocytes produce melanin, distinguishing them from the other cell types.

Question 14: Correct Answer: C) Testing the light source
Rationale: Testing the light source is essential to ensure proper visualization during the procedure. While calibrating the insufflator (Option A) and ensuring adequate CO2 supply (Option D) are important, they do not directly impact the immediate functionality of the endoscope. Sterilizing the endoscope (Option B) is a standard practice but not specific to ensuring equipment functionality. Testing the light source directly impacts the ability to visualize the surgical field.

Question 15: Correct Answer: B) To reduce patient discomfort
Rationale: Proper lubrication of a Foley catheter is essential to reduce patient discomfort during insertion. While preventing infection (A) and ensuring proper drainage (C) are important, they are not the primary reasons for lubrication. Maintaining catheter sterility (D) is crucial but unrelated to lubrication. Lubrication primarily minimizes friction, making the insertion process smoother and less painful for the patient.

Question 16: Correct Answer: B) Facial nerve (CN VII)
Rationale: The facial nerve (CN VII) is the cranial nerve that runs through the parotid gland and must be avoided during a parotidectomy. The trigeminal nerve (CN V) is involved in facial sensation, the glossopharyngeal nerve (CN IX) in taste and swallowing, and the vagus nerve (CN X) in autonomic functions. Only the facial nerve (CN VII) is directly at risk during this procedure, making it the correct answer.

Question 17: Correct Answer: B) Hip retractor set
Rationale: A hip retractor set is crucial for total hip arthroplasty to provide adequate exposure of the hip joint. An arthroscope (A) is used in arthroscopic procedures, a laparotomy sponge (C) is for open abdominal surgeries, and a bronchoscope (D) is used for examining the airways. Proper selection of instruments ensures the procedure can be performed efficiently and safely, minimizing complications.

Question 18: Correct Answer: B) Notify the surgeon and document the findings.
Rationale: The immediate action should be to notify the surgeon and document the findings, as the rash could indicate an allergic reaction, infection, or other complications. Applying a topical antibiotic (A) or antiseptic solution (D) without a proper diagnosis could exacerbate the issue. Administering an antihistamine (C) may mask symptoms without addressing the underlying cause.

Question 19: Correct Answer: B) Surgical instruments
Rationale: Surgical instruments are nondisposable items that must be immediately removed from the sterile field and properly decontaminated after surgery to prevent cross-contamination and ensure patient safety. Surgical drapes, gloves, and sponges are typically disposable and should be discarded appropriately. The immediate decontamination of surgical instruments is crucial to maintaining a sterile environment and preventing infections.

Question 20: Correct Answer: B) Ball-and-socket joint
Rationale: The hip joint is a ball-and-socket joint, which allows for a wide range of motion in multiple directions. This type of joint consists of the head of the femur fitting into the acetabulum of the pelvis. Hinge joints, like the elbow, allow for movement in one plane. Pivot joints, such as the atlantoaxial joint, allow for rotational movement. Saddle joints, like the thumb joint, allow for movement in two planes. Understanding joint types is essential for surgical interventions involving joint repair or replacement.

Question 21: Correct Answer: B) Patient's past surgical procedures
Rationale: Confirming the patient's past surgical procedures is essential because it provides critical information about previous complications, anesthesia reactions, and any surgical implants or alterations. Employment history, travel history, and educational background, while potentially relevant in other contexts, do not provide necessary medical information that could impact the current surgical procedure. Understanding past surgeries helps in planning and anticipating potential issues during the current operation.

Question 22: Correct Answer: C) Stop the procedure and post the laser warning sign immediately.
Rationale: The laser warning sign is crucial for ensuring the safety of all personnel by alerting them to the presence of a laser in use. Continuing without the sign (Options A and B) compromises safety, and ignoring it (Option D) is negligent. Stopping the procedure to post the sign (Option C) ensures compliance with safety protocols, preventing potential harm.

Question 23: Correct Answer: A) Diaphragm
Rationale: The diaphragm is the primary muscle responsible for inhalation. When it contracts, it flattens and increases the volume of the thoracic cavity, allowing air to be drawn into the lungs. While intercostal muscles assist in expanding the rib cage, they are secondary to the diaphragm. Abdominal muscles and pectoralis major are not primarily involved in the inhalation process. Therefore, the diaphragm is the correct answer due to its essential role in breathing.

Question 24: Correct Answer: A) Babcock forceps
Rationale: Babcock forceps are designed to grasp delicate tissues without causing damage, making them ideal for manipulating the gallbladder during a laparoscopic cholecystectomy. Kelly clamps are used for clamping large blood vessels or tissues, Maryland dissectors are used for dissecting and grasping tissues, and Allis forceps are used for grasping and holding tissues but are more traumatic compared to Babcock forceps. Therefore, Babcock forceps are the most appropriate choice for this procedure.

Question 25: Correct Answer: B) Balfour retractor
Rationale: The Balfour retractor is a self-retaining retractor, ideal for abdominal surgeries to keep the incision open without needing constant manual adjustment. The Army-Navy, Deaver, and Richardson retractors are hand-held and require an assistant to hold them in place, making them less suitable for this scenario. The Balfour retractor's self-retaining feature allows the surgical team to focus on the procedure without worrying about maintaining retraction manually.

Question 26: Correct Answer: B) To provide temporary support and stabilization
Rationale: The primary purpose of applying a splint during the intraoperative phase is to provide temporary support and stabilization to the affected area. Unlike a cast, which is used for complete immobilization, a splint allows for some movement and swelling. Compression to reduce swelling is not the main function of a splint, and it is not intended for permanent fixation.

Question 27: Correct Answer: A) To maintain intraocular pressure
Rationale: The primary function of the aqueous humor is to maintain intraocular pressure, which is crucial for the eye's shape and proper function. It also provides nutrients to the lens and cornea, but not the retina. Visual information transmission is the role of the optic nerve, and light control is managed by the iris.

Question 28: Correct Answer: D) Quaternary ammonium compounds
Rationale: Quaternary ammonium compounds are most commonly recommended for wiping down operating room furniture and surfaces due to their broad-spectrum antimicrobial activity and low toxicity. Alcohol-based disinfectants (A) are effective but can evaporate quickly and are flammable. Chlorine bleach solutions (B) are effective but can be corrosive and irritating. Phenolic disinfectants (C) are effective but can leave residues and are less commonly used in modern surgical settings. Quaternary ammonium compounds provide a balance of efficacy and safety.

Question 29: Correct Answer: C) Circumflex Artery
Rationale: The Circumflex Artery supplies oxygenated blood to the left atrium and the left ventricle. The Right Coronary Artery primarily supplies the right side of the heart. The Left Anterior Descending Artery supplies the front of the left ventricle. The Pulmonary Artery carries deoxygenated blood from the right ventricle to the lungs. Thus, the Circumflex Artery is the correct vessel for supplying the left atrium and left ventricle.

Question 30: Correct Answer: C) Acknowledge each instruction verbally as it is given.
Rationale: Verbally acknowledging each instruction ensures that the surgeon knows Sarah has heard and understood the directives, which is crucial in a fast-paced surgical environment. Waiting to ask for clarification (A) can lead to delays. Interrupting (B) can disrupt the flow of the procedure. Writing down instructions (D) is impractical during surgery and doesn't confirm immediate understanding.

Question 31: Correct Answer: C) Suggest a brief pause to review the surgical plan and discuss the options.
Rationale: Suggesting a brief pause to review the surgical plan and discuss the options ensures that all team members are on the same page, maintaining diplomacy and patient safety. Siding with one party (Options A and B) can create tension and undermine teamwork. Ignoring the disagreement (Option D) can lead to errors and compromise patient care.

Question 32: Correct Answer: A) Shoulder Roll
Rationale: A shoulder roll is used to extend the neck, providing optimal exposure of the thyroid gland and maintaining the airway during a thyroidectomy. The bean bag is used for stabilizing the patient in lateral positions, the bolster is for supporting limbs or the back, and the Wilson frame is primarily for spinal surgeries. Thus, the shoulder roll is the most appropriate device for this procedure.

Question 33: Correct Answer: B) Immediately update the preference card to include the new suture material.
Rationale: The correct action is to immediately update the preference card to ensure that the surgical team has the most current information, which helps in preparing the necessary supplies for future surgeries. Waiting until the end of the month (Option A) or only updating upon request (Option D) could lead to errors or delays. Discussing with the team (Option C) is good practice but does not replace the need for immediate update.

Question 34: Correct Answer: B) Gram-negative bacilli
Rationale: Gram-negative bacilli are often responsible for rapid onset infections due to their endotoxin production, which can cause a sudden fever. Gram-positive cocci can also cause infections but are less likely to produce such a rapid fever. Acid-fast bacilli, such as Mycobacterium tuberculosis, cause chronic infections. Spirochetes, like Treponema pallidum, are typically associated with syphilis, which has a different clinical presentation. Therefore, Gram-negative bacilli are the most likely cause in this scenario.

Question 35: Correct Answer: A) Sending emails to team members
Rationale: Sending emails is a direct and professional way for a CST to communicate important information and updates within the surgical team. While team-building games and simulation software

have their uses, they do not serve the primary function of communication. Browsing social media is not appropriate in a professional setting, making option A the correct answer.

Question 36: Correct Answer: C) Involving the parents in the preoperative preparation
Rationale: Involving the parents in the preoperative preparation is crucial as it helps reduce the child's anxiety and ensures better cooperation. While fasting (A) and antibiotics (D) are important, they are not specific to pediatric needs. Explaining in medical terms (B) can confuse and scare the child. Parental involvement provides emotional support and helps the child feel more secure.

Question 37: Correct Answer: B) Report the discrepancy to the surgeon immediately.
Rationale: Reporting the discrepancy to the surgeon immediately is crucial to ensure patient safety and prevent retained surgical items. Ignoring the discrepancy (A) or waiting until the end of the procedure (D) can lead to severe complications. Attempting to resolve the discrepancy independently (C) is not advisable as it may delay necessary interventions and lacks the collaborative approach required in surgical settings.

Question 38: Correct Answer: C) Increase the room temperature to 68°F.
Rationale: The optimal operating room temperature for adult patients undergoing lengthy surgeries is typically between 68°F and 73°F to prevent hypothermia. Increasing the temperature to 68°F helps maintain normothermia, reducing the risk of complications. Option A (75°F) is too warm and can cause discomfort for the surgical team. Option B (65°F) is too low and increases the risk of hypothermia. Option D (60°F) further exacerbates the risk of hypothermia.

Question 39: Correct Answer: D) Deep vein thrombosis (DVT)
Rationale: Deep vein thrombosis (DVT) is the least likely cause of a red, raised, and itchy rash. DVT typically presents with symptoms such as swelling, pain, and redness in the affected limb, not a rash. Allergic reactions to medication (A), surgical site infections (B), and contact dermatitis from adhesives (C) are all plausible causes of postoperative rashes, making them more likely explanations.

Question 40: Correct Answer: B) Staphylococcus aureus
Rationale: Staphylococcus aureus is a Gram-positive cocci and a frequent cause of surgical site infections. Escherichia coli is a Gram-negative rod, Pseudomonas aeruginosa is a Gram-negative rod, and Candida albicans is a yeast. The correct classification and pathogenicity of Staphylococcus aureus make it the most accurate answer, while the other options represent different classes of microorganisms that are not primarily associated with surgical site infections.

Question 41: Correct Answer: B) Keeping hands above waist level
Rationale: Keeping hands above waist level is crucial to maintain sterility, as it prevents contamination from lower, non-sterile areas. While wearing double gloves (A) and using sterile drapes (C) are important, they do not directly address the risk of contamination from hand movements. Wearing a surgical mask (D) is essential for preventing respiratory contamination but does not directly impact hand sterility.

Question 42: Correct Answer: B) Notify the supervisor and follow the facility's spill response protocol.
Rationale: The first step in the event of a chemical spill is to notify the supervisor and follow the facility's spill response protocol. This ensures that the spill is managed safely and effectively. Evacuating immediately (A) might not be necessary and could cause unnecessary disruption. Attempting to clean the spill (C) without proper knowledge and equipment could be dangerous. Ignoring the spill (D) is never acceptable as it poses a safety hazard.

Question 43: Correct Answer: B) Thyroid gland
Rationale: The thyroid gland secretes thyroxine (T4) and triiodothyronine (T3), which regulate the body's metabolic rate. The adrenal gland secretes hormones like cortisol and adrenaline, the pancreas secretes insulin and glucagon for blood glucose regulation, and the parathyroid gland secretes PTH for calcium regulation. Hence, the thyroid gland is the correct answer as it directly affects metabolic rate.

Question 44: Correct Answer: B) Safety straps
Rationale: Safety straps are essential in ensuring proper patient positioning during surgery, which helps avoid nerve damage and other positioning-related injuries. Anti-embolism stockings (A) prevent blood clots, ECG leads (C) monitor heart activity, and a thermal blanket (D) maintains body temperature, but none of these directly address the issue of proper positioning and nerve damage prevention, making safety straps the correct choice.

Question 45: Correct Answer: B) Cerebellum
Rationale: The cerebellum is primarily responsible for coordinating voluntary movements and maintaining balance. The cerebrum is involved in higher brain functions such as thought and action, the medulla oblongata controls autonomic functions like breathing and heart rate, and the thalamus acts as a relay station for sensory and motor signals to the cerebral cortex. Therefore, the cerebellum is the correct answer due to its specific role in motor control and balance.

Question 46: Correct Answer: B) Inform the anesthesiologist and the surgical team about Mrs. Smith's insulin status.
Rationale: Informing the anesthesiologist and the surgical team about Mrs. Smith's insulin status is crucial for managing her blood glucose levels during surgery, ensuring patient safety. Option A could lead to hypoglycemia, Option C minimizes the importance of insulin management, and Option D ignores a critical aspect of preoperative care.

Question 47: Correct Answer: C) Inform the surgical team and potentially reschedule the surgery
Rationale: If a patient has not adhered to

preoperative fasting guidelines, it is crucial to inform the surgical team and potentially reschedule the surgery to minimize the risk of aspiration during anesthesia. Options A, B, and D are incorrect because proceeding with surgery, administering a laxative, or allowing clear fluids could increase the risk of complications. The correct action ensures patient safety.

Question 48: Correct Answer: B) Ensuring the suture material is within its expiration date

Rationale: Ensuring the suture material is within its expiration date is crucial for maintaining sterility and integrity. Using non-sterile gloves (A), cutting with non-sterile scissors (C), and storing in a non-sterile environment (D) all compromise sterility. The expiration date ensures the material hasn't degraded and remains sterile.

Question 49: Correct Answer: C) Carbon dioxide

Rationale: Dr. Johnson's preference card specifies the use of carbon dioxide for insufflation during laparoscopic procedures due to its rapid absorption and minimal risk of gas embolism. Nitrous oxide (A) is not used due to its potential to support combustion. Oxygen (B) is not used for insufflation as it can cause combustion and is not absorbed as efficiently. Helium (D) is rarely used due to its high cost and limited availability. Therefore, carbon dioxide is the correct choice.

Question 50: Correct Answer: B) Assessing the patient's nutritional deficiencies

Rationale: Assessing the patient's nutritional deficiencies is crucial because bariatric patients often have underlying deficiencies that can affect healing and recovery. Ensuring proper nutrition preoperatively can reduce complications. While fasting (A) is important, it is standard for all surgeries. Weight loss history (C) and psychological readiness (D) are also important but secondary to addressing immediate nutritional needs.

Question 51: Correct Answer: D) Documenting it in the patient's chart and applying an allergy alert bracelet

Rationale: Best practice involves both documenting the allergy in the patient's chart and applying an allergy alert bracelet to ensure all team members are aware and can take appropriate precautions. Simply noting it in the chart or informing the surgeon verbally can lead to oversights. The bracelet serves as a constant, visible reminder.

Question 52: Correct Answer: B) Ovaries

Rationale: The ovaries are responsible for the production of estrogen and progesterone, which are crucial for regulating the menstrual cycle and supporting pregnancy. Option A is incorrect as the fallopian tubes transport the ova. Option C is incorrect because the uterus is where the fertilized egg implants and grows. Option D is incorrect as the cervix is the lower part of the uterus that opens into the vagina. Therefore, the correct structure for hormone production is the ovaries.

Question 53: Correct Answer: B) Verifying the shaver handpiece is properly connected to the power source.

Rationale: Verifying the shaver handpiece is properly connected to the power source is critical to ensure the device functions during surgery. While securing the shaver blade (A) and testing the suction (C) and irrigation (D) systems are important, they are secondary to ensuring the device is powered and operational. Without power, the shaver cannot function, making this the most crucial step.

Question 54: Correct Answer: C) Pass the instrument with the tips pointing towards the surgeon.

Rationale: The correct way to pass a Maryland dissector is with the tips pointing towards the surgeon to ensure the surgeon can immediately use the instrument without repositioning. Passing with tips upwards (A) or downwards (B) can cause delays or accidents. Passing with tips away from the surgeon (D) is incorrect as it requires the surgeon to adjust the instrument, leading to inefficiency and potential contamination.

Question 55: Correct Answer: B) Notify the surgeon immediately

Rationale: The most appropriate initial action is to notify the surgeon immediately, as a hematoma can indicate significant bleeding that may require surgical intervention. Applying a warm compress (A) or massaging the hematoma (C) can exacerbate the condition, and increasing IV fluids (D) does not address the underlying issue. Immediate surgeon notification ensures prompt evaluation and appropriate management.

Question 56: Correct Answer: B) Mediastinum

Rationale: The mediastinum is the central compartment of the thoracic cavity that separates the right and left pleural cavities. The diaphragm (A) separates the thoracic and abdominal cavities, pleural effusion (C) is a condition rather than a structure, and the pericardium (D) surrounds the heart. Thus, the mediastinum is the correct structure that separates the pleural cavities.

Question 57: Correct Answer: B) Thrombin

Rationale: Thrombin is a potent hemostatic agent used to control minor bleeding during surgeries. It works by converting fibrinogen to fibrin, thus promoting clot formation. Epinephrine is primarily a vasoconstrictor, silver nitrate is used for cauterization of small wounds, and acetic acid is not used for hemostasis. Thrombin is specifically designed for intraoperative hemostasis, making it the most appropriate choice.

Question 58: Correct Answer: C) Communicating with the surgical team about upcoming procedures

Rationale: The most critical step Sarah should take is communicating with the surgical team about upcoming procedures. This ensures she is aware of specific instrument needs and can prepare accordingly. While conducting weekly inventory checks (A) and relying on usage patterns (B) are helpful, they may not account for special requirements. Ordering extra instruments (D) can lead to unnecessary costs and storage issues. Communication ensures precise and efficient preparation.

Question 59: Correct Answer: B) By providing real-time updates on patient status

Rationale: Providing real-time updates on patient status is a key way computer technology enhances communication within a surgical team. This ensures that all team members are informed about the patient's condition and any changes during surgery. Automating procedures (A) and scheduling surgeries (D) without human intervention are not practical or safe. Replacing face-to-face meetings with emails (C) might reduce effective communication. Real-time updates facilitate timely decision-making and coordinated care.

Question 60: Correct Answer: B) Alveoli

Rationale: The alveoli are tiny air sacs in the lungs where gas exchange occurs. Oxygen diffuses into the blood, and carbon dioxide diffuses out. The bronchi and trachea are airways that conduct air to the lungs but do not participate in gas exchange. The pleura is a membrane surrounding the lungs, providing lubrication but not involved in gas exchange. Therefore, alveoli are the correct answer due to their direct role in gas exchange.

Question 61: Correct Answer: C) Pass the scalpel handle-first into the surgeon's hand

Rationale: The correct method for passing a scalpel is handle-first to ensure the surgeon can safely grasp it without risk of injury. Option A is incorrect as direct hand-to-hand passing increases the risk of accidental cuts. Option B is not ideal because it disrupts the workflow. Option D is dangerous as it presents the blade first, increasing the risk of injury.

Question 62: Correct Answer: C) Saphenous vein

Rationale: The saphenous vein is commonly harvested for use in coronary artery bypass grafting (CABG) due to its length and accessibility. The femoral vein is a deep vein in the thigh, the cephalic vein is located in the arm, and the jugular vein is in the neck. Understanding the appropriate vein for grafting is essential for surgical technologists to assist effectively in cardiovascular surgeries.

Question 63: Correct Answer: A) Use latex-free gloves and equipment.

Rationale: The correct action is to use latex-free gloves and equipment to prevent any allergic reaction. While informing the anesthesiologist (Option D) is important, it does not directly prevent exposure. Administering antihistamines (Option B) may help manage symptoms but does not eliminate the risk. Scheduling the surgery in a latex-free operating room (Option C) is ideal but not always feasible. The primary and most immediate action is to ensure all materials used are latex-free.

Question 64: Correct Answer: B) To keep the surgical field clear of debris and blood

Rationale: Irrigation is primarily used to keep the surgical field clear of debris and blood, ensuring better visibility for the surgeon. Cooling down instruments (A) is not the main purpose, sterilizing the site (C) is achieved through other means, and providing nutrients to the tissue (D) is not a function of irrigation. The primary goal is to maintain a clear operative field

for optimal surgical outcomes.

Question 65: Correct Answer: B) Actively listening to all team members and acknowledging their input.

Rationale: Actively listening to all team members and acknowledging their input (Option B) demonstrates effective diplomacy as it fosters an inclusive environment and encourages collaboration. Dominating the conversation (Option A) can stifle others' contributions. Avoiding difficult conversations (Option C) can lead to unresolved issues. Making decisions independently (Option D) can alienate team members. Effective diplomacy involves valuing and integrating diverse perspectives.

Question 66: Correct Answer: C) Maintaining the allograft in a sterile, cold saline solution

Rationale: Maintaining the allograft in a sterile, cold saline solution preserves its viability and prevents contamination. Keeping it at room temperature (A) can compromise its integrity. Dry heat sterilization (B) is inappropriate as it can damage the tissue. Exposing it to ambient air (D) increases the risk of contamination. Cold saline helps maintain the graft's cellular and structural integrity, ensuring its effectiveness during implantation.

Question 67: Correct Answer: B) Improved accuracy of patient data

Rationale: A key benefit of using electronic health records (EHRs) in surgical research is the improved accuracy of patient data. EHRs ensure that data is up-to-date and easily accessible, which enhances research quality. Increased patient wait times (A) and higher costs of data storage (C) are not benefits, and reduced need for surgical instruments (D) is unrelated to EHRs.

Question 68: Correct Answer: A) Hand the instrument to the surgeon herself and then assist John.

Rationale: The best approach is for Sarah to hand the instrument to the surgeon herself to avoid any delay and then assist John. This maintains the efficiency of the operation and supports the new team member. Ignoring John (B) or pressuring him (C) could lead to mistakes, and suggesting a break (D) is unnecessary and could disrupt the procedure.

Question 69: Correct Answer: B) Allowing the drape to touch non-sterile surfaces

Rationale: Allowing the drape to touch non-sterile surfaces compromises the sterile field, increasing the risk of infection. Handling the drape with sterile gloves (A), using a drape with adhesive edges (C), and covering the entire surgical site (D) are all correct practices that help maintain sterility. Avoiding contact with non-sterile surfaces is essential to ensure the integrity of the sterile field.

Question 70: Correct Answer: C) Iliac crest

Rationale: The iliac crest is a common site for harvesting autografts due to its rich supply of cancellous bone, which is ideal for grafting. While the tibia and femur can also be used, they are less common and typically provide less cancellous bone. The scapula is not a standard site for bone graft harvesting. This makes the iliac crest the most suitable and commonly used site for autografts in bone grafting procedures.

Question 71: Correct Answer: B) To verify the effectiveness of the sterilization process

Rationale: Biological indicators are used to verify the effectiveness of the sterilization process by using highly resistant bacterial spores. This ensures that the sterilization process is capable of killing all forms of microbial life. Measuring temperature, ensuring the sterilizer is not overloaded, and monitoring humidity levels are important but do not directly confirm the efficacy of the sterilization process.

Question 72: Correct Answer: B) Use the closed glove technique

Rationale: The closed glove technique is the best practice for ensuring sterility while donning gloves after gowning, as it keeps the hands covered by the gown sleeves, reducing the risk of contamination. Option A is incorrect as the open glove technique is used when not wearing a gown. Option C is plausible but less commonly used. Option D is incorrect as bare hands would compromise sterility.

Question 73: Correct Answer: A) Axillary lymph nodes

Rationale: The primary lymphatic drainage site for the right breast is the axillary lymph nodes. This is because the majority of the lymph from the breast drains into the axillary lymph nodes. Inguinal lymph nodes are associated with the lower extremities, cervical lymph nodes with the head and neck, and popliteal lymph nodes with the lower leg, making them incorrect options.

Question 74: Correct Answer: B) Use of bipolar electrosurgery

Rationale: Bipolar electrosurgery is highly effective for achieving hemostasis during laparoscopic cholecystectomy due to its precision and ability to coagulate tissue without extensive thermal spread. Topical thrombin (A) is more suitable for surface bleeding, bone wax (C) is used primarily in orthopedic procedures, and a tourniquet (D) is inappropriate for laparoscopic procedures. Bipolar electrosurgery provides controlled coagulation, minimizing collateral damage and ensuring effective hemostasis.

Question 75: Correct Answer: A) Common bile duct

Rationale: The common bile duct is most at risk of injury during the dissection of dense adhesions around the gallbladder due to its close proximity. The hepatic artery and portal vein are also nearby but are less likely to be damaged unless the dissection extends beyond the gallbladder area. The cystic duct is involved in the procedure but is not as critical as the common bile duct, which can lead to severe complications if injured.

Question 76: Correct Answer: B) Open the suture package and place it on the sterile field.

Rationale: The correct first step is to open the suture package and place it on the sterile field. This ensures the suture remains sterile and ready for use. Passing the suture directly to the surgeon (A) or cutting it to length (C) before opening the package could compromise sterility. Threading the suture onto a needle holder (D) is a subsequent step, not the initial one.

Question 77: Correct Answer: B) It minimizes thermal damage to surrounding tissues.

Rationale: The primary advantage of using a CO2 beam coagulator is that it minimizes thermal damage to surrounding tissues due to its precise control and limited depth of penetration. Option A is incorrect because deep tissue penetration is not a characteristic of CO2 beam coagulators. Option C is incorrect as cost-effectiveness varies and is not the primary advantage. Option D is incorrect because while it may reduce infection risk, this is not the primary advantage. ---

Question 78: Correct Answer: B) Notify the surgeon and prepare emergency medications.

Rationale: The immediate action is to notify the surgeon and prepare emergency medications, as this ensures that the patient receives prompt and appropriate treatment. Administering epinephrine (A) should be done by the anesthesiologist or surgeon. Increasing oxygen flow (C) is supportive but not sufficient alone. Stopping the procedure and calling for an anesthesiologist (D) delays immediate intervention. The correct approach prioritizes rapid communication and preparation for emergency treatment.

Question 79: Correct Answer: C) Topical hemostatic agents

Rationale: Topical hemostatic agents are primarily used to control diffuse oozing from capillaries and small vessels by promoting clot formation at the site of bleeding. Suturing (A) and ligation (D) are more suitable for larger vessels, while hemostatic clips (B) are used for specific vessel occlusion. Topical agents like gelatin sponges or oxidized cellulose are ideal for capillary oozing.

Question 80: Correct Answer: B) 121-134°C

Rationale: The recommended temperature range for steam sterilization in an autoclave is 121-134°C. This range ensures effective microbial destruction. Options A and D are incorrect as they are in Fahrenheit, not Celsius, and do not meet the necessary temperature for sterilization. Option C exceeds the recommended range, risking damage to instruments.

Question 81: Correct Answer: B) Pass the needle holder with the needle pointing away from the surgeon

Rationale: Passing the needle holder with the needle pointing away from the surgeon minimizes the risk of accidental injury. Option A is incorrect because it increases the risk of needle stick injuries. Option C disrupts the surgical flow and is not efficient. Option D is unsafe as it disregards proper needle orientation, increasing the risk of injury.

Question 82: Correct Answer: A) Lower risk of disease transmission

Rationale: Synthetic bone grafts are advantageous because they eliminate the risk of disease transmission, which is a concern with autografts and allografts. While options B) and C) might seem plausible, synthetic grafts generally do not have higher osteogenic potential or faster integration compared to natural grafts. Option D) is incorrect because the surgical time is not significantly reduced by using synthetic grafts.

Question 83: Correct Answer: C) Pre-cleaning instruments thoroughly before sterilization

Rationale: Pre-cleaning instruments thoroughly before sterilization is crucial to remove any organic material that can inhibit the sterilization process. Using a high concentration of sterilizing agent (A) is not relevant to flash sterilization. Wrapping instruments tightly (B) is not recommended as it can impede steam penetration. Placing instruments in a dry container (D) is less critical than ensuring they are clean, making option C the correct choice.

Question 84: Correct Answer: C) Chemical-resistant gloves

Rationale: Chemical-resistant gloves are most critical when dealing with a chemical spill to protect the skin from harmful substances. Surgical masks and sterile gloves do not provide adequate protection against chemicals, and a lead apron is irrelevant in this context. Proper PPE is crucial for ensuring safety and preventing contamination or injury.

Question 85: Correct Answer: A) To prevent deep vein thrombosis (DVT)

Rationale: Sequential compression devices (SCDs) are primarily used to prevent deep vein thrombosis (DVT) by promoting venous return and reducing venous stasis. While they do not directly reduce pain, enhance wound healing, or maintain body temperature, they play a critical role in preventing postoperative complications related to blood clots.

Question 86: Correct Answer: A) To prevent the patient from falling off the operating table

Rationale: The primary purpose of a safety strap is to secure the patient to the operating table to prevent falls and ensure stability during surgery. While maintaining sterility (Option B) and monitoring vital signs (Option C) are crucial, they are not the functions of a safety strap. Providing comfort (Option D) is secondary to the safety and stability the strap ensures.

Question 87: Correct Answer: B) Immediately inform the surgeon and halt the procedure until the issue is resolved.

Rationale: The correct action is to immediately inform the surgeon and halt the procedure until the grounding issue is resolved to prevent electrical burns or other injuries. Continuing the surgery (Option A) or adjusting the grounding pad without informing the surgeon (Option C) could lead to severe patient harm. Ignoring the issue (Option D) is unsafe and unprofessional.

Question 88: Correct Answer: B) To maintain an accurate patient medical record

Rationale: Accurately reporting the amount of medication and solution used is crucial for maintaining an accurate patient medical record, which is essential for postoperative care and future medical reference. While proper billing (A), inventory management (C), and preventing theft (D) are important, they are secondary to the primary goal of ensuring patient safety and continuity of care through accurate medical records.

Question 89: Correct Answer: B) Alveoli

Rationale: The alveoli are tiny air sacs within the lungs where the exchange of oxygen and carbon dioxide occurs. Unlike the bronchi and bronchioles, which primarily serve as air passageways, the alveoli have thin walls that allow for efficient gas exchange. The trachea is the main airway but does not participate in gas exchange. Thus, alveoli are the correct answer due to their specialized structure and function.

Question 90: Correct Answer: B) Electrocautery

Rationale: Electrocautery is the most appropriate thermal method for achieving hemostasis during a laparoscopic cholecystectomy. It uses electrical current to generate heat, effectively coagulating blood vessels. Cryotherapy (A) is used for freezing tissues, not for immediate hemostasis. Laser coagulation (C) can be used but is less common and more complex. Ultrasonic scalpel (D) is effective for cutting and coagulation but is not as commonly used for direct hemostasis of vessels like the cystic artery.

Question 91: Correct Answer: C) Supine

Rationale: The supine position is most commonly used for abdominal surgeries as it provides optimal access to the abdominal cavity. The lithotomy position is typically used for gynecological and urological procedures. The prone position is used for surgeries on the back or posterior aspect of the body. Trendelenburg position, where the body is laid flat on the back with the feet higher than the head, is used to improve venous return but not specifically for abdominal access.

Question 92: Correct Answer: C) Discard the vial and obtain a new one with a clear label.

Rationale: The correct action is to discard the vial and obtain a new one with a clear label to ensure patient safety and proper medication administration. Administering the medication based on a partially visible label (Option A) or asking the surgeon to verify (Option B) can lead to errors. Consulting the circulating nurse (Option D) is not as definitive as discarding and replacing the vial, which ensures the label is fully legible and accurate.

Question 93: Correct Answer: B) Ensuring the stapler is properly aligned with the incision

Rationale: Ensuring the stapler is properly aligned with the incision is crucial to avoid improper wound closure and potential complications. While loading the stapler (A) and handing it to the surgeon (C) are important, they do not directly impact the precision of the stapling. Removing the staples (D) is a post-operative task, not intraoperative. Proper alignment ensures effective wound closure, reducing the risk of infection and promoting better healing.

Question 94: Correct Answer: B) Breast cancer

Rationale: The BRCA1 and BRCA2 gene mutations are most commonly linked to an increased risk of breast cancer. These genes are responsible for repairing DNA damage, and their mutations can lead to uncontrolled cell growth in breast tissue. While

BRCA mutations can also increase the risk of ovarian and prostate cancers, they are most strongly associated with breast cancer. Lung and colon cancers are not typically linked to BRCA mutations.

Question 95: Correct Answer: B) Administering prophylactic antibiotics

Rationale: Administering prophylactic antibiotics is crucial for immunocompromised patients to prevent postoperative infections due to their weakened immune systems. While hydration (A), surgery timing (C), and nutrition (D) are important, they do not directly address the heightened risk of infection. Prophylactic antibiotics specifically target this increased vulnerability, making it the most critical consideration.

Question 96: Correct Answer: B) The power cord connection.

Rationale: The first step in troubleshooting an ESU that stops working is to check the power cord connection. Ensuring that the unit is properly plugged in can quickly resolve the issue. While grounding pad placement (A) and ESU settings (C) are important, they are secondary checks. Checking the patient's vital signs (D) is crucial for patient safety but does not directly address the equipment malfunction.

Question 97: Correct Answer: C) Uterine Artery

Rationale: The uterine artery is the correct vessel to clamp to control the blood supply to the uterus during a hysterectomy. The renal artery (A) supplies the kidneys, the pulmonary artery (B) carries blood from the heart to the lungs, and the femoral artery (D) supplies blood to the lower limb. Correct identification of the uterine artery is essential for minimizing blood loss during the procedure.

Question 98: Correct Answer: C) To inhibit the growth of certain microorganisms while allowing others to grow

Rationale: Selective culture media contain agents that inhibit the growth of certain bacteria while promoting the growth of others, making it easier to isolate specific types of microorganisms. Enhancing growth of all microorganisms (A) and providing a nutrient-rich environment (D) are not selective. Differentiation (B) is achieved by differential media, not selective media.

Question 99: Correct Answer: C) Replace the flickering light before the surgery begins.

Rationale: Replacing the flickering light before the surgery begins ensures consistent and reliable lighting throughout the procedure, which is critical for the surgical team's performance. Ignoring the flickering light (A) or attempting to fix it during surgery (B) can compromise the surgical field's visibility and patient safety. Using a flashlight (D) is impractical and inadequate for surgical lighting needs. Therefore, ensuring all lights are functioning correctly before surgery is essential for maintaining a safe and effective operating environment.

Question 100: Correct Answer: B) Hemostatic clips

Rationale: Hemostatic clips are the most effective mechanical method for achieving hemostasis in laparoscopic procedures, especially for controlling arterial bleeding. Electrocautery (A) is not a mechanical method but an electrical one. Topical thrombin (C) and fibrin sealant (D) are chemical agents, not mechanical methods. Hemostatic clips provide immediate and reliable control of bleeding by mechanically occluding the vessel.

Question 101: Correct Answer: B) Ensuring adequate hydration

Rationale: Ensuring adequate hydration is crucial for reducing the risk of postoperative delirium in elderly patients. Dehydration can exacerbate cognitive dysfunction and lead to delirium. Administering high doses of sedatives can increase the risk, while increasing physical activity and providing detailed surgical information, although beneficial, do not directly address the hydration status, which is a key factor in preventing delirium.

Question 102: Correct Answer: C) Compress the bulb of the Jackson-Pratt drain before securing the cap.

Rationale: Compressing the bulb creates a vacuum necessary for effective suction. Options A and B are incorrect as they do not pertain to the Jackson-Pratt drain's function. Option D is incorrect because it fails to create the needed vacuum for drainage.

Question 103: Correct Answer: B) Checking the camera's white balance and focus.

Rationale: Ensuring the camera's white balance and focus are correct is crucial for clear visualization during the procedure. While sterilization (A), battery charge (C), and cable connection (D) are important, they do not directly affect the camera's ability to provide a clear image. Proper white balance and focus ensure accurate color representation and sharpness, which are essential for the surgeon's visual guidance.

Question 104: Correct Answer: C) Parathyroid hormone (PTH)

Rationale: Parathyroid hormone (PTH) is crucial for regulating calcium levels in the blood by increasing calcium absorption in the intestines, reabsorption in the kidneys, and releasing calcium from bones. Insulin regulates blood glucose levels, cortisol is involved in stress response and metabolism, and thyroxine regulates metabolism. Thus, PTH is the correct answer as it directly influences calcium homeostasis.

Question 105: Correct Answer: B) Fold the drapes inward to contain any contaminants.

Rationale: Folding the drapes inward helps to contain any contaminants and prevent them from spreading. Option A is incorrect because the sterile field is no longer needed postoperatively. Option C is incorrect as placing drapes on the floor is not a sterile practice. Option D is incorrect because shaking the drapes can spread contaminants and is unsafe.

Question 106: Correct Answer: A) Pass the hemostat with the ratchets closed.

Rationale: The correct method is to pass the hemostat with the ratchets closed to ensure the surgeon can immediately use it without adjusting the instrument. Passing it with the ratchets open (B) could delay the procedure. Tips pointing towards the technologist (C) or the patient (D) can cause injury or contamination.

Question 107: Correct Answer: A) Periodically check the retractor's tension and adjust as needed.

Rationale: Periodically checking the retractor's tension and adjusting as needed ensures that the surgical field remains properly exposed and reduces the risk of tissue damage. Option B is incorrect as retractors may need repositioning. Option C is incorrect because different tissues may require different retractors. Option D is incorrect as the surgical technologist should assist in maintaining retractors to allow the surgeon to focus on the procedure.

Question 108: Correct Answer: B) Inform the circulating nurse and test the insufflator.

Rationale: The correct action is to inform the circulating nurse and test the insufflator. Testing the insufflator ensures it is functioning properly, which is crucial for maintaining pneumoperitoneum during laparoscopic procedures. Ignoring the issue (Option A) or waiting for the surgeon (Option C) can delay the surgery and compromise patient safety. Using a different insufflator without testing (Option D) also poses a risk as it may not be functioning correctly.

Question 109: Correct Answer: B) Keeping the autograft moist with saline solution

Rationale: Keeping the autograft moist with saline solution is essential to maintain its viability and prevent desiccation. Sterilizing with high heat (A) or using an autoclave (C) would damage the living cells in the graft. Freezing the autograft (D) is not standard practice and could affect cell viability. Therefore, maintaining moisture with saline is the correct approach.

Question 110: Correct Answer: A) Deltoid

Rationale: The deltoid muscle is primarily responsible for the abduction of the arm at the shoulder joint. The biceps brachii mainly flexes the elbow and supinates the forearm, while the triceps brachii extends the elbow. The latissimus dorsi is involved in the adduction, extension, and internal rotation of the shoulder. Therefore, the deltoid is the correct answer as it specifically facilitates arm abduction.

Question 111: Correct Answer: A) Reduced thermal damage to surrounding tissues

Rationale: CO2 beam coagulators are highly precise, minimizing thermal damage to surrounding tissues, which is crucial for patient recovery. Unlike options B, C, and D, which are incorrect, CO2 beam coagulators actually reduce the risk of infection, blood loss, and recovery time due to their precision and efficiency in coagulating tissues.

Question 112: Correct Answer: A) Conducting a preoperative checklist

Rationale: Conducting a preoperative checklist is the most important step in ensuring that all necessary supplies are available for a surgical procedure. This systematic approach helps to verify that nothing is overlooked. Consulting with the anesthesiologist (B) and reviewing the patient's chart (C) are important for patient care but do not directly ensure the availability

of supplies. Sterilizing the instruments (D) is crucial for infection control but is a separate process from verifying supply availability.

Question 113: Correct Answer: A) Hernia

Rationale: A hernia is the abnormal protrusion of an organ or tissue through the structure that usually contains it. Adhesions are bands of scar tissue that bind together normally separate anatomical structures. A fistula is an abnormal connection between two body parts, such as organs or vessels. An abscess is a collection of pus that has built up within the tissue of the body. Thus, hernia is the correct answer as it directly describes the condition of abnormal protrusion.

Question 114: Correct Answer: B) To confirm the implant is the correct one for the specific surgical procedure

Rationale: Verifying the type and size of an implantable item with the surgeon ensures that the correct implant is used for the specific surgical procedure, which is crucial for the success of the surgery and patient safety. Options A, C, and D are important but secondary considerations. Ensuring insurance coverage, availability, and sterilization are essential, but the primary concern is the appropriateness of the implant for the procedure.

Question 115: Correct Answer: B) Use a smoke evacuation system

Rationale: The most appropriate immediate action is to use a smoke evacuation system to remove the smoke from the surgical site, ensuring safety and visibility. Increasing insufflation pressure (A) does not address smoke removal. Opening the operating room doors (C) could introduce contaminants. Increasing oxygen flow (D) is unrelated to smoke evacuation and could pose a fire risk. Smoke evacuation systems are designed specifically for this purpose, making option B the correct choice.

Question 116: Correct Answer: C) Ensure the retractor is not under excessive tension

Rationale: Maintaining a retractor without excessive tension is crucial to prevent tissue damage and ensure optimal visibility for the surgeon. Frequent adjustments (A) can be disruptive, and cleaning with saline (B) is not typically necessary unless contamination occurs. Replacing the retractor every 30 minutes (D) is impractical and unnecessary. Proper tension management ensures that tissues are held apart effectively without causing harm, maintaining a clear surgical field.

Question 117: Correct Answer: B) Thoroughly clean and disinfect all surfaces and equipment.

Rationale: Thoroughly cleaning and disinfecting all surfaces and equipment (B) is crucial to prevent cross-contamination and infection. Quickly wiping down surfaces (A) is inadequate. Leaving cleaning to housekeeping staff (C) without ensuring thorough disinfection compromises safety. Filing patient records (D) is important but secondary to ensuring a sterile environment. Proper room turnover prioritizes patient safety through thorough disinfection.

Question 118: Correct Answer: B) Femoral artery

Rationale: The femoral artery is the major blood vessel supplying blood to the lower extremities. The brachial artery supplies the upper arm, the radial artery supplies the forearm and hand, and the carotid artery supplies the head and neck. Therefore, while the other options are plausible, they do not supply the lower extremities, making the femoral artery the correct answer.

Question 119: Correct Answer: D) Testes

Rationale: The testes are responsible for the production of sperm and the hormone testosterone. The epididymis (A) stores and matures sperm, the seminal vesicle (B) produces seminal fluid, and the prostate gland (C) secretes prostate fluid, a component of semen. Understanding the distinct functions of these structures is crucial for surgical technologists in procedures involving the male reproductive system.

Question 120: Correct Answer: B) Encrypting sensitive information before transmission

Rationale: Encrypting sensitive information before transmission ensures that only authorized personnel can access the data, maintaining confidentiality. Shared login credentials (A) compromise security, and public forums (C) expose sensitive information to unauthorized individuals. Solely relying on verbal communication (D) is impractical and can lead to information loss or misinterpretation. Encryption is a key practice for protecting patient and departmental data.

Question 121: Correct Answer: B) Using a steam autoclave cycle specifically designed for delicate instruments.

Rationale: The most appropriate method for sterilizing laparoscopic instruments is using a steam autoclave cycle designed for delicate instruments. This ensures that the instruments are sterilized without damage. Option A does not provide sterilization, only disinfection. Option C is insufficient for sterilization, and Option D, while a sterilization method, is not suitable for delicate instruments and may cause damage.

Question 122: Correct Answer: A) Arterial bleeding

Rationale: Bright red blood is indicative of arterial bleeding due to its high oxygen content. Venous bleeding (Option B) appears darker due to lower oxygen levels. Capillary bleeding (Option C) is usually slow and oozing, not bright red. Coagulated blood (Option D) is dark and clotted, not bright red. Recognizing the color difference is crucial for prompt and appropriate intervention.

Question 123: Correct Answer: A) Suggest extending the incision for better access.

Rationale: Extending the incision provides better access and visualization of the retrocecal appendix, facilitating its removal. Converting to a laparoscopic approach (Option B) is not practical mid-procedure. Providing a longer instrument set (Option C) may help but is secondary to gaining better access. Stopping the procedure (Option D) is unnecessary when the anomaly can be managed surgically with an extended incision.

Question 124: Correct Answer: C) Remove and segregate nondisposable instruments.

Rationale: The first step after surgery is to remove and segregate nondisposable instruments to ensure they are not accidentally discarded and can be properly cleaned and sterilized. Removing drapes (A) and disposing of sharps (B) should follow, and wiping down the surgical lights (D) is part of the room turnover process, not immediate postoperative care.

Question 125: Correct Answer: B) Electrocautery

Rationale: Electrocautery is the most commonly used thermal method for achieving hemostasis during laparoscopic surgery due to its effectiveness and precision. Cryotherapy is less commonly used in laparoscopic procedures as it is more suited for surface lesions. Laser coagulation is effective but less common due to its cost and complexity. The ultrasonic scalpel is used for cutting and coagulation but is less common than electrocautery for primary hemostasis.

Question 126: Correct Answer: A) Linear cutter stapler

Rationale: The linear cutter stapler is specifically designed for gastrointestinal surgeries, including bowel anastomosis, as it cuts and staples simultaneously, ensuring a secure and precise closure. Skin staplers are for external skin closure, ligating clip appliers are for vessel ligation, and hemorrhoidal staplers are for rectal procedures, making them unsuitable for bowel anastomosis.

Question 127: Correct Answer: B) Verify the specimen with the surgeon.

Rationale: The first step is to verify the specimen with the surgeon to ensure correct identification. This prevents errors in labeling and processing. Labeling the container (Option A) and placing the specimen in formalin (Option C) come after verification. Documenting the specimen (Option D) is also important but occurs later in the process. Verification ensures accuracy and prevents misidentification.

Question 128: Correct Answer: C) Wait until the end of the explanation to ask clarifying questions.

Rationale: Waiting until the end of the explanation to ask clarifying questions demonstrates active listening and respect for the speaker. It ensures that you have heard the entire plan before seeking clarification, which can prevent misunderstandings. Nodding and making eye contact (A) shows engagement but does not ensure understanding. Interrupting (B) can disrupt the flow of information and taking notes without eye contact (D) may miss non-verbal cues.

Question 129: Correct Answer: B) Use the computer in the operating room to access the EHR directly.

Rationale: Using the computer in the operating room to access the EHR directly is the most efficient and accurate method to retrieve the patient's allergy information. This ensures real-time access to up-to-date data. Asking the circulating nurse (A) or waiting for a break (C) can lead to delays and potential miscommunication, while calling the medical records department (D) is time-consuming and less reliable.

Question 130: Correct Answer: B) Directly enter the

follow-up appointment into the hospital's scheduling software.

Rationale: Directly entering the follow-up appointment into the hospital's scheduling software ensures that the appointment is accurately recorded and immediately visible to all relevant staff. Writing a note (A) and calling the patient (C) can lead to delays and errors. Asking the surgeon (D) is not efficient and may lead to miscommunication. Using the scheduling software streamlines the process and ensures accuracy.

Question 131: Correct Answer: A) To maintain a clear view of the surgical site

Rationale: The primary purpose of irrigation during surgery is to maintain a clear view of the surgical site by removing blood and debris. This is crucial for the surgeon to perform the procedure accurately. Option B is incorrect because increasing temperature is not a goal of irrigation. Option C is partially correct but not the primary purpose. Option D is incorrect as irrigation does not address air embolism risk.

Question 132: Correct Answer: B) Quadriceps

Rationale: The quadriceps muscle group, located at the front of the thigh, is primarily responsible for knee extension. The hamstrings, located at the back of the thigh, are responsible for knee flexion. The gastrocnemius, a calf muscle, is involved in plantar flexion of the foot, and the gluteus maximus is primarily responsible for hip extension. Therefore, the quadriceps are the correct answer for knee extension.

Question 133: Correct Answer: D) Wearing jewelry during the wash.

Rationale: Wearing jewelry during a medical hand wash should be avoided as it can harbor bacteria and compromise aseptic technique. Option A is correct as using antimicrobial soap is essential. Option B is correct as keeping hands above elbows while rinsing prevents contamination. Option C is correct as turning off the faucet with a clean paper towel maintains hand hygiene.

Question 134: Correct Answer: C) Gel pads and positioning devices

Rationale: Gel pads and positioning devices are most appropriate for preventing pressure ulcers during lengthy surgical procedures by redistributing pressure and providing cushioning. Sequential compression devices (A) and anti-embolism stockings (B) are primarily used to prevent DVT, while a pulse oximeter (D) monitors oxygen saturation. Only gel pads and positioning devices directly address the risk of pressure ulcers, ensuring patient comfort and safety during extended periods of immobility.

Question 135: Correct Answer: B) Mediastinum

Rationale: The mediastinum is the central compartment of the thoracic cavity that separates the right and left pleural cavities. The diaphragm separates the thoracic and abdominal cavities, not the pleural cavities. Pleural effusion is a condition involving fluid accumulation, not a structure. The pulmonary ligament is a fold of pleura that helps support the lungs but does not separate the pleural cavities. Therefore, the correct answer is B)

Mediastinum.

Question 136: Correct Answer: C) The microscope's objective lenses

Rationale: The objective lenses are delicate and crucial for the microscope's functionality, requiring careful handling to avoid scratches or misalignment. While the light bulb (A) and arm (D) are also important, they are more robust. The base (B) is sturdy and less susceptible to damage. Proper care of the objective lenses ensures the microscope maintains its precision and effectiveness for future procedures.

Question 137: Correct Answer: B) Inform the surgeon and prepare for potential conversion to an open procedure.

Rationale: The most appropriate initial action is to inform the surgeon and prepare for potential conversion to an open procedure. This ensures that the surgeon is aware of the situation and can take necessary steps to control the bleeding. Increasing suction power (A) does not address the source of bleeding. Administering IV fluids (C) is important but secondary to controlling the bleeding. Applying pressure (D) may help but is not the first step in managing significant blood loss.

Question 138: Correct Answer: C) Notify the supervisor and follow the facility's protocol for near-expiration items.

Rationale: Notifying the supervisor and following the facility's protocol ensures that near-expiration items are managed appropriately, aligning with cost containment processes. Using the drapes immediately (A) or storing them for future use (D) may not comply with safety standards. Discarding them (B) without proper assessment can lead to unnecessary waste.

Question 139: Correct Answer: C) Encouraging early mobilization and physical therapy

Rationale: Encouraging early mobilization and physical therapy is crucial to prevent complications such as deep vein thrombosis (DVT) and to promote joint function after a total knee replacement. While applying ice packs (A) and monitoring for infection (D) are important, they do not address the risk of immobility. Administering anticoagulants (B) is also important but must be combined with mobilization for optimal outcomes. Early mobilization is key to preventing multiple postoperative complications.

Question 140: Correct Answer: B) Drape the microscope with a sterile cover before positioning it.

Rationale: Draping the microscope with a sterile cover before positioning it is crucial to maintain sterility. Positioning the microscope before draping (Option A) risks contamination. Adjusting the focus before draping (Option C) is unnecessary and can compromise sterility. Cleaning with disinfectant (Option D) is important but does not replace the need for sterile draping. Ensuring the microscope remains sterile is vital to prevent surgical site infections.

Question 141: Correct Answer: A) To reduce blood loss by constricting blood flow to the surgical site

Rationale: The primary purpose of using a pneumatic tourniquet is to reduce blood loss by constricting blood flow to the surgical site. This allows for a clearer surgical field and minimizes bleeding. Option B is incorrect because expanding blood vessels would increase blood flow. Option C is incorrect as maintaining a sterile field is achieved through other means. Option D is incorrect because a tourniquet restricts, not promotes, blood circulation.

Question 142: Correct Answer: C) Bean bag positioner

Rationale: The bean bag positioner is ideal for laparoscopic cholecystectomy as it molds to the patient's body, providing stability and comfort while preventing movement. Arm boards (A) and shoulder braces (B) are not suitable for this procedure as they are primarily used for arm and shoulder stabilization. Stirrups (D) are used for gynecological or urological procedures, making them inappropriate for this scenario.

Question 143: Correct Answer: B) Production of exotoxins

Rationale: Clostridium perfringens causes gas gangrene primarily through the production of exotoxins, which lead to tissue necrosis and gas production. Endotoxins are associated with Gram-negative bacteria, while biofilm production is a mechanism for chronic infections but not specifically gas gangrene. Spore production allows Clostridium perfringens to survive in harsh conditions but is not the direct cause of gas gangrene. Understanding these mechanisms is essential for diagnosing and treating infections effectively.

Question 144: Correct Answer: A) Living Will

Rationale: A Living Will is a type of advanced directive that outlines a patient's preferences for medical treatment if they become incapacitated. Informed Consent and Surgical Consent are related to specific procedures, while a Discharge Summary details the care provided during hospitalization. Therefore, only a Living Will addresses the patient's wishes in situations where they cannot communicate.

Question 145: Correct Answer: A) Administering a broad-spectrum antibiotic immediately before the surgery.

Rationale: Administering a broad-spectrum antibiotic immediately before surgery is crucial for immunocompromised patients to minimize the risk of infection. While fasting (Option B) is important for anesthesia safety, it does not directly reduce infection risk. A high-protein diet (Option C) and vitamin C supplements (Option D) may support general health but are not specific measures to prevent surgical infections in immunocompromised patients.

Question 146: Correct Answer: D) Contact dermatitis from adhesive dressings

Rationale: Contact dermatitis from adhesive dressings is a common cause of postoperative rashes, typically presenting within 24-48 hours. Allergic reactions to surgical drapes and antibiotics are less common and usually present differently.

Infection at the surgical site would more likely present with additional symptoms such as fever, redness, and swelling, not just a rash. Therefore, D is the most plausible cause.

Question 147: Correct Answer: C) Place in a designated container for transport to decontamination

Rationale: Nondisposable surgical instruments should be placed in a designated container for transport to decontamination to prevent contamination and ensure proper sterilization. Soaking in saline solution (A) can cause corrosion, rinsing with sterile water (B) is insufficient for decontamination, and wiping with a dry cloth (D) does not remove bioburden. Proper handling ensures patient safety and instrument longevity.

Question 148: Correct Answer: C) Accessing patient records only when necessary for patient care.

Rationale: Accessing patient records only when necessary for patient care demonstrates adherence to HIPAA by ensuring that patient information is used appropriately and only by those involved in the patient's care. In contrast, sharing information with an uninvolved colleague, discussing details publicly, and leaving records unattended all violate HIPAA guidelines by risking unauthorized access to sensitive patient information.

Question 149: Correct Answer: B) Cortisol

Rationale: The pituitary gland regulates cortisol production through ACTH. Post-surgery, cortisol levels can drop, leading to adrenal insufficiency. Insulin (A) and glucagon (D) are related to pancreatic function, and thyroxine (C) is related to thyroid function, making them less immediate concerns in this context. Monitoring cortisol levels is crucial to avoid complications such as Addisonian crisis.

Question 150: Correct Answer: B) Polypropylene

Rationale: Polypropylene is a non-absorbable, synthetic suture material that is less likely to harbor bacteria compared to natural fibers like silk. It is ideal for contaminated wounds as it minimizes infection risk. Silk (A) is a natural fiber and can increase infection risk. Chromic gut (C) is absorbable and not ideal for contaminated wounds. Polyglycolic acid (D) is absorbable and can also increase infection risk in contaminated wounds.

CST Exam Practice Questions [SET 7]

Question 1: Which of the following is a key benefit of utilizing computer technology for interdepartmental communication in a surgical setting?
A) Reduces the need for face-to-face interactions
B) Increases the speed of information transfer
C) Eliminates the need for written documentation
D) Ensures complete privacy of patient information

Question 2: Which instrument is primarily used for clamping blood vessels during a surgical procedure?
A) Metzenbaum scissors
B) Kocher forceps
C) Hemostat
D) Babcock forceps

Question 3: During a laparoscopic cholecystectomy on a patient named John, the surgeon encounters diffuse oozing from the liver bed. Which chemical agent is most appropriate to achieve hemostasis in this scenario?
A) Epinephrine
B) Thrombin
C) Silver nitrate
D) Protamine sulfate

Question 4: During a surgical procedure, the electrosurgical unit (ESU) suddenly stops working. As the Certified Surgical Technologist, what is the first step you should take to troubleshoot the issue?
A) Check the patient's grounding pad for proper placement.
B) Replace the ESU with a new unit immediately.
C) Verify that the ESU is plugged into a functional electrical outlet.
D) Call for the biomedical technician to inspect the ESU.

Question 5: During an orthopedic surgery on a 60-year-old patient named Mrs. Johnson, the patient experiences a sudden drop in blood pressure and oxygen saturation. What should the surgical technologist do first in this emergency situation?
A) Administer intravenous fluids to the patient.
B) Alert the anesthesia provider and assist in stabilizing the patient.
C) Increase the oxygen flow rate to the patient.
D) Prepare for an immediate blood transfusion.

Question 6: Which of the following is the most appropriate action when preparing the surgical site on a patient with a known allergy to iodine?
A) Use an iodine-based antiseptic with caution
B) Use an alcohol-based antiseptic
C) Use a chlorhexidine-based antiseptic
D) Skip the antiseptic preparation

Question 7: During the initial phase of the surgical scrub, what is the recommended duration for scrubbing each finger, hand, and forearm?
A) 10 seconds each.
B) 30 seconds each.
C) 1 minute each.
D) 2 minutes each.

Question 8: Which of the following is a critical step when assisting with a circular stapler during colorectal surgery?
A) Ensuring the anvil is properly positioned
B) Clamping the stapler tightly before firing
C) Using the stapler to ligate major arteries
D) Removing the stapler immediately after firing

Question 9: During a laparoscopic cholecystectomy, the surgeon notices that the patient's gallbladder is inflamed and filled with stones. What is the most likely diagnosis for this condition?
A) Cholecystitis
B) Hepatitis
C) Pancreatitis
D) Gastritis

Question 10: During a laparoscopic cholecystectomy on Mr. Johnson, the surgeon asks you to place the bovie pad. Where should you place the bovie pad to ensure optimal safety and effectiveness?
A) On the patient's chest
B) On the patient's upper arm
C) On the patient's thigh
D) On the patient's lower back

Question 11: During the preoperative preparation for Mr. Smith's laparoscopic cholecystectomy, the surgical technologist notices that one of the sterile instrument trays has a broken seal. What should be the next step?
A) Use the tray as long as the instruments appear clean.
B) Resterilize the tray immediately and use it for the procedure.
C) Discard the tray and obtain a new sterile tray.
D) Cover the tray with a sterile drape and continue with the procedure.

Question 12: During a laparoscopic procedure, a fire ignites inside the patient's abdomen. What is the most appropriate immediate action?
A) Remove the laparoscope and close the incision
B) Irrigate the area with saline
C) Disconnect the insufflation tubing
D) Increase the flow of CO2

Question 13: Which of the following is a critical step when testing an endoscopic camera system

before surgery?
A) Ensuring the camera is fully charged
B) Checking the white balance
C) Verifying the type of endoscope used
D) Confirming the patient's identity

Question 14: Which of the following structures is primarily responsible for filtering lymph and housing lymphocytes?
A) Thymus
B) Spleen
C) Lymph nodes
D) Tonsils

Question 15: During a laparoscopic cholecystectomy on Ms. Smith, the surgical technologist notices that the insufflation tubing is leaking CO2. What should be the immediate course of action?
A) Replace the leaking tubing and continue the procedure.
B) Inform the surgeon and replace the tubing immediately.
C) Reduce the CO2 flow to minimize the leak.
D) Continue the procedure as the leak is minimal.

Question 16: During an intraoperative procedure, what is the primary responsibility of the surgical technologist when monitoring the use of medications and solutions?
A) Administering medications directly to the patient
B) Ensuring all medications and solutions are labeled correctly
C) Deciding on the dosage of medications to be used
D) Prescribing medications as needed

Question 17: What is the recommended method for hair removal at the surgical site to minimize the risk of surgical site infections (SSIs)?
A) Shaving with a razor
B) Depilatory creams
C) Clipping with electric clippers
D) Waxing

Question 18: Which of the following structures is primarily responsible for the production of cerebrospinal fluid (CSF)?
A) Choroid plexus
B) Pineal gland
C) Pituitary gland
D) Medulla oblongata

Question 19: What is the appropriate method for disposing of contaminated drapes after surgery in compliance with Standard Precautions?
A) Place them in a regular trash bin.
B) Place them in a biohazard bag.
C) Rinse them before disposal.
D) Place them in a linen hamper.

Question 20: Which of the following is NOT typically included in a surgeon's preference card?

A) Specific suture materials
B) Patient's insurance information
C) Preferred draping techniques
D) Instrument setup instructions

Question 21: What is the correct action for a surgical technologist to take if they notice a discrepancy in the medication dosage during an intraoperative procedure?
A) Ignore the discrepancy and continue with the procedure
B) Adjust the dosage themselves
C) Immediately inform the surgeon or anesthesiologist
D) Document the discrepancy after the procedure is completed

Question 22: Which of the following methods is most effective for sterilizing heat-sensitive surgical instruments?
A) Autoclaving
B) Ethylene oxide gas
C) Dry heat sterilization
D) Boiling

Question 23: John, a Certified Surgical Technologist, is preparing for an orthopedic surgery. After completing the surgical scrub, what is the next appropriate step to maintain sterility?
A) Donning sterile gloves immediately after scrubbing
B) Allowing hands to air dry completely before donning gloves
C) Keeping hands above waist level and away from the body
D) Rinsing hands with sterile water before drying

Question 24: When coordinating additional equipment for a surgery, which of the following is the best practice to ensure equipment readiness?
A) Storing all equipment in a central location
B) Regularly updating the equipment inventory
C) Labeling equipment with the date of last use
D) Conducting a preoperative equipment checklist

Question 25: Mrs. Smith, who recently had a cholecystectomy, is experiencing increased pain and swelling at the surgical site, along with a noticeable amount of fresh blood on the dressing. What is the most appropriate action for the surgical technologist to take?
A) Administer pain medication and monitor the site.
B) Elevate the affected area and apply ice.
C) Reinforce the dressing and contact the surgeon immediately.
D) Document the findings and continue with routine postoperative care.

Question 26: Which of the following is considered an abnormal postoperative finding that requires immediate reporting?
A) Elevated temperature of 100.4°F (38°C) for the first 24 hours
B) Persistent vomiting and inability to retain fluids

C) Bruising around the incision site
D) Mild pain controlled with prescribed analgesics

Question 27: Sarah, a surgical technologist, is responsible for ensuring that all surgical instruments are properly sterilized. What is the most critical step she should take to verify the sterilization process?
A) Visually inspect the instruments for cleanliness.
B) Check the sterilization indicator tape for color change.
C) Rely on the sterilization cycle completion signal.
D) Assume instruments are sterile if the autoclave was used.

Question 28: Which of the following is the most appropriate first step when conducting research using computer technology in a surgical setting?
A) Collecting data from previous surgeries
B) Formulating a research question
C) Analyzing statistical data
D) Reviewing literature

Question 29: During an abdominal surgery on a patient named Ms. Davis, the surgeon instructs you to use suction. What is the main reason for using suction in this scenario?
A) To prevent the patient from feeling pain
B) To remove excess fluids and maintain a clear surgical field
C) To increase the patient's blood pressure
D) To sterilize the surgical site

Question 30: What is the primary purpose of participating in a postoperative case debrief?
A) To evaluate the patient's overall health condition
B) To review the surgical procedure and identify areas for improvement
C) To discuss the patient's discharge plan
D) To determine the next surgical case

Question 31: Sarah, a surgical technologist, is preparing to mix a solution for irrigation during a procedure. What is the most crucial action she must take before mixing the solution?
A) Check the expiration date on the solution bottle.
B) Ask the surgeon how much solution is needed.
C) Label the solution container with the date and time.
D) Verify the solution type and concentration with the circulating nurse.

Question 32: 1 A 45-year-old patient named Mr. Johnson is undergoing surgery for a suspected bacterial infection. The surgical team collects a sample for culture. Which of the following is the most critical factor to ensure accurate identification of the pathogen?
A) Immediate refrigeration of the sample
B) Proper labeling and documentation
C) Using a sterile container
D) Transporting the sample within 24 hours

Question 33: During a postoperative case debrief, which aspect is most crucial to discuss to enhance future surgical procedures?
A) The duration of the surgery
B) The instruments used during the procedure
C) Any unexpected events or complications that occurred
D) The patient's preoperative condition

Question 34: During a cystoscopy on Mrs. Smith, the surgeon encounters difficulty visualizing the left ureteral orifice. Which anatomical landmark should the surgical technologist suggest to help locate the left ureteral orifice?
A) Trigone of the bladder
B) Urethral sphincter
C) Bladder dome
D) Anterior vaginal wall

Question 35: When should a surgical technologist revise a surgeon's preference card?
A) After every surgical procedure
B) When there is a change in the surgeon's technique or equipment preference
C) At the end of each month
D) Only when instructed by the surgeon

Question 36: Which of the following actions should a sterile team member take to maintain sterility while gloving?
A) Touch the outside of the glove with bare hands
B) Use the closed-glove technique
C) Use the open-glove technique
D) Adjust the glove fit by touching the outside

Question 37: During a laser surgery involving Mr. Smith, the surgical team decides to use helium as a cooling agent. What is the primary reason for using helium in this context?
A) Helium is less expensive than other gases.
B) Helium has a high thermal conductivity.
C) Helium is heavier than air, providing better cooling.
D) Helium enhances the laser's cutting precision.

Question 38: During a preoperative team briefing, the anesthesiologist, Dr. Johnson, suggests a different approach to anesthesia management than what was initially planned. The surgical team appears divided on the decision. As a Certified Surgical Technologist, what is the best course of action to facilitate effective group dynamics and decision-making?
A) Support the anesthesiologist's suggestion without question.
B) Encourage an open discussion where all team members can voice their opinions.
C) Side with the majority opinion to avoid conflict.
D) Remain silent and follow whatever decision is made by the lead surgeon.

Question 39: During a surgical procedure on a 45-year-old patient named John, the surgeon needs

to identify the primary lymphatic drainage of the right upper limb. Which lymph nodes should the surgical technologist anticipate being involved?
A) Inguinal lymph nodes
B) Axillary lymph nodes
C) Cervical lymph nodes
D) Popliteal lymph nodes

Question 40: During a cesarean section for a patient named Mrs. Davis, the surgical technologist and circulator are performing counts. When should the final count be performed?
A) Before the uterus is closed.
B) After the skin incision is closed.
C) Before the skin incision is closed.
D) After the patient is transferred to the recovery room.

Question 41: During a cystoscopy on Mrs. Johnson, the surgeon requests a Foley catheter to be prepared for insertion. Which of the following is a critical step in the preparation of the Foley catheter?
A) Inflate the balloon before insertion to check for leaks.
B) Lubricate the catheter tip with sterile jelly.
C) Cut the catheter to the desired length before insertion.
D) Attach the drainage bag to the catheter before insertion.

Question 42: Emily, a patient undergoing abdominal surgery, has just had her wound closed. As a surgical technologist, what is the most appropriate type of dressing to apply to her wound site to promote healing and prevent infection?
A) Non-adhesive dressing with a sterile gauze pad.
B) Adhesive bandage directly on the wound.
C) Transparent film dressing.
D) Non-sterile cotton dressing.

Question 43: During a phacoemulsification procedure, what is the primary function of the ultrasound technology used?
A) To create a clear visual field for the surgeon
B) To emulsify and remove the cataractous lens
C) To maintain intraocular pressure
D) To deliver medication to the eye

Question 44: During a total knee arthroplasty on a patient named Mrs. Smith, the surgeon requests the tourniquet to be deflated. What should be your primary concern as the Certified Surgical Technologist at this moment?
A) Ensuring the surgical site is irrigated with antibiotic solution.
B) Monitoring the patient's blood pressure closely.
C) Preparing for potential increased bleeding.
D) Checking the sterility of the instruments.

Question 45: What is the most effective action a

surgical technologist can take to prevent a retained surgical item (RSI) during an operation?
A) Double-checking the instrument count at the end of the procedure.
B) Ensuring all instruments are accounted for before the incision is closed.
C) Relying on the surgeon's memory to account for all instruments.
D) Using radiopaque sponges and instruments.

Question 46: During surgery, dark red blood is observed. What is the most likely source of this bleeding?
A) Arterial bleeding
B) Venous bleeding
C) Capillary bleeding
D) Hemolysed blood

Question 47: During an open appendectomy, the patient, Ms. Davis, experiences sudden cardiac arrest. What is the most appropriate action for the surgical technologist to take?
A) Begin chest compressions immediately.
B) Ensure the sterile field is maintained while the team resuscitates.
C) Hand the surgeon the defibrillator pads.
D) Call for additional help and prepare the crash cart.

Question 48: What is the first step a surgical technologist should take when removing drapes from a patient postoperatively?
A) Remove the drapes quickly to minimize patient exposure.
B) Ensure all instruments and sharps are accounted for before removing drapes.
C) Remove the drapes while the patient is still under anesthesia.
D) Fold the drapes inward to contain any contaminants.

Question 49: During a laparoscopic cholecystectomy on a patient named Mr. Johnson, the surgeon asks you to irrigate the operative site. What is the primary purpose of this irrigation?
A) To maintain the sterility of the surgical instruments
B) To clear the operative field of blood and debris
C) To cool down the surgical instruments
D) To reduce the risk of postoperative infection

Question 50: According to national disaster plan protocols, what is the first action a CST should take when a disaster is declared?
A) Report to the operating room
B) Check the availability of surgical instruments
C) Report to the designated assembly area
D) Contact family members

Question 51: When preparing the C-arm for a surgical procedure, which of the following steps is essential to ensure proper aseptic technique?
A) Positioning the C-arm before the patient is draped
B) Draping the C-arm with a sterile cover

C) Cleaning the C-arm with alcohol wipes
D) Ensuring the C-arm is plugged in and operational

Question 52: After a cholecystectomy, Mrs. Johnson reports severe abdominal pain, fever, and a yellowish drainage from her surgical site. As a Certified Surgical Technologist, what should you do next?
A) Reassure Mrs. Johnson that these symptoms are normal post-surgery.
B) Advise Mrs. Johnson to take over-the-counter pain medication.
C) Report these symptoms immediately to the surgeon.
D) Suggest Mrs. Johnson apply a warm compress to the surgical site.

Question 53: Sarah, a Certified Surgical Technologist, notices that the sterilization indicator tape on a set of instruments has not changed color after autoclaving. What should be her next step?
A) Use the instruments since they were in the autoclave.
B) Re-run the sterilization cycle with a new indicator tape.
C) Check the autoclave settings and run a biological indicator test.
D) Use a chemical disinfectant on the instruments before use.

Question 54: What is the primary advantage of using an autograft in surgical procedures?
A) Reduced risk of immune rejection
B) Lower cost compared to allografts
C) No need for a secondary surgical site
D) Faster healing time compared to synthetic grafts

Question 55: During a total knee arthroplasty on a 60-year-old patient named Mary, the surgical team notices oozing from the bone surface. Which hemostatic method is most appropriate to manage this situation?
A) Bone wax
B) Tourniquet application
C) Suture ligation
D) Electrocautery

Question 56: During the preoperative assessment of Ms. Smith, the nurse notes that she has a history of allergic reactions to certain skin products. What is the best approach for hair removal in her case?
A) Shaving with a razor
B) Using depilatory cream
C) Clipping with electric clippers
D) Waxing

Question 57: During a cholecystectomy procedure on Mr. Smith, the surgeon decides to make an incision that provides the best access to the gallbladder. Which type of incision is most appropriate for this procedure?
A) Pfannenstiel incision
B) McBurney incision
C) Kocher incision
D) Midline incision

Question 58: What is the primary role of a Certified Surgical Technologist (CST) during an organ procurement procedure?
A) To perform the organ removal surgery independently
B) To assist the surgical team by providing necessary instruments and maintaining a sterile field
C) To decide which organs are suitable for transplantation
D) To transport the organs to the recipient hospital

Question 59: During a surgical procedure to remove a kidney stone from Mr. Johnson's left ureter, the surgeon requests the surgical technologist to identify the anatomical structure that lies anterior to the left ureter. Which structure should the surgical technologist identify?
A) Inferior vena cava
B) Descending aorta
C) Left renal vein
D) Left adrenal gland

Question 60: Which of the following is the most appropriate initial action when a surgical technologist notices excessive bleeding at the surgical site during the postoperative period?
A) Apply direct pressure to the site.
B) Increase the patient's IV fluid rate.
C) Administer a blood transfusion immediately.
D) Notify the surgeon immediately.

Question 61: What is the primary responsibility of a Certified Surgical Technologist (CST) when it comes to maintaining surgical instruments?
A) Sterilizing instruments after each use
B) Ordering new instruments when needed
C) Ensuring instruments are available and functional before surgery
D) Disposing of used instruments

Question 62: During a spinal fusion surgery for Ms. Davis, the surgeon requests a specific type and size of pedicle screws. What should the Certified Surgical Technologist do to ensure the correct implant is provided?
A) Select the screws based on the inventory list.
B) Confirm the screw type and size with the surgical preference card.
C) Verify the screw type and size with the surgeon before passing them.
D) Rely on the surgical assistant to confirm the screw type and size.

Question 63: While setting up the sterile field for Ms. Johnson's knee arthroscopy, the surgical technologist accidentally brushes against the

sterile drape with a non-sterile sleeve. What should be done next?
A) Continue with the procedure as the contact was minimal.
B) Replace the sterile drape with a new one.
C) Cover the contaminated area with a sterile towel.
D) Notify the surgeon and proceed as instructed.

Question 64: Which of the following actions should a CST prioritize when following the national disaster plan protocol in a mass casualty event?
A) Secure all surgical instruments
B) Ensure personal safety and report to the designated area
C) Start performing surgeries immediately
D) Take charge of the hospital's emergency operations center

Question 65: Sarah, a surgical technologist, is preparing for a surgery involving a patient with a high risk of bloodborne pathogens. Which of the following PPE items should be donned first?
A) Gloves
B) Gown
C) Mask
D) Goggles

Question 66: What is the primary reason for verifying a patient's identity and surgical site before the procedure begins?
A) To ensure the surgical team is aware of the patient's preferences.
B) To comply with hospital policy and avoid legal issues.
C) To prevent wrong-site, wrong-procedure, and wrong-patient surgeries.
D) To make the patient feel more comfortable and secure.

Question 67: In which patient position is the patient placed on their side with the lower leg flexed and the upper leg straight, commonly used for renal surgeries?
A) Fowler's
B) Lateral
C) Sims'
D) Jackknife

Question 68: What is the primary mechanism by which the harmonic scalpel achieves hemostasis during surgical procedures?
A) Electrical cauterization
B) Ultrasonic vibration
C) Laser ablation
D) Radiofrequency energy

Question 69: Which of the following structures is responsible for initiating the electrical impulse that triggers the heartbeat?
A) Atrioventricular (AV) node
B) Sinoatrial (SA) node

C) Bundle of His
D) Purkinje fibers

Question 70: What is the primary purpose of using a ground fault circuit interrupter (GFCI) in the operating room?
A) To prevent electrical fires
B) To maintain a constant voltage supply
C) To protect against electrical shock
D) To regulate the flow of electricity

Question 71: During a postoperative case debrief, the surgical team discusses an unexpected intraoperative complication that occurred with Mr. Johnson's laparoscopic cholecystectomy. What is the primary purpose of this debrief?
A) To assign blame for the complication.
B) To identify areas for improvement and prevent future occurrences.
C) To document the complication for legal purposes.
D) To determine the financial impact of the complication.

Question 72: During a laparoscopic cholecystectomy, the surgeon decides to use a laser to dissect the gallbladder from the liver bed. What is the primary advantage of using laser technology in this procedure?
A) Reduced risk of infection
B) Increased precision in tissue dissection
C) Lower cost compared to traditional methods
D) Faster recovery time for the patient

Question 73: 4 During an appendectomy on Ms. Smith, the surgical technologist is tasked with handling instruments that have come into contact with the patient's appendix, which is infected. What is the best practice to prevent the spread of infection?
A) Place the contaminated instruments on a separate sterile tray.
B) Immediately sterilize the instruments in the autoclave.
C) Use the contaminated instruments for the rest of the procedure.
D) Isolate the contaminated instruments and inform the circulating nurse.

Question 74: What is the primary reason for avoiding live vaccines in immunocompromised patients during the preoperative period?
A) They may cause dehydration
B) They can lead to severe infections
C) They interfere with anesthesia
D) They increase the risk of bleeding

Question 75: During a thyroidectomy on a patient named Ms. Smith, the surgeon needs to achieve hemostasis on the thyroid gland. Which method is most suitable for this purpose?
A) Electrocautery
B) Application of bone wax

C) Use of a pneumatic tourniquet
D) Application of a pressure dressing

Question 76: During a laparoscopic cholecystectomy on Mr. Smith, the surgical team notices that the insufflator is not maintaining the desired pneumoperitoneum pressure. As the Certified Surgical Technologist, what is the most appropriate initial step to troubleshoot this equipment malfunction?
A) Increase the flow rate of CO2.
B) Check for leaks in the tubing and connections.
C) Replace the insufflator with a new one.
D) Adjust the patient's position.

Question 77: During a surgery involving the removal of a malignant tumor in the abdomen, the surgeon asks about the role of the thoracic duct. What should the surgical technologist explain?
A) The thoracic duct drains lymph from the right upper quadrant of the body.
B) The thoracic duct drains lymph from the entire body except the right upper quadrant.
C) The thoracic duct drains lymph only from the lower extremities.
D) The thoracic duct drains lymph from the head and neck region.

Question 78: Mary, a 60-year-old patient, is being transported to the operating room for a total knee replacement. What is the most important consideration for the Certified Surgical Technologist during this process?
A) Ensure Mary has removed all jewelry and dentures before transport.
B) Allow Mary to bring her personal belongings to the operating room for comfort.
C) Verify that Mary has received her preoperative medications before transport.
D) Confirm Mary's identity and surgical site with the preoperative checklist.

Question 79: During a laparoscopic cholecystectomy on a patient named Mr. Smith, the surgeon asks you to prepare the wound site for closure. Which of the following steps is most critical to ensure proper wound healing and prevent infection?
A) Apply sterile gloves before handling the dressings.
B) Use a non-sterile dressing to cover the wound site.
C) Ensure the wound site is dry before applying the dressing.
D) Apply an antiseptic solution directly to the dressing.

Question 80: During an intraoperative procedure, the surgical team is using an argon laser to coagulate bleeding vessels. What is the primary advantage of using an argon laser in this context?
A) Argon lasers provide deeper tissue penetration.
B) Argon lasers are highly absorbed by hemoglobin.
C) Argon lasers are less expensive than other lasers.
D) Argon lasers have a longer wavelength than CO2

lasers.

Question 81: A 60-year-old female patient named Mary is experiencing difficulty swallowing, weight loss, and a chronic cough. Imaging reveals a mass in the lower esophagus. What is the most likely diagnosis?
A) Esophageal varices
B) Achalasia
C) Esophageal carcinoma
D) Gastroesophageal reflux disease (GERD)

Question 82: During a knee arthroscopy on a patient named John, the surgeon asks you to identify the muscle group responsible for extending the knee. Which muscle group should you identify?
A) Hamstrings
B) Quadriceps
C) Gastrocnemius
D) Soleus

Question 83: Which of the following is the most critical safety measure to implement when using a laser in the operating room to prevent accidental exposure?
A) Wearing lead aprons
B) Using laser-specific eyewear
C) Applying sterile drapes
D) Ensuring proper ventilation

Question 84: Which of the following steps is crucial when preparing a Foley catheter for insertion to ensure sterility and proper function?
A) Lubricating the catheter tip before donning sterile gloves
B) Testing the balloon by inflating it with sterile water
C) Cutting the catheter to the desired length
D) Inserting the catheter without checking for balloon integrity

Question 85: Which of the following is the most appropriate step to ensure effective suctioning during the removal of drapes and other equipment from the patient postoperatively?
A) Use a Yankauer suction tip to clear the surgical site.
B) Use a Poole suction tip for deep abdominal suctioning.
C) Use a Frazier suction tip for fine, precise suctioning.
D) Use a bulb syringe for general suctioning.

Question 86: Which of the following is the most crucial step to ensure patient safety when transferring a patient from the operating table to the stretcher?
A) Ensuring the patient is fully awake before transfer
B) Securing all IV lines and catheters
C) Using a transfer board or sheet
D) Confirming the patient's identity

Question 87: Emily, a surgical technologist, is responsible for updating the electronic health records (EHR) with the details of a recent surgery. Which of the following actions best demonstrates effective interdepartmental communication?
A) Updating the EHR and sending a notification to the relevant departments
B) Updating the EHR and assuming other departments will check it
C) Verbally informing the nurse in charge without updating the EHR
D) Writing the details on a paper chart and placing it in the patient's file

Question 88: 1 Which type of microorganism is responsible for causing tuberculosis?
A) Virus
B) Bacterium
C) Fungus
D) Protozoa

Question 89: During the postoperative cleanup after a surgery on Ms. Smith, the surgical technologist accidentally drops a contaminated scalpel. What should the technologist do to comply with Standard Precautions?
A) Pick up the scalpel with gloved hands and place it in a sharps container.
B) Use a mechanical device or tool to pick up the scalpel and dispose of it in a sharps container.
C) Leave the scalpel on the floor for the cleaning staff to handle.
D) Wrap the scalpel in a sterile cloth before disposing of it.

Question 90: Which of the following is the most critical parameter to monitor continuously during an intraoperative procedure to ensure patient safety?
A) Blood pressure
B) Respiratory rate
C) Oxygen saturation
D) Body temperature

Question 91: Which of the following is a critical step when documenting the amount of solution used during a surgical procedure?
A) Estimating the amount based on visual inspection
B) Recording the amount immediately after the procedure
C) Relying on the surgeon's memory for the exact amount
D) Documenting only the initial amount prepared

Question 92: Which of the following is a common sign of postoperative bleeding that a surgical technologist should report?
A) Decreased heart rate.
B) Elevated blood pressure.
C) Increased drainage in the surgical drain.
D) Improved skin color.

Question 93: During a research study on postoperative infection rates, a surgical technologist named Alex is tasked with entering patient data into a computer system. Which of the following actions should Alex prioritize to ensure data integrity and accuracy?
A) Entering data as quickly as possible to meet deadlines
B) Double-checking each entry for accuracy before submission
C) Using abbreviations to save time
D) Relying on memory for patient details

Question 94: During a surgical procedure, a surgical technologist named Alex notices that the surgeon is about to use a piece of equipment that has not been properly sterilized. What should Alex do in this situation to adhere to ethical and legal practices?
A) Ignore the issue to avoid disrupting the procedure.
B) Inform the circulating nurse immediately.
C) Wait until after the procedure to report the issue.
D) Sterilize the equipment himself without informing anyone.

Question 95: Which frequency range is typically used in intraoperative ultrasound for optimal imaging resolution?
A) 1-3 MHz
B) 3-5 MHz
C) 7-15 MHz
D) 20-30 MHz

Question 96: Which of the following is a primary cause of fire in the operating room?
A) Electrical equipment malfunction
B) Sterile field contamination
C) Improper hand hygiene
D) Inadequate patient positioning

Question 97: Sarah, a Certified Surgical Technologist, encounters a chemical spill in the storage area. What is the correct sequence of actions she should take?
A) Report the spill to the supervisor, contain the spill, and then clean it up.
B) Contain the spill, report it to the supervisor, and then clean it up.
C) Clean up the spill immediately, report it to the supervisor, and then contain it.
D) Evacuate the area, report the spill to the supervisor, and then contain it.

Question 98: During the preoperative assessment, Mr. Smith informs the surgical technologist that he has an advanced directive specifying that he does not want any life-sustaining treatment if he becomes incapacitated. What should the surgical technologist do next?
A) Ignore the advanced directive and proceed with the preoperative preparations.
B) Notify the surgeon and ensure the advanced

directive is included in the patient's medical record.
C) Advise Mr. Smith to discuss the advanced directive with his family members.
D) Cancel the surgery until further clarification is obtained from the hospital administration.

Question 99: During the transfer of Ms. Smith from the operating table to the stretcher post-surgery, the surgical technologist notices that the patient is still under the effects of anesthesia. What is the appropriate action to take?
A) Proceed with the transfer quickly to minimize time under anesthesia.
B) Ensure the patient's head is supported to maintain airway patency.
C) Wake the patient up before transferring to ensure cooperation.
D) Transfer the patient without any additional support to avoid delays.

Question 100: Which of the following chemical agents is most commonly used to achieve hemostasis during surgical procedures?
A) Epinephrine
B) Heparin
C) Silver Nitrate
D) Thrombin

Question 101: While preparing for a complex ophthalmic surgery on Mrs. Smith, the surgical technologist must ensure the operating microscope is correctly draped. Which of the following is the best practice for draping the microscope?
A) Use a sterile drape that is large enough to cover the entire microscope.
B) Use multiple small sterile drapes to cover different parts of the microscope.
C) Use a non-sterile drape and then cover it with a sterile cloth.
D) Use a sterile drape only on the parts of the microscope that will be touched.

Question 102: During a gastric bypass surgery on a patient named Maria, the surgeon asks for a circular stapler. What is the most critical factor to verify before passing the stapler to the surgeon?
A) Ensure the stapler is loaded with the correct size staples.
B) Confirm the stapler is within the expiration date.
C) Verify the anvil is properly attached and the stapler is correctly assembled.
D) Check if the stapler has been used in a previous surgery.

Question 103: When performing an anastomosis of the bowel, which stapling device is most commonly used to ensure a secure and leak-proof connection?
A) Skin stapler
B) Linear cutter stapler
C) Ligating clip applier

D) Hemorrhoidal stapler

Question 104: John, a surgical technologist, is responsible for documenting the surgical count before and after a procedure. Which method should he use to ensure accuracy and efficiency in documentation?
A) Write the count on a whiteboard in the operating room.
B) Enter the count into the computerized surgical count system.
C) Memorize the count and verbally report it to the surgeon.
D) Record the count on a paper chart and file it after the procedure.

Question 105: Maria, a 30-year-old female, presents with symptoms of weight gain, fatigue, and cold intolerance. Her lab results show elevated TSH and low T3 and T4 levels. What is the most likely diagnosis?
A) Hyperthyroidism
B) Hypothyroidism
C) Addison's Disease
D) Cushing's Syndrome

Question 106: During the preparation of an autograft for a soft tissue repair, the surgical technologist must ensure the graft is handled properly. What is the most critical consideration in handling the autograft?
A) Minimizing the time the graft is exposed to air
B) Ensuring the graft is exposed to UV light for sterilization
C) Wrapping the graft in a dry, sterile cloth
D) Using alcohol to clean the graft before implantation

Question 107: When assisting in the application of a cast, what is the most crucial step to ensure proper limb alignment?
A) Ensuring the limb is clean and dry
B) Applying padding evenly
C) Positioning the limb correctly before the cast hardens
D) Using the correct type of casting material

Question 108: During a laparoscopic cholecystectomy on a patient named Mr. Smith, the surgeon requests an additional 500 mL of normal saline to be administered. As the surgical technologist, what is the most appropriate action to take?
A) Administer the saline without confirming the dosage.
B) Confirm the dosage with the circulating nurse before administration.
C) Administer the saline after the surgeon's verbal order.
D) Wait for a written order before administering the saline.

Question 109: The surgical team is preparing Mr.

Johnson for an abdominal surgery. The surgeon requests hair removal from the surgical site. Which of the following methods is considered the safest and most effective for preoperative hair removal?
A) Shaving with a razor
B) Depilatory cream
C) Clipping with electric clippers
D) Waxing

Question 110: During a laryngectomy procedure on Mrs. Smith, the surgical team must be cautious to avoid damaging which of the following nerves to prevent vocal cord paralysis?
A) Hypoglossal nerve
B) Vagus nerve
C) Recurrent laryngeal nerve
D) Glossopharyngeal nerve

Question 111: Maria, a surgical technologist, is required to complete her annual continuing education credits. Which of the following is the most efficient method for Maria to track her progress and ensure she meets the requirements?
A) Keep a handwritten log of completed courses.
B) Use the hospital's online continuing education tracking system.
C) Rely on email confirmations from course providers.
D) Check with her supervisor periodically.

Question 112: During the postoperative assessment of Mr. Johnson, a patient who underwent an appendectomy, the surgical technologist notices a significant amount of blood soaking through the dressing at the surgical site. What should be the immediate action taken by the surgical technologist?
A) Apply a new dressing over the existing one.
B) Reinforce the dressing and notify the surgeon immediately.
C) Remove the dressing and inspect the wound.

D) Wait for the next scheduled assessment to report the finding.

Question 113: During the preoperative preparation of a patient named Mrs. Johnson for a knee arthroscopy, the surgical technologist must ensure the surgical site is properly prepared. Which of the following actions should be avoided to maintain a sterile field?
A) Using sterile gloves while applying the antiseptic solution.
B) Shaving the surgical site immediately before the procedure.
C) Allowing the antiseptic solution to dry completely before draping.
D) Using a single-use applicator for the antiseptic solution.

Question 114: What is the safest practice when dealing with electrical equipment in a wet environment within a surgical suite?
A) Use equipment with frayed cords only if it is essential
B) Ensure all electrical equipment is properly grounded
C) Operate electrical devices with wet hands if wearing gloves
D) Place electrical devices directly on wet surfaces to avoid tripping hazards

Question 115: 8 A surgical patient named Ms. Lee is being treated for a wound infection. The lab identifies the pathogen as Staphylococcus aureus. What is the primary virulence factor that allows this microorganism to evade the host immune system?
A) Endotoxin
B) Exotoxin
C) Capsule
D) Protein A

ANSWER WITH DETAILED EXPLANATION SET [7]

Question 1: Correct Answer: B) Increases the speed of information transfer

Rationale: Utilizing computer technology significantly increases the speed of information transfer, ensuring timely and efficient communication between departments. While reducing face-to-face interactions (A) and eliminating written documentation (C) may be secondary benefits, they are not the primary advantage. Ensuring complete privacy (D) is crucial but not guaranteed solely by computer technology. Therefore, the key benefit is the increased speed of information transfer, which enhances overall workflow and patient care.

Question 2: Correct Answer: C) Hemostat

Rationale: Hemostats are specifically designed for clamping blood vessels to control bleeding during surgery. Metzenbaum scissors are used for cutting delicate tissues, Kocher forceps are used for grasping tough tissue, and Babcock forceps are used for holding soft tissue without causing damage. The hemostat's design and function make it the correct choice for clamping blood vessels, unlike the other instruments which serve different purposes.

Question 3: Correct Answer: B) Thrombin

Rationale: Thrombin is a potent hemostatic agent that converts fibrinogen to fibrin, facilitating clot formation and achieving hemostasis. Epinephrine (A) is primarily a vasoconstrictor, not a hemostatic agent. Silver nitrate (C) is used for cauterizing superficial wounds, not for internal hemostasis. Protamine sulfate (D) is an antidote for heparin overdose, not a hemostatic agent. Thus, thrombin is the most appropriate choice for achieving hemostasis in the liver bed during surgery.

Question 4: Correct Answer: C) Verify that the ESU is plugged into a functional electrical outlet.

Rationale: The first step in troubleshooting an ESU that stops working is to verify that it is plugged into a functional electrical outlet. This is a basic principle of electrical safety and ensures that the issue is not due to a simple power supply problem. Checking the patient's grounding pad (A) and calling for the biomedical technician (D) are secondary steps if the power supply is confirmed. Replacing the ESU (B) is premature without initial troubleshooting.

Question 5: Correct Answer: B) Alert the anesthesia provider and assist in stabilizing the patient.

Rationale: The correct action is to alert the anesthesia provider and assist in stabilizing the patient. The anesthesia provider is responsible for managing the patient's vital signs and can quickly address the drop in blood pressure and oxygen saturation. Administering IV fluids (A) and increasing oxygen flow (C) are secondary actions that the anesthesia provider may decide to take. Preparing for a blood transfusion (D) is premature without further assessment.

Question 6: Correct Answer: C) Use a chlorhexidine-based antiseptic

Rationale: For patients with a known allergy to iodine, a chlorhexidine-based antiseptic is the most appropriate alternative. Option A is incorrect as using iodine-based antiseptics on allergic patients can cause severe reactions. Option B is partially correct but alcohol-based antiseptics are not as effective alone. Option D is incorrect as skipping antiseptic preparation increases the risk of infection.

Question 7: Correct Answer: B) 30 seconds each.

Rationale: The recommended duration for scrubbing each finger, hand, and forearm during the initial phase of the surgical scrub is 30 seconds. This ensures adequate removal of transient microorganisms. Option A is too short to be effective, while options C and D are unnecessarily long and not typically recommended in standard guidelines. Scrubbing for 30 seconds strikes a balance between efficacy and efficiency in reducing microbial load.

Question 8: Correct Answer: A) Ensuring the anvil is properly positioned

Rationale: Proper positioning of the anvil in a circular stapler is crucial for creating a secure and leak-proof anastomosis in colorectal surgery. Clamping the stapler tightly (B) and removing it immediately after firing (D) are important but secondary steps. Using the stapler to ligate major arteries (C) is incorrect, as circular staplers are not designed for vascular ligation. Correct anvil positioning ensures the integrity and functionality of the anastomosis.

Question 9: Correct Answer: A) Cholecystitis

Rationale: Cholecystitis is the inflammation of the gallbladder, often caused by gallstones obstructing the cystic duct. Hepatitis involves liver inflammation, pancreatitis affects the pancreas, and gastritis involves stomach lining inflammation. The presence of gallstones and inflammation in the gallbladder makes cholecystitis the most accurate diagnosis.

Question 10: Correct Answer: C) On the patient's thigh

Rationale: The bovie pad should be placed on a large, well-vascularized muscle mass such as the thigh to ensure optimal electrical grounding and minimize the risk of burns. Placing it on the chest (A) or upper arm (B) may not provide sufficient muscle mass and could increase the risk of burns. The lower back (D) is also not ideal due to potential interference with spinal structures and insufficient muscle mass.

Question 11: Correct Answer: C) Discard the tray and obtain a new sterile tray.

Rationale: The correct action is to discard the tray and obtain a new sterile tray. A broken seal compromises the sterility of the instruments, posing a risk of infection. Using the tray (A), resterilizing it immediately (B), or covering it with a sterile drape (D) are not acceptable practices as they do not guarantee sterility and patient safety.

Question 12: Correct Answer: B) Irrigate the area with saline

Rationale: Irrigating the area with saline (B) is the immediate action to extinguish the fire inside the patient's abdomen. Removing the laparoscope and closing the incision (A) would trap the fire inside. Disconnecting the insufflation tubing (C) and increasing the flow of CO2 (D) are not effective immediate actions to extinguish the fire. Saline irrigation directly addresses the fire while ensuring patient safety.

Question 13: Correct Answer: B) Checking the white balance

Rationale: Checking the white balance is crucial to ensure accurate color representation during endoscopic procedures. This step ensures that tissues and structures appear in their true colors, aiding in accurate diagnosis and treatment. Ensuring the camera is charged (A) is important but secondary, verifying the endoscope type (C) is necessary but not specific to camera testing, and confirming patient identity (D) is a separate preoperative step.

Question 14: Correct Answer: C) Lymph nodes

Rationale: Lymph nodes are small, bean-shaped structures that filter lymph and house lymphocytes, which are crucial for immune response. The thymus is involved in T-cell maturation, the spleen filters blood and recycles old red blood cells, and tonsils are lymphoid tissues that guard against ingested or inhaled pathogens. Therefore, lymph nodes are the primary structures for filtering lymph and housing lymphocytes, making option C the correct answer.

Question 15: Correct Answer: B) Inform the surgeon and replace the tubing immediately.

Rationale: The correct action is to inform the surgeon and replace the tubing immediately to maintain proper insufflation and prevent complications. Simply replacing the tubing without informing the surgeon (Option A) or reducing the CO2 flow (Option C) does not address the root cause. Continuing the procedure with a leak (Option D) can compromise the surgical field and patient safety.

Question 16: Correct Answer: B) Ensuring all medications and solutions are labeled correctly

Rationale: The primary responsibility of the surgical technologist is to ensure all medications and solutions are labeled correctly to prevent medication errors and ensure patient safety. Administering medications (A) and prescribing medications (D) are responsibilities of the surgeon or anesthesiologist, while deciding on the dosage (C) is also outside the scope of the surgical technologist's duties.

Question 17: Correct Answer: C) Clipping with electric clippers

Rationale: Clipping with electric clippers is the recommended method for hair removal at the surgical site because it minimizes skin abrasions, which can reduce the risk of surgical site infections. Shaving with a razor can cause micro-abrasions, increasing infection risk. Depilatory creams can cause skin irritation and allergic reactions. Waxing is not recommended due to the potential for skin trauma and subsequent infection.

Question 18: Correct Answer: A) Choroid plexus

Rationale: The choroid plexus is primarily responsible for the production of cerebrospinal fluid (CSF). It consists of a network of capillaries and specialized ependymal cells found in the ventricles of the brain. The pineal gland, pituitary gland, and medulla oblongata have different functions unrelated to CSF production. The pineal gland regulates sleep-wake cycles, the pituitary gland secretes hormones, and the medulla oblongata controls autonomic functions.

Question 19: Correct Answer: B) Place them in a biohazard bag.

Rationale: Contaminated drapes must be placed in a biohazard bag to prevent the spread of infection and ensure safe disposal. Regular trash bins (Option A) do not provide adequate containment for biohazardous materials. Rinsing them (Option C) can spread contaminants, and placing them in a linen hamper (Option D) is inappropriate as it is meant for reusable linens, not contaminated disposables.

Question 20: Correct Answer: B) Patient's insurance information

Rationale: A surgeon's preference card typically includes details such as specific suture materials, preferred draping techniques, and instrument setup instructions to ensure the surgical team is well-prepared. Patient's insurance information is not relevant to the surgical procedure and is therefore not included in the preference card. This information is managed separately by administrative staff. Options A, C, and D are all relevant to the surgical process and are included in the preference card.

Question 21: Correct Answer: C) Immediately inform the surgeon or anesthesiologist

Rationale: The correct action is to immediately inform the surgeon or anesthesiologist of any discrepancy in medication dosage. Ignoring the discrepancy (A) or adjusting the dosage themselves (B) can lead to serious patient harm. Documenting the discrepancy after the procedure (D) is important but secondary to immediate communication to ensure patient safety.

Question 22: Correct Answer: B) Ethylene oxide gas

Rationale: Ethylene oxide gas is the most effective method for sterilizing heat-sensitive surgical instruments because it operates at lower temperatures and can penetrate complex instrument structures. Autoclaving and dry heat sterilization require high temperatures that can damage heat-sensitive instruments, while boiling is not a reliable sterilization method as it does not eliminate all types of microorganisms.

Question 23: Correct Answer: C) Keeping hands above waist level and away from the body

Rationale: Keeping hands above waist level and away from the body after scrubbing prevents contamination from non-sterile surfaces. Donning sterile gloves immediately after scrubbing without drying can lead to contamination. Air drying is not practical; hands should be dried with a sterile towel. Rinsing hands with sterile water before drying is unnecessary if proper scrubbing technique is followed.

Question 24: Correct Answer: D) Conducting a preoperative equipment checklist

Rationale: Conducting a preoperative equipment checklist ensures that all necessary equipment is present, functional, and ready for use. While storing equipment centrally (A), updating inventory (B), and labeling (C) are useful practices, they do not guarantee immediate readiness. The checklist is a proactive step that verifies the equipment status just before surgery, ensuring no last-minute issues arise.

Question 25: Correct Answer: C) Reinforce the dressing and contact the surgeon immediately.

Rationale: Reinforcing the dressing and contacting the surgeon immediately is essential to address potential complications from postoperative bleeding. Administering pain medication (Option A) does not address the bleeding. Elevating the area and applying ice (Option B) may help with swelling but not with active bleeding. Documenting and continuing routine care (Option D) neglects the urgency of the situation. Immediate surgeon notification is critical for prompt intervention.

Question 26: Correct Answer: B) Persistent vomiting and inability to retain fluids

Rationale: Persistent vomiting and inability to retain fluids are abnormal postoperative findings that may indicate complications such as ileus or bowel obstruction and require immediate reporting. An elevated temperature within the first 24 hours can be a normal inflammatory response, bruising around the incision site is typically expected, and mild pain controlled with prescribed analgesics is a normal postoperative occurrence.

Question 27: Correct Answer: B) Check the sterilization indicator tape for color change.

Rationale: The most critical step is to check the sterilization indicator tape for color change, as it provides a visual confirmation that the sterilization parameters were met. Option A is insufficient as cleanliness does not guarantee sterility. Option C, while important, does not confirm the effectiveness of sterilization. Option D is incorrect as it assumes sterility without verification, which could lead to using non-sterile instruments.

Question 28: Correct Answer: B) Formulating a research question

Rationale: The most appropriate first step in conducting research is formulating a research question. This step provides a clear focus and direction for the study. Collecting data, analyzing statistical data, and reviewing literature are subsequent steps that depend on having a well-defined research question. Without a research question, the research lacks purpose and direction, making it difficult to proceed effectively.

Question 29: Correct Answer: B) To remove excess fluids and maintain a clear surgical field

Rationale: The main reason for using suction during surgery is to remove excess fluids and maintain a clear surgical field, which is crucial for the surgeon's visibility and precision. Preventing pain (A) is managed by anesthesia, not suction. Increasing blood pressure (C) and sterilizing the site (D) are not functions of suction.

Question 30: Correct Answer: B) To review the surgical procedure and identify areas for improvement

Rationale: The primary purpose of a postoperative case debrief is to review the surgical procedure and identify areas for improvement. This helps in enhancing future surgical outcomes and team performance. Option A is incorrect as evaluating the patient's overall health condition is done during postoperative care, not specifically in a debrief. Option C is incorrect as discussing the discharge plan is part of patient management, not the debrief. Option D is incorrect as determining the next surgical case is unrelated to the debrief process.

Question 31: Correct Answer: D) Verify the solution type and concentration with the circulating nurse.

Rationale: Verifying the solution type and concentration with the circulating nurse ensures the correct solution is used, preventing potential complications. Checking the expiration date (A) is important but secondary to verification. Asking the surgeon (B) about the quantity does not address the solution's correctness. Labeling the container (C) should be done after verification and mixing.

Question 32: Correct Answer: C) Using a sterile container

Rationale: Using a sterile container is crucial to prevent contamination, which can lead to false results. While proper labeling and documentation (B) and timely transportation (D) are also important, they do not prevent contamination. Immediate refrigeration (A) is not always necessary for all types of cultures and can sometimes be inappropriate. Thus, using a sterile container ensures the integrity of the sample, making it the most critical factor.

Question 33: Correct Answer: C) Any unexpected events or complications that occurred

Rationale: Discussing any unexpected events or complications that occurred during the surgery is crucial for enhancing future procedures. This allows the team to learn from these events and implement strategies to avoid them in the future. Option A is less critical as the duration of the surgery is a metric but not as impactful as addressing complications. Option B, while important, is secondary to understanding complications. Option D, the patient's preoperative condition, is relevant but not the focus of the debrief.

Question 34: Correct Answer: A) Trigone of the bladder

Rationale: The trigone of the bladder is a triangular area on the bladder floor where the ureteral orifices and the internal urethral orifice are located. This landmark helps in identifying the ureteral orifices. The urethral sphincter (B) and bladder dome (C) are not relevant landmarks for locating the ureteral orifices. The anterior vaginal wall (D) is not part of the bladder anatomy and does not aid in locating the ureteral orifices.

Question 35: Correct Answer: B) When there is a change in the surgeon's technique or equipment preference

Rationale: A surgical technologist should revise a surgeon's preference card when there is a change in the surgeon's technique or equipment preference. This ensures that the surgical team is always prepared with the correct tools and supplies. Options A and C are impractical and unnecessary, while option D is too restrictive, as proactive updates are essential for optimal surgical outcomes.

Question 36: Correct Answer: B) Use the closed-glove technique

Rationale: The closed-glove technique is used to maintain sterility by ensuring that the hands do not touch the outside of the gloves. Touching the outside of the glove with bare hands (Option A) and adjusting the glove fit by touching the outside (Option D) can contaminate the gloves. The open-glove technique (Option C) is less commonly used in the operating room and does not provide the same level of sterility as the closed-glove technique.

Question 37: Correct Answer: B) Helium has a high thermal conductivity.

Rationale: Helium is used as a cooling agent in laser surgeries primarily due to its high thermal conductivity, which efficiently dissipates heat generated by the laser. Option A is incorrect as cost is not the primary factor. Option C is incorrect because helium is lighter than air. Option D is incorrect as helium does not enhance cutting precision but aids in cooling.

Question 38: Correct Answer: B) Encourage an open discussion where all team members can voice their opinions.

Rationale: Encouraging open discussion (Option B) fosters teamwork, ensures all perspectives are considered, and leads to a well-informed decision. Blindly supporting one suggestion (Option A) or siding with the majority (Option C) may overlook critical insights, and remaining silent (Option D) does not contribute to effective group dynamics.

Question 39: Correct Answer: B) Axillary lymph nodes

Rationale: The axillary lymph nodes are the primary lymphatic drainage for the right upper limb. Inguinal lymph nodes drain the lower limbs and pelvis, cervical lymph nodes drain the head and neck, and popliteal lymph nodes drain the lower leg. Understanding the correct lymphatic drainage pathways is crucial for surgical planning and avoiding complications.

Question 40: Correct Answer: C) Before the skin incision is closed.

Rationale: The final count should be performed before the skin incision is closed to ensure no instruments or sponges are left inside the patient. Option A is incorrect because the count should be done after the uterus is closed but before the skin. Option B is incorrect as the count must be done before the skin closure. Option D is incorrect because it is too late to perform the final count after the patient is in the recovery room.

Question 41: Correct Answer: B) Lubricate the catheter tip with sterile jelly.

Rationale: Lubricating the catheter tip with sterile jelly reduces friction and eases insertion, minimizing patient discomfort and risk of urethral injury. Option A is incorrect because inflating the balloon before insertion can damage the catheter. Option C is

incorrect as catheters are pre-sized and should not be cut. Option D is incorrect because the drainage bag is typically attached after the catheter is inserted and secured.

Question 42: Correct Answer: A) Non-adhesive dressing with a sterile gauze pad.

Rationale: A non-adhesive dressing with a sterile gauze pad is the most appropriate for promoting healing and preventing infection in a postoperative wound. This type of dressing is gentle on the wound and allows for absorption of exudate. Option B is incorrect as adhesive bandages can cause trauma to the wound upon removal. Option C is incorrect because transparent film dressings are not ideal for wounds with heavy exudate. Option D is incorrect as non-sterile dressings can introduce contaminants.

Question 43: Correct Answer: B) To emulsify and remove the cataractous lens

Rationale: The primary function of ultrasound technology in phacoemulsification is to emulsify and remove the cataractous lens. This is achieved by using ultrasonic vibrations to break up the lens into small fragments, which are then aspirated out of the eye. Options A, C, and D are incorrect as they do not describe the primary role of ultrasound in this procedure. Creating a clear visual field, maintaining intraocular pressure, and delivering medication are important but secondary functions.

Question 44: Correct Answer: C) Preparing for potential increased bleeding.

Rationale: When the tourniquet is deflated, there is a risk of increased bleeding as blood flow returns to the surgical site. The primary concern should be to prepare for this potential increased bleeding. Irrigating with antibiotic solution (A) and monitoring blood pressure (B) are important but secondary to managing bleeding. Checking instrument sterility (D) is a routine task but not immediately critical at this moment.

Question 45: Correct Answer: B) Ensuring all instruments are accounted for before the incision is closed.

Rationale: Ensuring all instruments are accounted for before the incision is closed is the most effective preventative action to avoid RSIs. While double-checking counts and using radiopaque materials are helpful, they are supplementary. Relying on the surgeon's memory is unreliable. Thus, a thorough count before closing ensures no items are left inside the patient.

Question 46: Correct Answer: B) Venous bleeding

Rationale: Dark red blood is typically associated with venous bleeding, which is deoxygenated. Arterial bleeding (Option A) would be bright red due to high oxygen content. Capillary bleeding (Option C) is generally slow and oozing, not dark red. Hemolysed blood (Option D) refers to ruptured red blood cells, which is not a typical source of bleeding observed during surgery. Therefore, dark red blood most likely indicates venous bleeding.

Question 47: Correct Answer: D) Call for additional help and prepare the crash cart.

Rationale: The surgical technologist should call for

additional help and prepare the crash cart, ensuring that all necessary resuscitation equipment is available. Beginning chest compressions (A) is not the technologist's role. Maintaining the sterile field (B) is secondary to patient survival. Handing the defibrillator pads (C) is important but follows calling for help and preparing the crash cart. The correct action ensures that the team has the resources needed for effective resuscitation.

Question 48: Correct Answer: B) Ensure all instruments and sharps are accounted for before removing drapes.

Rationale: The first step in removing drapes postoperatively is to ensure all instruments and sharps are accounted for to prevent any retained surgical items. Option A is incorrect as removing drapes quickly can lead to contamination. Option C is incorrect because drapes should be removed after ensuring the patient is stable. Option D, while important, is not the first step in the process.

Question 49: Correct Answer: B) To clear the operative field of blood and debris

Rationale: The primary purpose of irrigation during surgery is to clear the operative field of blood and debris, which provides the surgeon with a clear view and helps in precise surgical maneuvers. While maintaining sterility (A) and reducing infection risk (D) are important, they are not the primary reasons for intraoperative irrigation. Cooling instruments (C) is not relevant in this context.

Question 50: Correct Answer: C) Report to the designated assembly area

Rationale: When a disaster is declared, the first action a CST should take is to report to the designated assembly area as per the hospital's disaster plan. This ensures they are accounted for and can receive further instructions. Reporting to the operating room (A) or checking instruments (B) are not immediate priorities. Contacting family members (D) is important but should be done after reporting to the assembly area.

Question 51: Correct Answer: B) Draping the C-arm with a sterile cover

Rationale: Draping the C-arm with a sterile cover is essential to maintain aseptic technique and prevent contamination during surgery. Positioning the C-arm before draping (Option A) is important but does not address aseptic technique. Cleaning with alcohol wipes (Option C) is necessary but insufficient alone. Ensuring the C-arm is operational (Option D) is crucial for functionality but not related to aseptic technique.

Question 52: Correct Answer: C) Report these symptoms immediately to the surgeon.

Rationale: Severe abdominal pain, fever, and yellowish drainage are signs of a potential postoperative infection or complication. These symptoms are not normal and require immediate medical attention. Options A and D are incorrect because they downplay the severity of the symptoms. Option B is incorrect as over-the-counter pain medication does not address the underlying issue. Reporting to the surgeon ensures timely intervention, preventing further complications.

Question 53: Correct Answer: C) Check the autoclave settings and run a biological indicator test.

Rationale: Sarah should check the autoclave settings and run a biological indicator test to ensure the autoclave is functioning correctly. Using the instruments (A) or re-running the cycle with a new tape (B) without verifying the autoclave's functionality is unsafe. Using a chemical disinfectant (D) does not replace the need for proper sterilization. Running a biological indicator test confirms the sterility of the instruments.

Question 54: Correct Answer: A) Reduced risk of immune rejection

Rationale: The primary advantage of using an autograft is the reduced risk of immune rejection since the tissue is harvested from the patient's own body. This minimizes the likelihood of an immune response. While options B and D may seem plausible, they do not address the primary advantage. Option C is incorrect because an autograft typically does require a secondary surgical site for tissue harvesting.

Question 55: Correct Answer: A) Bone wax

Rationale: Bone wax is specifically designed to control bleeding from bone surfaces by physically blocking the bleeding channels. Tourniquet application (B) is used to control blood flow to the entire limb but is not specific to bone surface bleeding. Suture ligation (C) is not applicable for diffuse bone bleeding. Electrocautery (D) is less effective on bone surfaces compared to bone wax, which provides immediate and localized hemostasis.

Question 56: Correct Answer: C) Clipping with electric clippers

Rationale: For patients with a history of allergic reactions to skin products, clipping with electric clippers is the best approach as it avoids the use of chemicals that could cause irritation or allergic reactions. Shaving with a razor (Option A) can lead to cuts and infections. Depilatory creams (Option B) can cause allergic reactions. Waxing (Option D) can cause skin trauma and is not recommended.

Question 57: Correct Answer: C) Kocher incision

Rationale: The Kocher incision, made subcostally on the right side, provides optimal access to the gallbladder and biliary tree, making it ideal for cholecystectomy. The Pfannenstiel incision is used for pelvic surgeries, the McBurney incision for appendectomies, and the midline incision for general abdominal access. While the other incisions are plausible, they do not offer the best access to the gallbladder specifically.

Question 58: Correct Answer: B) To assist the surgical team by providing necessary instruments and maintaining a sterile field

Rationale: The primary role of a CST during an organ procurement procedure is to assist the surgical team by providing necessary instruments and maintaining a sterile field. This ensures the procedure is conducted efficiently and safely. Option A is incorrect because CSTs do not perform surgeries independently. Option C is incorrect as the suitability of organs is determined by the transplant team. Option D is incorrect because organ transportation is typically handled by specialized personnel.

Question 59: Correct Answer: C) Left renal vein
Rationale: The left renal vein lies anterior to the left ureter. This anatomical relationship is crucial for avoiding vascular injury during ureteral surgeries. The inferior vena cava (A) and descending aorta (B) are not in the correct anatomical position relative to the left ureter. The left adrenal gland (D) is superior to the kidney and does not lie anterior to the left ureter.

Question 60: Correct Answer: D) Notify the surgeon immediately.
Rationale: Notifying the surgeon immediately is crucial because the surgeon can assess the situation and determine the appropriate intervention. Applying direct pressure (A) may be necessary but should follow the surgeon's assessment. Increasing IV fluids (B) and administering a blood transfusion (C) are interventions that require a physician's order and should not be the initial actions taken by a surgical technologist.

Question 61: Correct Answer: C) Ensuring instruments are available and functional before surgery
Rationale: The primary responsibility of a CST in maintaining surgical instruments is to ensure they are available and functional before surgery. While sterilizing instruments (A) and ordering new ones (B) are important, they are secondary to the immediate need for functional instruments during surgery. Disposing of used instruments (D) is not a typical duty of a CST. Ensuring availability and functionality directly impacts surgical efficiency and patient safety.

Question 62: Correct Answer: C) Verify the screw type and size with the surgeon before passing them.
Rationale: Verifying the screw type and size with the surgeon ensures the correct implant is used, aligning with best practices for patient safety. Option A is incorrect as the inventory list may not reflect the specific needs of the surgery. Option B is incorrect because the preference card may not always be updated. Option D is incorrect as the technologist must take direct responsibility for the verification process.

Question 63: Correct Answer: B) Replace the sterile drape with a new one.
Rationale: The correct action is to replace the sterile drape with a new one. Any contact with non-sterile items compromises the sterility of the field. Continuing with the procedure (A), covering the area with a sterile towel (C), or notifying the surgeon without taking immediate corrective action (D) do not ensure the maintenance of a sterile environment, which is crucial for preventing infections.

Question 64: Correct Answer: B) Ensure personal safety and report to the designated area
Rationale: In a mass casualty event, a CST should prioritize ensuring personal safety and reporting to the designated area. This allows them to receive instructions and be deployed effectively. Option A is incorrect as securing instruments is secondary.

Option C is incorrect because surgeries are performed based on triage and not immediately. Option D is incorrect because CSTs do not take charge of the emergency operations center; this is typically managed by higher-level administrative personnel.

Question 65: Correct Answer: C) Mask
Rationale: The mask should be donned first to protect the respiratory tract from potential exposure to bloodborne pathogens. This is crucial as the respiratory tract is a primary entry point for pathogens. Option A (gloves) and B (gown) are donned later to protect the body and hands. Option D (goggles) should be donned after the mask to ensure the eyes are protected without compromising the mask's fit.

Question 66: Correct Answer: C) To prevent wrong-site, wrong-procedure, and wrong-patient surgeries.
Rationale: Verifying a patient's identity and surgical site is crucial to prevent wrong-site, wrong-procedure, and wrong-patient surgeries, which are serious and preventable errors. While complying with hospital policy (Option B) and making the patient feel comfortable (Option D) are important, they are secondary to ensuring patient safety. Ensuring the surgical team is aware of patient preferences (Option A) does not address the critical safety aspect of verification. The primary reason is to ensure patient safety and prevent surgical errors.

Question 67: Correct Answer: B) Lateral
Rationale: The lateral position is used for renal surgeries and involves placing the patient on their side with the lower leg flexed and the upper leg straight. Fowler's position is a semi-sitting position used for respiratory or cardiac conditions. Sims' position is used for rectal examinations and enemas. The jackknife position is used for rectal and certain spinal surgeries. The lateral position provides the best access to the kidney area compared to the other positions.

Question 68: Correct Answer: B) Ultrasonic vibration
Rationale: The harmonic scalpel achieves hemostasis primarily through ultrasonic vibration, which generates mechanical energy to cut and coagulate tissue simultaneously. Unlike electrical cauterization (A), laser ablation (C), or radiofrequency energy (D), the harmonic scalpel uses high-frequency ultrasonic waves to denature proteins, leading to coagulation without significant thermal damage to surrounding tissues. This makes it a precise and effective tool in surgical procedures.

Question 69: Correct Answer: B) Sinoatrial (SA) node
Rationale: The sinoatrial (SA) node, located in the right atrium, is the primary pacemaker of the heart, initiating the electrical impulse that triggers the heartbeat. The atrioventricular (AV) node, Bundle of His, and Purkinje fibers are part of the conduction pathway but do not initiate the impulse. The AV node delays the impulse, the Bundle of His transmits it to the ventricles, and the Purkinje fibers distribute it throughout the ventricles. The SA node's role is unique and crucial for setting the heart's rhythm.

Question 70: Correct Answer: C) To protect against

electrical shock

Rationale: The primary purpose of a ground fault circuit interrupter (GFCI) is to protect against electrical shock by quickly cutting off power when a ground fault is detected. Unlike option A, which focuses on fire prevention, option B, which deals with voltage regulation, and option D, which concerns electricity flow, GFCIs are specifically designed to enhance electrical safety by preventing shock hazards.

Question 71: Correct Answer: B) To identify areas for improvement and prevent future occurrences.

Rationale: The primary purpose of a postoperative case debrief is to identify areas for improvement and prevent future occurrences of similar complications. This process promotes a culture of safety and continuous improvement. Assigning blame (Option A) is counterproductive, documenting for legal purposes (Option C) is secondary, and determining financial impact (Option D) is not the main focus during a debrief.

Question 72: Correct Answer: B) Increased precision in tissue dissection

Rationale: The primary advantage of using laser technology in a laparoscopic cholecystectomy is increased precision in tissue dissection. Lasers allow for more accurate cutting and coagulation, reducing damage to surrounding tissues. While reduced risk of infection (A) and faster recovery time (D) are benefits, they are secondary to the precision offered by lasers. Lower cost (C) is incorrect as laser technology is generally more expensive.

Question 73: Correct Answer: D) Isolate the contaminated instruments and inform the circulating nurse.

Rationale: The best practice is to isolate the contaminated instruments and inform the circulating nurse to prevent cross-contamination. Placing them on a separate tray (Option A) or using them (Option C) risks further contamination. Immediate sterilization (Option B) is impractical during the procedure. Isolating and informing ensures proper handling and reduces infection risk.

Question 74: Correct Answer: B) They can lead to severe infections

Rationale: Live vaccines can lead to severe infections in immunocompromised patients because their immune systems are unable to effectively combat the attenuated pathogens. Dehydration (A), interference with anesthesia (C), and increased bleeding risk (D) are not directly related to the risks posed by live vaccines. The primary concern is the potential for severe infections, making this the most critical reason for avoidance.

Question 75: Correct Answer: A) Electrocautery

Rationale: Electrocautery is the most suitable method for achieving hemostasis on the thyroid gland due to its precision and effectiveness. Bone wax (B) is used for bone bleeding, not soft tissue. A pneumatic tourniquet (C) is inappropriate for this type of surgery. A pressure dressing (D) is not effective for immediate intraoperative hemostasis.

Question 76: Correct Answer: B) Check for leaks in the tubing and connections.

Rationale: The most appropriate initial step is to check for leaks in the tubing and connections. Leaks are a common cause of pressure loss in insufflators. Increasing the flow rate (A) or replacing the insufflator (C) are more drastic measures that should only be considered after confirming there are no leaks. Adjusting the patient's position (D) is unrelated to the issue of maintaining pneumoperitoneum pressure.

Question 77: Correct Answer: B) The thoracic duct drains lymph from the entire body except the right upper quadrant.

Rationale: The thoracic duct is the largest lymphatic vessel and drains lymph from the entire body except the right upper quadrant, which is drained by the right lymphatic duct. Options A, C, and D are incorrect as they misrepresent the regions drained by the thoracic duct, which include the left side of the head, neck, chest, abdomen, and both lower extremities.

Question 78: Correct Answer: D) Confirm Mary's identity and surgical site with the preoperative checklist.

Rationale: Confirming Mary's identity and surgical site with the preoperative checklist (Option D) is crucial to prevent wrong-site surgery and ensure patient safety. While removing jewelry and dentures (Option A) and verifying preoperative medications (Option C) are important, they are secondary to confirming identity and surgical site. Allowing personal belongings (Option B) is inappropriate and could introduce contaminants into the sterile environment.

Question 79: Correct Answer: C) Ensure the wound site is dry before applying the dressing.

Rationale: Ensuring the wound site is dry before applying the dressing is crucial to prevent infection and promote proper healing. Moisture can harbor bacteria, leading to infection. While applying sterile gloves (Option A) is important, it is not the most critical step. Using a non-sterile dressing (Option B) is incorrect as it increases infection risk. Applying antiseptic solution directly to the dressing (Option D) is less effective than ensuring the wound site is dry.

Question 80: Correct Answer: B) Argon lasers are highly absorbed by hemoglobin.

Rationale: Argon lasers are highly absorbed by hemoglobin, making them ideal for coagulating bleeding vessels. This property allows for precise control of bleeding with minimal damage to surrounding tissues. Option A is incorrect because argon lasers do not provide deeper tissue penetration compared to other lasers. Option C is a misconception; cost varies by equipment and usage. Option D is incorrect as argon lasers have a shorter wavelength compared to CO2 lasers.

Question 81: Correct Answer: C) Esophageal carcinoma

Rationale: Esophageal carcinoma often presents with symptoms such as difficulty swallowing, weight loss, and chronic cough, along with imaging showing a mass in the esophagus. Esophageal varices typically present with bleeding, achalasia with difficulty swallowing but without a mass, and GERD with heartburn and regurgitation. The presence of a mass in the lower esophagus strongly suggests esophageal carcinoma, distinguishing it from the other conditions.

Question 82: Correct Answer: B) Quadriceps

Rationale: The quadriceps muscle group is responsible for extending the knee. The hamstrings are responsible for knee flexion, the gastrocnemius assists in plantar flexion of the foot, and the soleus also aids in plantar flexion. Correctly identifying the quadriceps ensures accurate anatomical knowledge crucial for assisting in knee surgeries.

Question 83: Correct Answer: B) Using laser-specific eyewear

Rationale: Laser-specific eyewear is essential to protect the eyes from accidental exposure to laser beams, which can cause severe damage. Lead aprons are used for radiation protection, sterile drapes prevent infection, and proper ventilation controls airborne contaminants but does not specifically address laser safety. Thus, laser-specific eyewear is the most critical measure.

Question 84: Correct Answer: B) Testing the balloon by inflating it with sterile water

Rationale: Testing the balloon by inflating it with sterile water is crucial to ensure it functions properly and does not leak. This step ensures patient safety and prevents complications. Option A is incorrect as lubrication should be done after donning sterile gloves. Option C is incorrect because cutting the catheter can compromise its sterility and function. Option D is incorrect as not checking the balloon can lead to insertion issues and patient discomfort.

Question 85: Correct Answer: A) Use a Yankauer suction tip to clear the surgical site.

Rationale: The Yankauer suction tip is specifically designed for effective suctioning of the surgical site, providing a wide bore for rapid removal of fluids. The Poole suction tip is more suited for deep abdominal cavities, the Frazier suction tip is used for fine, precise suctioning in neurosurgery, and a bulb syringe is generally not used for surgical suctioning. The Yankauer tip ensures thorough clearing of the surgical area, minimizing the risk of fluid accumulation and infection.

Question 86: Correct Answer: C) Using a transfer board or sheet

Rationale: Using a transfer board or sheet is essential to ensure patient safety during transfer, as it provides stability and minimizes the risk of injury. While securing IV lines and catheters (B) is important, it is not the most crucial step. Ensuring the patient is fully awake (A) and confirming the patient's identity (D) are also necessary but do not directly impact the physical safety during the transfer process.

Question 87: Correct Answer: A) Updating the EHR and sending a notification to the relevant departments

Rationale: Updating the EHR and sending a notification to the relevant departments ensures that all necessary parties are informed in a timely manner. This method leverages computer technology for efficient communication. Assuming others will check the EHR or relying solely on verbal or paper communication can lead to missed information and delays in patient care.

Question 88: Correct Answer: B) Bacterium

Rationale: Tuberculosis is caused by the bacterium Mycobacterium tuberculosis. Unlike viruses, fungi, and protozoa, bacteria are single-celled organisms that can cause diseases such as tuberculosis. Viruses require a host cell to replicate, fungi are eukaryotic organisms that can cause infections like athlete's foot, and protozoa are single-celled eukaryotes that cause diseases like malaria. Thus, the correct answer is bacterium.

Question 89: Correct Answer: B) Use a mechanical device or tool to pick up the scalpel and dispose of it in a sharps container.

Rationale: Using a mechanical device or tool to pick up the scalpel (Option B) minimizes the risk of injury and contamination, ensuring compliance with Standard Precautions. Picking up the scalpel with gloved hands (Option A) still poses a risk of injury. Leaving the scalpel on the floor (Option C) is unsafe and non-compliant. Wrapping the scalpel in a sterile cloth (Option D) does not address the need for proper disposal in a sharps container.

Question 90: Correct Answer: C) Oxygen saturation

Rationale: Monitoring oxygen saturation is crucial as it provides immediate information about the patient's respiratory and circulatory status, ensuring adequate oxygen delivery to tissues. While blood pressure, respiratory rate, and body temperature are also important, they do not offer as direct an indication of oxygenation status. Misconceptions may arise from focusing solely on these other parameters, but oxygen saturation directly reflects the patient's ability to oxygenate blood, making it the most critical.

Question 91: Correct Answer: B) Recording the amount immediately after the procedure

Rationale: Recording the amount immediately after the procedure ensures accuracy and prevents errors due to memory lapses or estimation. Visual inspection (A) and relying on memory (C) are prone to inaccuracies, while documenting only the initial amount (D) ignores any additional usage, leading to incomplete records.

Question 92: Correct Answer: C) Increased drainage in the surgical drain.

Rationale: Increased drainage in the surgical drain is a common sign of postoperative bleeding and should be reported. Decreased heart rate (A) and elevated blood pressure (B) are not typical signs of bleeding; in fact, bleeding often causes increased heart rate and decreased blood pressure. Improved skin color (D) is generally a positive sign and not indicative of bleeding.

Question 93: Correct Answer: B) Double-checking each entry for accuracy before submission

Rationale: Double-checking each entry ensures data integrity and accuracy, which are crucial for reliable research outcomes. Entering data quickly (A) can lead to errors, using abbreviations (C) might cause misinterpretations, and relying on memory (D) increases the risk of inaccuracies. Ensuring accuracy before submission minimizes errors and maintains the credibility of the research.

Question 94: Correct Answer: B) Inform the circulating nurse immediately.

Rationale: Alex should inform the circulating nurse immediately to ensure patient safety and adhere to ethical and legal practices. Ignoring the issue (Option A) or waiting until after the procedure (Option C) could put the patient at risk of infection. Sterilizing the equipment himself (Option D) without informing anyone bypasses the proper protocol and does not address the immediate risk to the patient.

Question 95: Correct Answer: C) 7-15 MHz

Rationale: The frequency range of 7-15 MHz is typically used in intraoperative ultrasound to achieve optimal imaging resolution of soft tissues. Lower frequencies (1-3 MHz and 3-5 MHz) provide deeper penetration but less resolution, making them less suitable for detailed intraoperative imaging. Option D (20-30 MHz) is incorrect as it is too high and would not penetrate tissues effectively, limiting its use in surgical settings.

Question 96: Correct Answer: A) Electrical equipment malfunction

Rationale: Electrical equipment malfunction is a primary cause of fires in the operating room due to the high usage of electronic devices. Sterile field contamination (B) and improper hand hygiene (C) are infection control issues, not fire hazards. Inadequate patient positioning (D) is related to patient safety but does not directly cause fires. Therefore, understanding and maintaining electrical safety protocols is crucial in preventing operating room fires.

Question 97: Correct Answer: B) Contain the spill, report it to the supervisor, and then clean it up.

Rationale: The correct sequence is to first contain the spill to prevent it from spreading, then report it to the supervisor for further instructions, and finally clean it up following proper protocols. Cleaning up immediately (Option C) without containment can lead to further hazards. Evacuating the area (Option D) is not necessary unless the spill poses an immediate danger. Reporting first (Option A) delays the crucial step of containment.

Question 98: Correct Answer: B) Notify the surgeon and ensure the advanced directive is included in the patient's medical record.

Rationale: The correct action is to notify the surgeon and ensure the advanced directive is included in the patient's medical record. This ensures that the patient's wishes are respected throughout the surgical process. Ignoring the directive (Option A) is unethical and illegal. Advising Mr. Smith to discuss it with family (Option C) is not the surgical technologist's responsibility. Canceling the surgery (Option D) is unnecessary and could delay necessary treatment.

Question 99: Correct Answer: B) Ensure the patient's head is supported to maintain airway patency.

Rationale: Ensuring the patient's head is supported to maintain airway patency is crucial when the patient is still under the effects of anesthesia. This prevents airway obstruction and ensures the patient's safety

during the transfer. Option A is incorrect as rushing can lead to mistakes and injuries. Option C is incorrect because waking the patient before transferring can cause disorientation and potential harm. Option D is incorrect as additional support is necessary to prevent complications during the transfer.

Question 100: Correct Answer: D) Thrombin

Rationale: Thrombin is a potent hemostatic agent used to promote blood clotting during surgical procedures. It acts by converting fibrinogen to fibrin, forming a stable clot. Epinephrine is primarily a vasoconstrictor, Heparin is an anticoagulant, and Silver Nitrate is used for cauterization rather than hemostasis. Thus, Thrombin is the most effective and appropriate choice for achieving hemostasis.

Question 101: Correct Answer: A) Use a sterile drape that is large enough to cover the entire microscope.

Rationale: Using a sterile drape large enough to cover the entire microscope ensures comprehensive sterility. Multiple small drapes (Option B) can leave gaps and risk contamination. A non-sterile drape covered with a sterile cloth (Option C) does not ensure full sterility. Draping only parts that will be touched (Option D) overlooks the need for complete sterility. Full coverage with a sterile drape is essential to maintain a sterile field throughout the procedure.

Question 102: Correct Answer: C) Verify the anvil is properly attached and the stapler is correctly assembled.

Rationale: Ensuring the anvil is properly attached and the stapler is correctly assembled is crucial for the device to function correctly and avoid complications. While loading the correct size staples (A) and confirming the expiration date (B) are important, they are secondary to proper assembly. Checking if the stapler has been used previously (D) is irrelevant if it has been reprocessed correctly.

Question 103: Correct Answer: B) Linear cutter stapler

Rationale: The linear cutter stapler is specifically designed for creating anastomoses in the bowel, providing a secure and leak-proof connection. Skin staplers (A) are used for external skin closure, not internal anastomosis. Ligating clip appliers (C) are used for vessel ligation, not bowel anastomosis. Hemorrhoidal staplers (D) are specialized for hemorrhoid surgery and are not suitable for bowel anastomosis.

Question 104: Correct Answer: B) Enter the count into the computerized surgical count system.

Rationale: Entering the count into the computerized surgical count system ensures accuracy and efficiency, providing a reliable and traceable record. Writing on a whiteboard (A) or memorizing and verbally reporting (C) increases the risk of errors. Recording on a paper chart (D) is less efficient and can lead to documentation discrepancies.

Question 105: Correct Answer: B) Hypothyroidism

Rationale: Elevated TSH and low T3 and T4 levels indicate hypothyroidism, where the thyroid gland is underactive. Hyperthyroidism (A) would show low

TSH and high T3 and T4. Addison's Disease (C) involves adrenal insufficiency, not thyroid function. Cushing's Syndrome (D) is characterized by excessive cortisol, unrelated to the thyroid. Hypothyroidism explains Maria's symptoms of weight gain, fatigue, and cold intolerance.

Question 106: Correct Answer: A) Minimizing the time the graft is exposed to air
Rationale: Minimizing the time the graft is exposed to air is crucial to prevent contamination and desiccation. Exposing the graft to UV light (B) or using alcohol (D) would damage the tissue. Wrapping the graft in a dry cloth (C) would lead to desiccation. Therefore, reducing air exposure time is the most critical consideration.

Question 107: Correct Answer: C) Positioning the limb correctly before the cast hardens
Rationale: The most crucial step in ensuring proper limb alignment when applying a cast is positioning the limb correctly before the cast hardens. While cleanliness, even padding, and the correct casting material are important, they do not directly affect the alignment. Proper positioning ensures that the bone heals correctly, which is essential for optimal recovery.

Question 108: Correct Answer: B) Confirm the dosage with the circulating nurse before administration.
Rationale: The correct action is to confirm the dosage with the circulating nurse before administration. This ensures that the correct amount is administered and adheres to the protocol of double-checking medication and solution use. Administering without confirmation (A) or solely based on the surgeon's verbal order (C) can lead to errors. Waiting for a written order (D) may cause unnecessary delays in the procedure.

Question 109: Correct Answer: C) Clipping with electric clippers
Rationale: Clipping with electric clippers is the safest and most effective method for preoperative hair removal as it minimizes the risk of skin abrasions and infections. Shaving with a razor (Option A) can cause micro-abrasions, increasing infection risk. Depilatory creams (Option B) can cause skin irritation and allergic reactions. Waxing (Option D) is not recommended due to the potential for skin trauma and infection.

Question 110: Correct Answer: C) Recurrent laryngeal nerve
Rationale: The recurrent laryngeal nerve innervates the vocal cords and is crucial for their movement. Damage to this nerve during a laryngectomy can result in vocal cord paralysis. The hypoglossal nerve controls tongue movements, the vagus nerve has broader parasympathetic functions, and the glossopharyngeal nerve affects swallowing and taste. Hence, the recurrent laryngeal nerve is the correct answer due to its direct role in vocal cord function.

Question 111: Correct Answer: B) Use the hospital's online continuing education tracking system.
Rationale: Using the hospital's online continuing education tracking system (B) is the most efficient method as it provides real-time updates and centralized tracking. Handwritten logs (A) and email confirmations (C) can be prone to errors and misplacement. Periodic checks with a supervisor (D) are less efficient and may not provide timely updates. Therefore, B is the most reliable and efficient option.

Question 112: Correct Answer: B) Reinforce the dressing and notify the surgeon immediately.
Rationale: Reinforcing the dressing and notifying the surgeon immediately is crucial to manage potential postoperative bleeding effectively. Applying a new dressing over the existing one (Option A) may delay necessary intervention. Removing the dressing (Option C) could exacerbate bleeding. Waiting for the next scheduled assessment (Option D) is inappropriate as it delays critical care. Immediate notification ensures timely medical intervention.

Question 113: Correct Answer: B) Shaving the surgical site immediately before the procedure.
Rationale: Shaving the surgical site immediately before the procedure should be avoided as it can cause microabrasions, increasing the risk of infection. Option A is correct as sterile gloves prevent contamination. Option C is correct because the antiseptic must dry to be effective. Option D is correct as single-use applicators prevent cross-contamination.

Question 114: Correct Answer: B) Ensure all electrical equipment is properly grounded
Rationale: Proper grounding of electrical equipment is crucial for safety, especially in wet environments, as it prevents electrical shock. Option A is unsafe as frayed cords can lead to electrical hazards. Option C is incorrect; wet hands increase the risk of shock despite wearing gloves. Option D is also incorrect; placing devices on wet surfaces increases the risk of electrical shock.

Question 115: Correct Answer: D) Protein A
Rationale: Protein A is a primary virulence factor of Staphylococcus aureus that binds to the Fc region of antibodies, preventing opsonization and phagocytosis. Endotoxins are associated with Gram-negative bacteria, not Staphylococcus aureus. Exotoxins are secreted proteins that can cause damage but are not primarily involved in immune evasion. Capsules are more commonly associated with bacteria like Streptococcus pneumoniae. Thus, Protein A is the correct answer for Staphylococcus aureus.